Put On Your Parky Face
(Expanded Edition)

Bill Schmalfeldt

I0475147

THE LEGAL STUFF

Visit my website at http://www.billschmalfeldt.com

Printed in the United States of America

First Printing of Expanded Version, April 2011
Second Printing of Expanded Version, November 2011

ISBN-13: 978-1456458546
ISBN-10: 145645854X

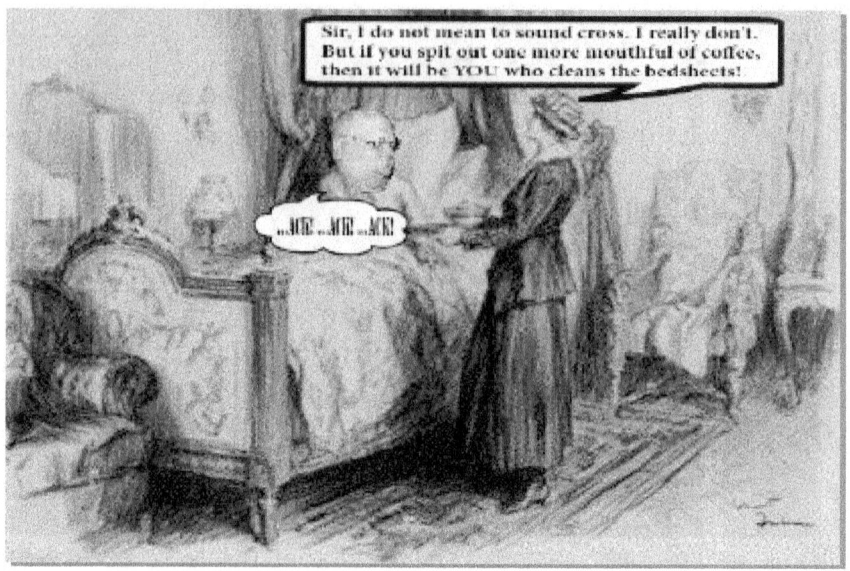

FOREWORD FOR REVISED VERSION

When I was first diagnosed with Parkinson's disease back in 2000, I used to lie awake some nights wondering what it would be like to experience the later stages of Parkinson's disease, the freezing-of-gait, executive dysfunction, postural instability, dyskinesia and stuff like that. Face it, when you're 45 years old it's really hard to imagine what it's going to be like when you can't walk at your former rate of speed. What's it going to be like when you can't control your motions? What's it going to be like when you freeze up as you walk?

Since my first edition of this book, I've begun to experience the whole gamut of what Parkinson's disease has to offer.

THIS IS WHY I WROTE THIS BOOK! THIS IS WHY I SHARE THESE EXPERIENCES!!!

Other books by other PD patients seem to either be religious treatises on how God will lift you through any trial and tribulation, to depressing tomes by people who lost their wives, lost their jobs and went as far as putting the barrel of the gun in their mouths but stopped themselves before redecorating the bedroom wallpaper.

You see books and blogs by other folks, especially those who are newly diagnosed, that are full of joyful optimism about how "they have PD but PD doesn't have them." And that's right! And that's good! But you do NOT see many books or blogs written by people who have had PD for more than a decade. You rarely see books or blogs written by folks who are into Stage IV of the PD Hoehn and Yahr scale. You rarely see patient books or blogs written by someone who is really feeling the effects of the disease who feels medical science has done just about all it can for him.

I will not be maudlin. I will not be downhearted. I will not be defeated. I will not be like the idiot Gunther von Hagens of "Body Works" fame who has had this thing for two years and has announced, therefore, he figures he has seven years left to live.

I will write about my experiences so that you, especially if you're newly diagnosed or love someone who is, will have some semblance of a clue of how one person and his loving caregiver handled things as they happened. PD affects us all differently. Me, for instance… I am largely without tremor. Rarely had it except for one day recently when I had a really bad shake going on in both hands… it was gone the next day.

I will not downplay the disease's effect on me. I will not write rosy descriptions about how "it's all in God's loving hands and he will lead me as he will." I will not post pretty little poems and pictures of pretty little flowers. I will be honest with you. In some cases, brutally honest!

I will tell you about how some mornings taking a crap is like trying to push wet driftwood through your ass and other days you're sitting at your desk trying to get some work done and suddenly -- *poopie*! Diaper changing time!

I will tell you about how some days each step comes with great difficulty.

I will tell you about the times when I fall, the times when I drool in public, the times when I befoul myself in public, the times I cough up all over the table because part of what I was swallowing went into my windpipe instead of my food tube, the times when I try to speak on the phone and sound like Porky Pig, the times when I'm speaking directly to a person and can… not… make… my… mouth… say… the… word… I… want… to… say.

I want you to KNOW Mr. Parkinson's! I want you to CARE about Mr. Parkinson's! I want you to reach into your pockets, if you are able, and DONATE to the Parkinson's disease charity of your choice. I want you… I NEED you to help science find a cure for this damn thing.

But I will not be defeated. I will not be broken. As long as I am able, I will write about my experience. The bad as well as the good.

If you want flowers, go to a florist.

If you want the truth about living with advanced Parkinson's disease, welcome to my book!

DEDICATION FOR THE REVISED VERSION

What a piece of work is a man, how noble in reason, how infinite in faculties, in form and moving how express and admirable, in action how like an angel, in apprehension how like a god! the beauty of the world, the paragon of animals—and yet, to me, what is this quintessence of dust?

Hamlet, Act II, Scene II, Page 3

William Shakespeare

I know the Bard wasn't writing about, and Hamlet wasn't speaking about Parkinson's disease here. But this verse came to my mind after today's round of physical therapy.

What an ASTOUNDING piece of machinery we are. Whether created by a benevolent God or formed by chance through one cosmic accident after another, what a WONDERFUL thing the human brain is. Wonderful, mystifying, marvelous and terrifying all at once.

I think of all the people on the planet, going about their daily business. Going here and there without giving the slightest thought to the tenuous nature of the delicate, silky spider web that keeps their brain functioning properly. So many things that can go wrong, so many things that DO go wrong on a daily basis to millions of people, whether through their own actions or by no fault of their own.

Riding with my wife to the mall today, I saw people walking, holding hands with their children, taking long, striding steps. Do they realize what's INVOLVED in that? Of course they don't. I never considered it before being diagnosed with Parkinson's. Neither did you.

Think about it now. Think of the various balance of chemicals your brain is supposed to produce on a moment-by-moment basis. Something gets a little out of kilter, not enough serotonin, perhaps, and you get depressed. You can't sleep. Or you sleep too much. You either see a doctor to replace the lost chemical, to enhance the receptors in the brain to fool it into thinking it's getting MORE of the lost chemical than it actually is. Or you ignore it, the depression gets worse, you sink into a dark melancholy, and in the worst case, you end your own life.

Dopamine is one of those tenuous, delicate spider webs upon which the smooth movement of the body depends. When you consider it pragmatically, what is the body if not solely for the purpose of getting the brain from place to place? To keep the heart beating so that oxygenated blood can keep your brain alive, so that the nutrients you absorb keep all the working parts of the machine working so they can follow the orders your brain gives to them. Your eyes and ears and nose and tongue and skin transfer vital information to your brain which will then decide how the body should react to whatever stimulus it is you are feeling so you'll know whether or not to flee from the stimulus or to embrace and seek more of it.

Dopamine is what makes that part of the body work so smoothly. By the time you start to notice "something ain't right" in Parkinson's disease, around 80 percent of the cells in your brain that make this vital chemical have already died, no longer able to create this all-important neurotransmitter, this "lube oil" that allows impulses created by your brain to jump from nerve ending to nerve ending from the point of origination in your brain ("Move left foot!") to the muscles the brain is attempting to command, (muscles in leg contract causing foot to move in accordance to the orders it receives), back to the brain (Message received, foot has moved.)

When you walk, do you THINK about it? Of course you don't! Who does? Other than making the conscious decision to walk faster or to run or to stop because the "Don't Walk" sign is lighted, the act of taking normal step after normal step is something that doesn't cross your mind. And why should it? Your BRAIN is controlling it. That part of your mid-brain that regulates everything, it sends out the dopamine that is absorbed by the dopamine receptors on the neurons in your brain and the signal transmits smoothly, without conscious effort.

When the dopamine is gone, so is that fluidity of movement.

In advanced Parkinson's disease, speaking for myself, I still do not think about every step I take. Because my brain is no longer producing sufficient amounts of that "lube oil" to ensure smooth transfer of brain impulses from neuron to neuron, the muscles that control the motion of my legs do not get the correct instructions. Imagine sitting at the microphone at a radio base station. You send an order to a squadron of attack jets.

"DROP YOUR BOMBS ON THE MUNITIONS DUMP, BUT BE CAREFUL BECAUSE THERE IS A SCHOOL HOUSE AND A HOSPITAL WITHIN THE IMMEDIATE AREA."

Because the message you sent is garbled in transmission, what the jet pilots hear is…

"DROP… BOMBS ON… SCHOOL… AND… HOSPITAL… AREA."

Tragedy ensues.

In Parkinson's disease, for whatever reason, different parts of the brain react in different ways to this lack of dopamine. You can take a dopamine substitute, like a levodopa/carbidopa combination, that synthesizes into dopamine when it crosses the blood/brain barrier. But that only lasts for so long and after years of this treatment, your brain betrays you by accepting the dopamine replacement and causing you to twist and writhe uncontrollably with dyskinesia.

You can electrically stimulate a part of the brain called the subthalamic nucleus to jam the erratic signal it gives out when it doesn't get the dopamine it wants. That smooths out your movement to a degree, relaxes the rigid muscles somewhat. But it's not a cure.

And then, there are the parts of your brain that do not react to the dopamine replacement. Why? Nobody knows yet. Balance. Gait. Speech. Swallowing. For some reason, they are resistant to dopaminergic treatment. Take all the levodopa your doctor prescribes, get yourself some deep brain stimulation. It does a lot of good in the areas where it can help. It does nothing in the areas it can't help.

I think back to this morning's physical therapy. I was on the treadmill. We had it going 2mph. While holding on to the hand rails, I am able to take long, striding steps. Why? Because the mid-brain is receiving the signal from my hands that we are holding on to something secure and are not likely to fall. The mid-brain sends out a signal that all is well and normal stepping is possible. I let go of the hand rail. The mid-brain loses that "safety signal" and orders the legs to take smaller steps to maintain my balance. Gone is the "heel/toe" step of a normal person. I am taking shorter, flat-footed steps.

The therapist slows the machine down to 1mph. I grab the bar. Without any conscious effort, I am now able to take long, graceful striding steps. It feels wonderful. I'm stretching muscles in the back of my thighs that don't get used regularly. He tells me to let go with one hand. There's not a whole lot of difference, except I can no longer take the longer, exaggerated, striding steps. The mid-brain feels confident that we're still holding on to something, but we're not as secure as we were.

The therapist tells me to let go of the rail one finger at a time.

Four fingers, not much change.

Three fingers, the steps get shorter, but we're still going heel/toe.

Two fingers, one finger…

The steps are shorter and shorter. I'm walking flat-footed.

Let go entirely.

The mid-brain believes we are unstable. Therefore, we must take short, Frankenstein-like halting steps. Flat-footed. And, at the slower speed, the difficulty is compounded by having to spend more time on each foot than we did at the higher speed.

Clomp! Clomp! Clomp! Clomp!

I focus. I concentrate. I try my level best to extend my stride and return to some semblance of the proper heel/toe step. My mid-brain acquiesces, but only a little. The stride increases, but it is a struggle. My thighs are tight. My muscles just will not stretch to allow it, because my mid-brain is still sending the signal that we are in danger of falling…

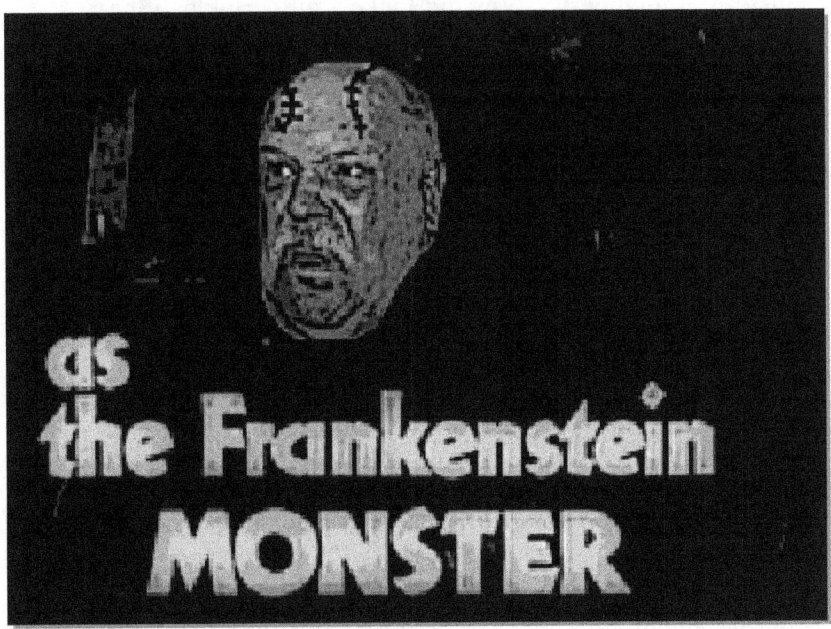

Until I grab the rail again. Then all is well. With no conscious effort at all, the stride lengthens, we return to the normal heel/toe stepping pattern.

Why does the mid-brain do this? Nobody knows. Why does my brain not send orders to my muscles to stop me from falling if I tip too far forward, backward, left or right? It probably does. But the muscles just don't receive the messages. Instead, they bomb the school and hospital.

Why does the lack of dopamine cause the frontal lobes of the brain to malfunction, leading to something called executive dysfunction and for up to 80 percent of us with Parkinson's, outright Parkinson's disease dementia? I'm a smart person. I'm as smart as I ever was, probably even smarter. So why, after taking ibuprofen for ankle pain last night, did I try to put the bottle cap onto the glass I drank the water from? "Cap no go THERE," my brain said. "Cap go on BOTTLE! Not GLASS!" Why have I, more than once, found myself looking in the mirror with my toothbrush in my left hand and a tube of Preparation H or some sort of antibiotic ointment or anti-itch cream in my right hand instead of toothpaste? Why did I take a pill, drink half the glass of water, dump the water on the counter before putting the glass into the sink? Why did I recently pull some labels (those long, sticky "size" labels you get on new sweat pants) and try to flush them in the toilet? Why did I try to flush an empty toilet paper roll? Why did I pour freshly ground coffee beans into my wife's cup instead of into the coffee machine's filter? Why did I think that a group of little ornaments dangling from our car's rear view mirror was a kid my wife was about to run over? Why did I once see a guy standing near the off ramp on the express way, only to have him vanish like a mirage when we got closer? Why do I depend on an audio alarm to remind me to take my pills? Why did I lay awake the other night because I couldn't remember the opening segment of "The William Tell Overture" — a piece of music I know as well as my own name — and have to get up, find a copy on iTunes and listen to it before I could get any rest, which it turned out I couldn't get anyway because I forgot to take my nightly sleep pills?

There's a lot of "why's" in the alphabet of Parkinson's disease. Does anyone have the answer key to this persistent quiz?

I share this info, not with a sense of sadness, not with a sense of regret, without the slightest hint of depression. I share it because it confirms something I learned too late in life. That is, what a wonderful machine we are, and how dependent we are on the tiniest things.

As the Bard of Avon wrote a page earlier in Scene II, Act II of Hamlet…

…for there is nothing either good or bad but thinking makes it so.

Or, to put it in the 21st Century vernacular…

It is what it is.

With that in mind, this expanded version of "Put On Your Parky Face" is dedicated to my former colleagues at the National Institutes of Health, Dr. P. David Charles and Dr. Peter Konrad at the Vanderbilt University Medical Center in Nashville, Dr. Stephen Grill at the Parkinson's & Movement Disorder Center of Maryland, and most of all to my caring angel, my life, my happiness, my eternal helper, sidekick, cheerleader and asskicker, my beloved wife Gail.

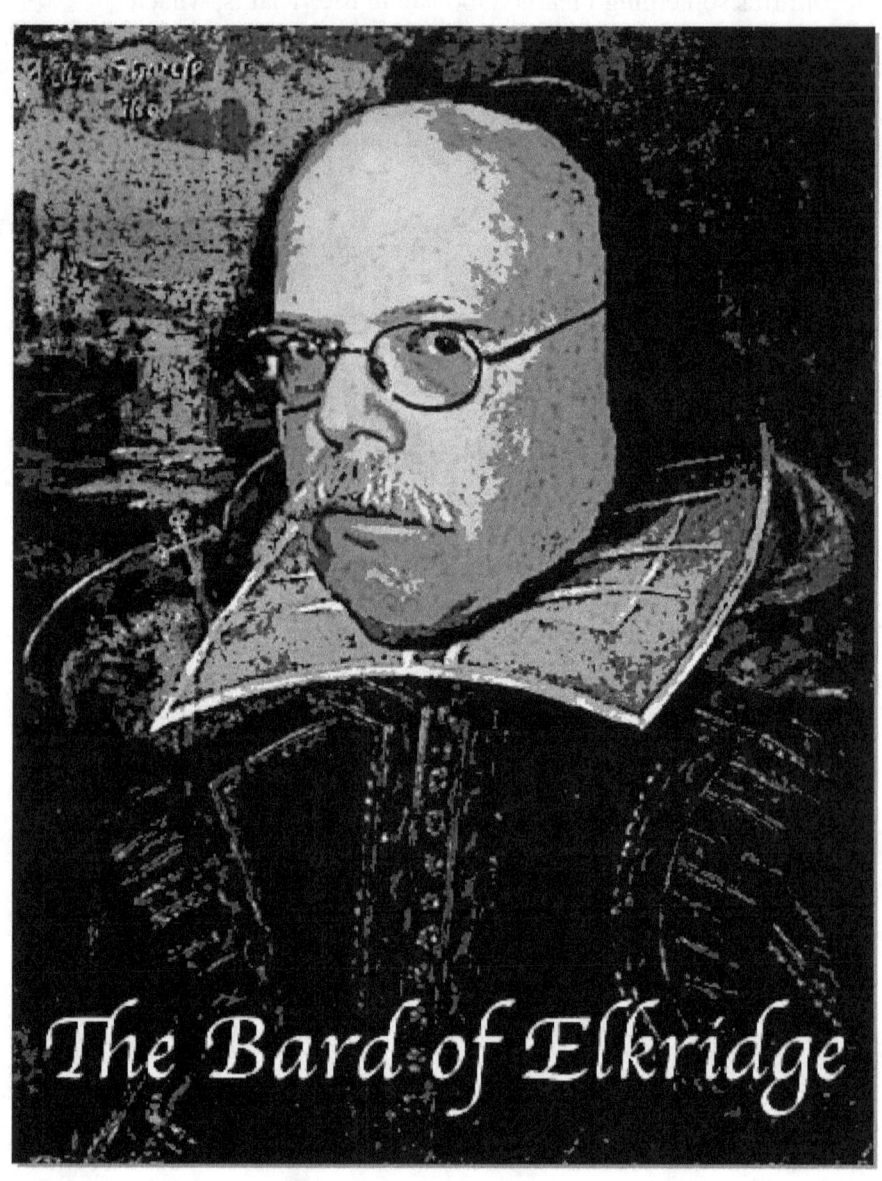

The Bard of Elkridge

If I chance to talk a little wild, forgive me…

William Shakespeare

Henry the Eighth, Act I, Scene IV

ORIGINAL FOREWORD

I'm Serving Notice!

It's time to stop being invisible.

It's time for people with Parkinson's disease – or "Parkies" – and their caregivers to raise their voices and say—Here we are! Look! We're here! There are 1,500,000 of us in the United States! There are 50,000 new members of our little fraternity every year!

And we're not just old people. We're getting younger and younger.

Not long ago, I was sitting and watching MSNBC. My eyes wandered to the crawler below the main screen and I saw the words "October is Breast Cancer Awareness Month."

We just got home from Milwaukee the previous day, visiting my 80- year old Mom who broke her leg—feisty old thing, we had to almost coerce her into going into rehab to get her strength built back up. While there, we saw the fountain at the art museum. The water was colored pink for Breast Cancer Awareness Month.

I watched my beloved Green Bay Packers lose in overtime that next day to the Washington Redskins. Everyone on the field was wearing pink to commemorate Breast Cancer Awareness Month. Even the referees had the pink ribbon behind the NFL logo on their hats.

Any given number of products advertised on TV promise donations to one Breast Cancer Awareness group or another. Here in the DC area, we just had our 3-day Susan G. Komen Breast Cancer Awareness Walk.

I pray that medical science someday finds a cure for this cruel disease which has affected family members and friends of mine.

But where is OUR "Breast Cancer Awareness Month?"

I know April is officially Parkinson's Disease Awareness Month. But where was the awareness? Where were the marches? Where were the calls for support? Where were the pleas for donations to organizations like the National Parkinson Foundation or the

American Parkinson's Disease Association or any ONE of the numerous PD awareness groups?

Where is OUR "awareness?"

Why are my fellow activist Parkies being met with blank faces and silence when they contact their local media outlets asking for a story, a feature, a report of SOME kind about Parkinson's disease?

My cynical opinion?

We don't have a "sexy" disease. There's nothing attractive about Parkinson's. We drool, we shake, we walk very slowly, we fall, we break our hips, we get pneumonia, we die. If this started happening to 20-year olds on a regular basis, you damn BETCHA it would start getting some serious media attention.

But Parkinson's is typically a disease of aging. It doesn't have the devastating quality of Alzheimer's where we keep our bodies but lose our minds. We keep our minds but lose our bodies.

We just don't have an ATTRACTIVE disease. The money demo in the TV world is the 25-40 year old group. Testing shows that these younger folks don't really like looking at older people anyway. Add some drool, some shaking, some shuffling, some slurred speech, and you have a real tune-out factor with these folks.

We're just not CUTE enough. Since this disease typically strikes after age 50, it's rough for Jerry Lewis to hold a telethon to get folks to cough up cash because they feel sorry for us. The typical, ill-informed reaction to someone with PD is NOT, "Oh, that person is sick. I want to do something to help." The reaction is, "Oh, that's an old person. I hope I don't get like that when I'm old."

We're just not TRAGIC enough... like a celebrity who jumps a horse over a hedge, falls and breaks his neck. We have our examples, of course, with young, vibrant, tragic Michael J. Fox. And we all know that Muhammad Ali no longer floats nor stings. And then, there's NBA star Brian Grant, but he hasn't really shown any signs of the disease yet. But we also have Janet Reno, who is still joke-fodder for the right wing. We have Yassar

Arafat, a dead terrorist. We have Billy Graham. Old. We had Pope John Paul II. Old. We had Adolf Hitler. Evil. So MJF carries the celebrity load, the "Champ" does what he can, and Brian Grant is just getting into the act. We don't have anyone from "Twilight" coming down with PD. No one from "Avatar." No one from "30 Rock."

Our shaking, drooling, shuffling, slurring, pooping and peeing ourselves, choking on food and drink, falling and slowness is seen by the uninformed as just a natural part of getting older.

Now, if we had a RESPONSIBLE media that could take its eye off the bottom line for a minute, we COULD get a good public service campaign going. I mean, they've got a good one for the ASPCA now with the sad doggies and kitties and folks are sending money THERE to help. But the media knows that sad doggies and kitties will move people. Shuffling, drooling, slurring older folks will just make people change the channel. Folks get SAD when doggies and kitties are mistreated and uncared for. Folks turn away when faced with images of middle-aged to elderly folks who pee their pants.

So what about it? What can we do? Why is it that no matter what kind of fuss we try to raise, it seems that Michael J. Fox and Muhammad Ali (and now Brian Grant) are the only people in America with Parkinson's disease—at least as far as the national media is concerned? Why is there no nationwide, concerted effort to raise awareness, to help you and the other wonderful organizations fund and find new and better treatments, and perhaps a cure for this horrible affliction? My own efforts—writing and self-publishing three books on the subject and donating 100% of author proceeds to research—have thus far netted just a bit over $200. I have widgets on my site where folks can donate directly. I volunteered for brain surgery, and now I'm trying to raise funds so that Vanderbilt can expand their Phase 1 clinical trial with 30 people to a nationwide Phase III clinical trial, multi-center, involving hundreds if not thousands of younger folks with PD. I feel like I've done my part, and God knows I want to do more.

But nobody knows who I am!

I can't snap my fingers and demand TV or print or web media coverage. Hell, I spent hundreds on press releases and they resulted in one live radio and two Internet radio interviews. I'm just a civil servant who gets funny looks in the grocery store because of my walk and the scars on my bald head.

Where's our Jerry Lewis? Where's our Susan G. Komen? Who can we find to lead us? Who can we find—someone with a national spotlight—who will draw attention to the 1 million of us in America with this disease, the 50,000 new cases that will be diagnosed this year, and next year, and the year after that and the year after that?

How do we draw attention to ourselves? Without seeming pathetic or whiny or demanding anything more than that which we are due – respect, and a serious effort to fund research efforts to help the various research organizations to find new and better treatments and someday, some blessed day, a cure.

Well, a journey of a thousand miles begins with a single step. I'll write a book about my experiences and hope that people read it. I hope that after they read it, they'll understand that we're PEOPLE. We may not be CUTE. We may not be CUDDLY! We don't ALL have tremor. (And tremor is HARDLY the worst thing about Parkinson's disease.) We're your fathers, your mothers, your aunts and uncles, your grannies and gramps. And as the "baby boom" population gets older, chances are we're your brothers, your sisters, your nieces, your nephews. Maybe even your children.

If you don't care about Parkinson's disease, I can give you 1.5 million reasons why you should. And if this year is like any other year, there will be 50-thousand new reasons by the end of this year.

So... I'm serving notice. I'm going to tell you one man's story about his decade with Parkinson's disease. I'm going to ask you to keep in mind that my experience is unique, since no two cases of PD will progress at the exact same rate or exhibit the exact same symptoms.

I'm going to teach you something by sharing my experience. I'll tell you about my nonchalant attitude towards the affliction for the first five years, my sudden awakening when I went to work for the federal government, my experience as a volunteer for experimental brain surgery in a clinical trial, and the events that led up to my deciding to retire from the federal government to devote my remaining time and strength to spreading the word – getting out awareness – about this second most prevalent of the neurodegenerative diseases. (Alzheimer's is still #1. And they get PLENTY of awareness.)

I'm hoping by my example, others will start talking about it. And that will cause others to talk about it. And then more. And more.

And before you know it – AWARENESS! People will UNDERSTAND this monster of a disease that steals the body but, by and large, leaves the mind. (The lights are off, but everyone is home.)

At least, I hope that's the result. Otherwise, October will continue to be Breast Cancer Awareness Month, while April slogs along as African American Women's Fitness Month, Amateur Radio Month, Autism Awareness Month, Cancer Control Month, Child Abuse Prevention Month, Confederate History Month, Emotional Overeating Awareness Month, Global Child Nutrition Month, Fresh Florida Tomatoes Month, Irritable Bowel Syndrome Month, National Child Abuse Prevention Month, National Pecan Month, and National Straw Hat Month.

Thank you for your time. Now, some history.

CHAPTER 1

I Was Once an Unaware Boob!

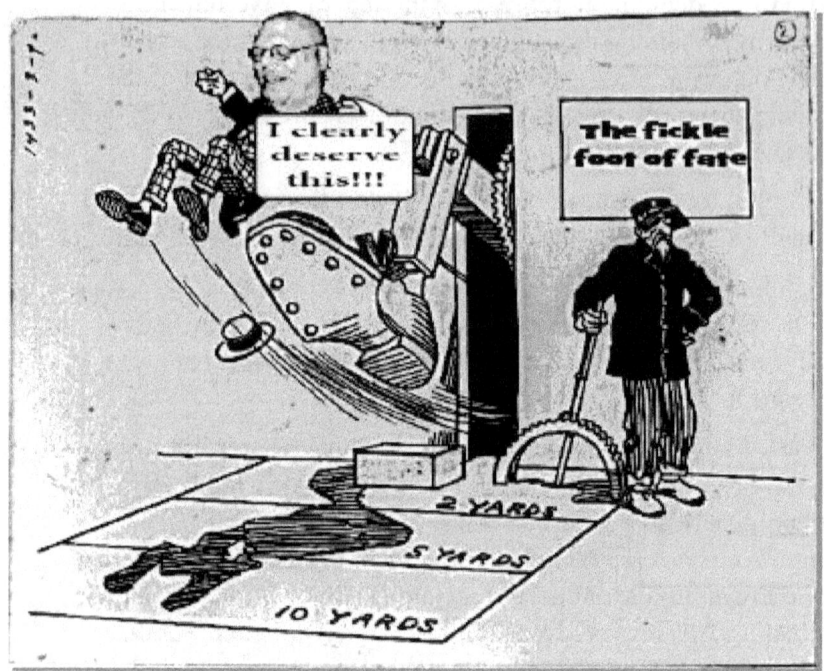

The table was set for lunch, although they called it "supper." I never understood that. To me the word "supper" was interchangeable with the word "dinner." But I didn't care what they called it. After a long, hot morning of hauling hay bales with my brother Bob and our friend Eric, I was hungry. And whatever what they called it, there sure was a lot of it! Hot fresh baked rolls with honey to slather over them. A huge bowl of boiled potatoes mashed with the peels still on them. Corn on the cob drizzled with melted butter. A pitcher of Kool-Aid that, for some reason, they called "nectar." And chicken! Heaping mounds of it. Hot, crispy, golden fried. Delicious!

A guy didn't make much money hauling hay bales on the Bornemann farm. A nickel per bale got divided three ways, and by the time the week was over if you had a few bucks you considered yourself lucky. That wasn't the point of the job anyway. The real purpose was to build up arm strength before football season. The little bit of money you got was just icing on the cake.

Oh, yeah. I forgot to mention the cake. A thick, two-layer yellow cake with vanilla frosting waited for dessert.

We may have been working for slave wages. But we ate like lords.

"Boys. Get you some chicken meat," Mrs. Bornemann said with a smile. She was a round, jolly woman with a large head covered in white curls. She loved to watch teenage boys eat. "Put some gravy on them 'taters," she commanded, gravy boat in hand, smothering the potatoes on my plate with rich, creamy goodness.

Mr. Bornemann ate in silence. He rarely spoke, and when he did it was usually to yell at us for lollygagging, meaning we weren't getting the bales from the field to the flatbed behind his trailer nearly fast enough. I believed Mr. Bornemann was deeply disappointed with the youth of the day. We clearly didn't understand the value of a hard day's work, accustomed as we were to sitting around on our

candy asses watching the color TV and listening to our rock and roll records on our stereos that our daddies bought for us with their hard-earned money. I'm sure he feared for the future of the America he loved, and I have no doubt that he resented having to pay us – let alone feed us.

"Get you some more chicken meat," Mrs. Bornemann said as I gnawed a drumstick to the cartilage. "Best meat's on the breast," she said and I wondered why such a grandmotherly woman had no kids of her own.

That question would be answered by a quick glance at her husband. A grim, thin man with a pointed nose and crooked neck, his eyes were small, set and mean. Sparse white hair covered the crest of his small head like an early winter snow flurry atop a grain silo. His tiny mouth was set in a concrete frown. He didn't look like he had a drop of blood to spare for something so frivolous as making love to a woman when there were CHORES to be done and CROPS to be raised and a HERD to take care of. Dammit.

There was another thing about him, too. He shook. I thought at first it was because of that ramshackle tractor he rode all day up and down, around and between the neat rows of evenly spaced alfalfa bales. But he shook even when the tractor was still and silent. His head and neck twitched and craned as if he were always trying to get a better look at something. His right arm seemed to have a mind of its own, as if it were trying to break free from its disagreeable owner and find a more hospitable, friendlier body with which to cleave. The only way he could drink his coffee was to hold the cup on the table top with both hands, dip his face down to the cup, and slurp.

He caught me watching him.

"Tend to your business!" he barked. I fixed my gaze on the half-eaten chicken breast on my plate.

"Eat some of these 'taters," Mrs. Bornemann said as she dropped a generous dollop of the spuds onto my brother's plate. "And you, Henry, stop barking at the boys."

"I'll bark at who I wanna," he muttered as he dipped his face back to the coffee cup. Bob and Eric regarded me, smiling the way boys smile when someone's in trouble and it's not them.

Mr. Bornemann picked up his napkin and I noticed that when he used his hand, it didn't shake. He dabbed at his lips and dropped the napkin back onto the table as his hand resumed its back and forth rhythm. He glared at Eric.

"You, boy. You said you can drive a tractor? When you're done, the three of you get back to where we left off. I'm gonna lay down awhile. No lollygagging."

But without him there to keep an eye on us, lollygag we did and how! As Eric drove the tractor, I grabbed bales and pitched them onto the flatbed at Bob who stacked them. And we laughed and laughed as we mocked Mr. Bornemann's voice, his appearance, his attitude, and mostly – his affliction.

"I wonder if he taught his dog to shake," I said. Bob laughed.

"That chicken we had today, ya think it was 'Shake 'n Bake'?" Eric guffawed and almost drove the tractor into a row of bales as he looked back.

"Betcha five bucks it was," he said. "Wanna shake on it?"

We laughed and laughed and laughed. The job only lasted a couple weeks more, but our fun at the expense of Mr. Bornemann's neurological condition lasted all summer.

Some years later, I began to understand the concept of Karma.

I do not have Parkinson's disease because I made fun of an old man and his shaking palsy. I got Parkinson's disease because a bunch of cells in a portion of my brain known as the substantia nigra (Latin for "black stuff") whose only job is to produce a neurotransmitting chemical called dopamine have decided, for whatever reason, to die. We don't know what killed them – as the popular bumper sticker of the late 1990s put it – shit happens. And I suppose it was in the late 1990s when shit started happening to ME! In late 1999, to be specific...

For about a year I had been dropping things with my right hand. This was not just your garden-variety clumsiness, of which I have always been something of a poster child. I would have something in my right hand – a glass, a cassette tape, a butter knife. Then, suddenly, I wouldn't have it. No tingling. No numbness. No warning. The hand would just "let go and let gravity."

By itself, no big deal. Nor, when taken separately, was I particularly concerned about the cramping in my thighs when I climbed stairs, the fact that I was inexplicably exhausted by the end of the day, or the shaking in my right hand when excited or stressed.

The thing that tipped the scales was when I was doing the morning talk show at a radio station in Naples, Florida, when I couldn't for the life of me remember the name of my co-host. We had been together for nearly four months. I called her by her first name at least three dozen times a day. She was my boss, for God's sake. And with the microphone open and a good part of southwest Florida tuned in, I stammered and fumbled and tried for all I was worth to remember just what in the hell her name was.

But I couldn't. So instead I grabbed a tape cartridge with a recorded public service announcement and told the audience we'd be taking a break. I dropped the tape right into the woman's coffee cup – whatever her name was. I picked it up and dropped it again. My hand shook like a leaf in the wind. I struggled to put the tape into the player, and stabbed at the "start" button, missing it.

Nanci (that was her name! Nanci! How in the hell do you forget a name like Nanci?) pushed my trembling hand out of the way and pushed the button. I turned off the mic. She looked at me and her forehead creased the way it did when I had just said something on the air that she knew would be the focus of a meeting with the station manager after the show.

"Would you please call a doctor," she said. The show was almost over so she offered to slide behind the control board and finish things off for the day. I went to my desk, pulling out my wallet as I walked. Once seated, I withdrew my insurance card and called the 800 number for "medical advice nurse." The nice lady on the phone asked me to describe my situation. I told her what I had noticed before and what had just happened.

"Are you near a hospital?" she asked. "Uh, yeah."

 "Go there," she said. "Right now. I don't want to alarm you, but what you are describing sounds like you might be in the early stages of a stroke."

"Oh. Right. Nothing alarming about that," I said.

"Don't drive," she said. "Call an ambulance."

"Right," I said. "Thank you." I hung up and called my wife. She said she'd be right there to pick me up and take me to the ER. I was not going to be hauled out of the radio station on a gurney, down the hallway of the office building, into the elevator, out into the parking lot, a topic of conversation, a focus of entertainment above and beyond the call of my duties as morning radio show host.

I sat at my desk and wondered if I'd notice or recognize any of the subtle signs of approaching and imminent death. Not that I'm a melodramatic sort. But I did have some time to kill.

The first thing they did in the ER was take my blood pressure. It was fine. They did an EKG. It was fine. Off to the CT scanner. The images were normal. I was admitted for observation – which was an odd thing to call it, since to my knowledge no one "observed" me. I lay in my hospital bed feeling fine – somewhat hungry, but otherwise fit. I watched TV, and every couple hours or so, someone would take my blood pressure.

The next morning, a neurologist came to visit me.

"Good news," he said. Those are the best two words a doctor can say. I smiled. "You didn't have a stroke. You don't have a tumor. But I think you do have a little something going on there."

A "little something", eh, I thought. Hell. I can deal with a "little" something.

"Do me a favor," he said. "Get out of bed and walk up and down the hallway for me."

"You're the doctor," I said. I got up, walked to the door, turned around and came back.

"One more time," he said. I complied.

"Why aren't you swinging your right arm?" he asked. I looked at my arm as I walked. It just kind of hung there. My left arm was moving back and forth, doing the work for both arms apparently.

"Damned if I know," I said. The doctor patted the edge of the bed. I walked over – this time forcing my right arm to do its damn job – and sat.

He told me to open and close my right hand fast as I could. Then the left. Then tap my right index finger and thumb. Then the left. Then he told me to put my right palm on my thigh and turn it over, like flipping a burger, over and over, fast as I could. I did. Then he told me to do the same thing, but this time while opening and closing my left hand as fast as I could.

That's when we came to a screeching halt. I couldn't do it. Not smoothly, anyway. I could do one or the other. But doing both required massive concentration.

"OK, here's the problem," he said. "Like I said, you didn't have a stroke, you don't have a tumor. So, you don't have anything that's going to kill you. But I think you might have Parkinson's disease."

"That's nice," I said. I knew a little bit about Parkinson's disease. Months earlier, actor Michael J. Fox had gone public with his own diagnosis. I admired him for doing so and marveled that one so young would have an old guy's disease.

"I'm going to suggest you see a special kind of neurologist," he said. "A movement disorder specialist. There's a great one in Miami, Dr. William Koller. If you'd like, I can set up an appointment."

I thanked him and explained that my insurance company required that I jump through their hoops before doing anything so drastic as seeing a specialist. I asked him to write down the doctor's name and I would try to work the system with the ultimate end of seeing this Dr. Koller he spoke so highly of.

My insurance company said I had to first see my family doctor. There was a problem with that. I didn't have a family doctor. My insurance didn't go into effect until three months after employment, which was just a month ago, and I hadn't needed a doctor until then.

But bureaucracy must be honored, so after being discharged from the hospital I scanned the insurance company's preferred provider list and picked out a family practitioner. I called for an appointment.

"And what is this appointment for," the appointment clerk asked.

"So I can see a neurologist," I explained.

"The doctor isn't a neurologist," she said patiently.

"I know that," I said, "but I need him to give me a referral to SEE a neurologist."

"How do you know you need to see a neurologist if you haven't even seen a family practitioner yet," she asked, that sweet "I'm talking to an idiot" tone in her voice.

I explained my situation and she set the appointment for a couple days later.

The doctor sat and listened as I described the events of the past several days. Then he shook his head. "I don't think it's Parkinson's," he said. "You're too young for that."

"You would think so," I said. "But look at Michael J. Fox..."
"Who's he?" the doctor asked. "Alex P. Keaton on 'Family Ties'. 'Back to the Future'..."

"Oh yeah," he said, the light of recognition finally burning. "That guy. But that has to be a rare case. Did seeing that on the news make you think you had PD too?"

"I thought I was having a stroke," I told him. "The neurologist at the hospital said he thought I had PD."

"Nah, you're too young," he said. But he agreed – at my insistence – to refer me to a neurologist.

A couple weeks later, the neurologist told me I was too young to have PD. He tested my reflexes, noticed some twitching in my calves and some hyper reflexes in my Achilles tendons.

"I don't think it's Parkinson's," he said in a thick accent – maybe Middle Eastern, I'm not sure. "But you might want to prepare yourself for the possibility that you may have Lou Gehrig's disease."

Oh! Fine! A fatal disease! MUCH better than Parkinson's, I thought. I told him I wanted a second opinion. We set up an appointment with one of his colleagues.

The next doctor told me I did not have ALS. We did all the testing I had done in the hospital room. Then he shut the door and sat down, leaning toward me with the air of a conspirator.

"What do you think it is?" he asked me.

"My money's still on Parkinson's Disease," I said.

"That's probably a good bet. But you know what? I'm an HMO doctor. And I'm going to be very honest with you. And if you repeat this to anyone, I will swear I never said it. OK?"

I assured him I was cool with it.

"I'm going to diagnose you with extrapyramidal syndrome. It's a catch-all phrase for a variety of conditions, including Parkinson's. If I pull the trigger on the PD diagnosis, it goes on my record. It's an expensive diagnosis. And it's the sort of thing the HMO looks at when they do the books at the end of the year. I don't want it on my record. What I will do, is refer you to the Parkinson's disease Foundation clinic in Miami. We'll let them pull the trigger. Any problem with that?"

Nope. Other than the corporate cowardice, I had no problem with that at all.

On January 31, 2000 I saw Dr. William Koller – the same doctor the neurologist at the ER in Naples wanted to send me to 90 days earlier. We did all the tests again. And he made the diagnosis.

"How do you feel about that?" he asked me. "Beats Lou Gehrig's Disease," I said.

He smiled and patted me on the shoulder. "Remember, Bill... it's not a death sentence. It's a life sentence."

Still, it was now official. A doctor—a preeminent one in the world of movement disorders—had just diagnosed me with Parkinson's disease. He gave me a sampler pack of Mirapex and a prescription for more when I got home.

My eyes focused on the road, I couldn't even hear the music on the radio.

"Parkinson's disease. Well, it's official."

Dr. Koller explained that it was very early in the disease process and that I likely had a number of "good years" ahead of me. How many? "No way to say for sure. It's different for everyone."

As the Everglades whizzed by on the left and right of the car, I did a survey of my current symptoms. The cramping, the dropping of stuff with my right hand, the occasional difficulty finding the right word. I tried to think ahead, wondering what the future would be like for me. Surely they'd find a cure for this thing by the time I would be disabled by it, right? Dr. Koller sure seemed optimistic about it. I mean, all this new stuff with embryonic stem cell research and all... whoever wins the 2000 election will SURELY allow federal funding to continue and they'll HAVE to have a cure for this thing five years from now, ten at the outside...

Well... we all saw how THAT turned out with President Bush ending federal funding to any new embryonic stem cell lines for eight years and then, once President Obama lifted the ban and research began in earnest, a left-over Reagan-appointed judge outlawed federal funding for ESCR again because of, what he called, a lack of available adoptable babies. After eight years in the wilderness, once again a clump of frozen cells in a petri dish had more rights than I did.

Ten years. A lot has been done. Not as much as I had hoped. But at the time, I didn't even know what to think about it all. Zipping across Alligator Alley, Parkinson's was a concept. A thing I knew that I had. But I had no idea.

No idea.

The first thing I did the next day was tell my radio listeners that I had been diagnosed. I explained that I looked fine and felt fine and you wouldn't know a thing was wrong if you didn't know what to look for, but that it was a progressive disease... it would get worse over the years, barring a cure, of course. I joined the Parkinson's Disease Association of Southwest Florida and even MC'ed some of their charity events. But I stopped going to the support meetings because I just didn't feel that sick! And frankly, being confronted with monthly reminders of what was waiting for me down the road – it was a bring down.

For our remaining time in Florida, I stayed on the Mirapex – well, at least until the side-effects caught up with me. I started falling asleep at stop lights. My wife, Gail, would watch my eyes for that "glazed over" look while I was driving and jolt me back into consciousness when such jolting was required. Eventually, Dr. Koller switched me to a low dosage of Sinemet, the gold-standard levodopa/carbidopa treatment for Parkinson's. And I felt fine! As I said, to look at me you wouldn't know there was a thing wrong.

We left Florida in 2001 when I was hired by XM Satellite Radio. I got a new neurologist. And HE didn't think there was a thing wrong with me. "Well, if Dr. Koller says you have PD, he's a pretty respected guy in the field, so I'll just have to bow to his diagnosis," one doctor said. "But I don't see a thing wrong with you." I explained the reason for that MIGHT just be because the medication was working, but that seemed to fall on deaf ears. In 2003, I began seeing a real movement disorder specialist, Dr. Susanne Goldstein at the Parkinson's Disease and Movement Disorder Center in Elkridge, Md. She confirmed the diagnosis, said my symptoms were still in the early stage, and she switched me from generic Sinemet to a new drug called Stalevo – it contains the levodopa/carbidopa combination of Sinemet, but adds a dose of entacapone which levels out the distribution of the levodopa into the blood brain barrier – or something like that.

Later in 2003, I left XM. I also lost my health insurance. I worked at a series of radio stations from 2003 until 2005 where health insurance was either not an option, or it was priced beyond my means. So for all that time, I went without medication.

In early 2005, I was hired as an information development specialist at the National Institutes of Health in Bethesda, Md. Not only did my financial situation improve, as a federal employee I had great benefits. I chose an insurance company and started seeing Dr. Goldstein again. Then my insurance company stopped listing Dr. Goldstein as an approved provider and I had to see the neurologist the company recommended.

The insurance company's neurologist told me he didn't think I had Parkinson's because I was much too young. He thought it was carpal tunnel syndrome.

When testing for carpal tunnel came back negative, he decided I had cervical spinal stenosis – a narrowing of the canal the spinal cord goes through in the neck.

I had an MRI and CT of the cervical spine, and yes, the spinal canal was narrower than it should be, but not so narrow as to cause the symptoms I was having.

So then he decided it must be some other condition I can't even remember the name of and it doesn't matter because I fired him during health insurance "open season" in 2006 and started seeing my previous movement disorder specialist. By this time I was walking very slowly, my whole body was stiff, and my balance was getting worse.

I had an appointment with her on February 1, 2007 and I related my frustration with the situation and the doctor I had been seeing the previous year. After doing the neurological tests she said, "With all due respect to your former neurologist, you DO seem to have Parkinson's disease—and a fairly classical case of it."

Yaaaay! I'm CLASSICAL!

She gave me samples of Stalevo 100 – this is a relatively new medication – a mixture of levodopa and carbidopa, and something called entacapone, which enhances the benefit of the levodopa. After the appointment I took one in the car.

Within 30 minutes...

I was standing up straight!

I was walking with a normal stride!

I actually had ARM SWING on my right side as I walked!

I made a vow to heaven above that if I ever have another child—I will name it STALEVO!

As I dug into my duties at the NIH, I began to look into the concept of clinical research, clinical trials where folks volunteer to be examined, try new drugs and participate in other ways to help scientists find new and better ways to treat disease. It was part of my job to write stories and record podcasts about the importance of clinical trials, and I felt guilty about having this "perfectly good disease" without being involved in such research.

Thus began the next part of the adventure.

CHAPTER 2

Volunteer for Brain Surgery? Why Not?

Searching for a clinical trial in which to involve myself, it seemed as if the studies there on the NIH Campus in Bethesda were not a good fit. Either I had to LITTLE Parkinson's (I wasn't sick enough), or I had too MUCH Parkinson's (I was already on dopamine therapy.)

So, I dug further. In my research on a story about clinical trials I noticed that a major university is conducting a study on people like me! Early stage PD patients who have had a positive response to medications. Age 50 to 65. Willing to undergo brain surgery.

Yup! That's ME!

The study—to see whether deep brain stimulation has a neuroprotective effect on early stage PD, meaning it might slow or stop the progression of PD.

I ran the idea past my neurologist—she said she thought the study was worthwhile. So I e-mailed for more info.

Of course, it wasn't as simple a matter as showing up, hopping onto the table and getting the operation. There was screening to be done. First, they had to see if I'm a nut case. (Who ELSE would volunteer for brain surgery, someone SANE???) Then they would need to take me off the meds for a week and poke, prod, and test me—on video. Then they would flip a metaphorical coin and I would either get the surgery—implantation of electrodes deep into my noodle—or go to the control group, where I just keep taking the meds.

This next section comes from a diary-style blog I kept during the screening process.

The First Trip to Nashville

February 16, 2007

I made it to Nashville.

Eleven hours in a car is a long time. It sucks when the FM part of your car radio doesn't work.

All the sports talk radio shows spent the day yesterday talking about former NBA player Tim Hardaway and why he hates gays.

Trees look very pretty in the sunlight with a coating of ice on them. The same cannot be said for highways. Thank God the roads were clean and dry.

I got here at about 5 p.m. Nashville time, which was about an hour after I was due to take my third Stalevo of the day. I staggered into the hotel lobby, happy that I had taken the time a few days ago to complete the "express check-in" thing on the hotel's website. It turned out to be a futile gesture as there was a tourist couple in front of me experiencing some sort of problem that took the sole clerk at the desk some 15 minutes to sort out. But once it was MY turn, check-in was a breeze!

Got to my room. Took a Stalevo. Got a bag of burgers. Watched a movie on Showtime. Fell asleep at 8:30.

Today, feeling more or less fresh, but with a sleep hangover. Meds don't seem to be working quite as well today. I've got a work laptop with me, so I'm connected to the office, checking e-mails, uploading sound files as I would ordinarily do on a Friday. Ain't technology GRAND?

At 1 p.m. local, I will meet with Dr. P. David Charles, neurologist, lead researcher on this study. At 2 p.m. I'll meet with Dr. Peter Konrad, the neurosurgeon who will become intimately acquainted with my brain if I enter the study and am selected for surgery. At 3 p.m. I will meet Dr. Stuart Finder, the medical ethicist, who will—I suppose—ensure to the satisfaction of all that I know what the risks are.

On Saturday I will meet with my book agent. Nice fella. Happens to have an office in Nashville. This will be our first face-to-face.

On Sunday I will swim in the hotel pool and otherwise vegetate.

Then on Monday, I go back to Vanderbilt University Medical Center to sign the consents—providing I don't chicken out first. That's what the 72 hour waiting period is all about, I suppose. It might sound good on Friday, but by Monday I might decide that I need this surgery like I need a hole in the head.

Two holes, actually. Then, on Tuesday, I will go home. LATER THAT DAY Such nice people, these doctors. Seriously!

Met first with a very pleasant young lady named Chandler Gill. She's the coordinator for the clinical trial. We discussed the protocol, why I want to take part, all the stuff you would expect would be discussed.

Then I met Dr. Charles. Nice guy. Youngish. Has identical twin sons. VERY optimistic about the research. He really did a great job explaining the theory behind the possibility of neuroprotection from DBS. And although it's just a theory—it makes great sense!

Then I met Dr. Konrad—who basically wrote the book on this procedure. He gave me a copy of the book. And he laid out the whole procedure, start to finish. Very steady hands. I like that. Clean fingernails, too!

Then I met Dr. Finder—and it was his job to ensure that I was fully informed and was making a wise decision based on my needs and expectations.

Very nice afternoon. We'll get back together on Monday and I'll sign the consents. Unless I chicken out. Which I won't.

Probably.

I Signed the Consent Forms!

February 19, 2007

Oh my God! What have I DONE? I SIGNED "THE CONSENT FORM!"

No! NO!!! NOOOOOOOO!!!!!!!

Heh! That was written for the benefit of the medical ethicist, Dr. Finder. The man was relentless! And that's just what you would want from someone whose job it is to make absolutely certain that YOU are absolutely certain that you are making a decision like this for the right reasons.

I'm sure. Absolutely. I'll explain.

A large part of my job as production manager of the National Institutes of Health Radio News Service is writing radio news stories and public service announcements about the importance of clinical research.

As a person suffering from a condition where research holds so much hope for a cure, I felt it would be hypocritical of me to not take an opportunity to participate in clinical research if presented with a chance to do so.

Also, think about the concept they're trying to prove with this particular clinical study into the safety and tolerability of deep brain stimulation in early Parkinson's disease. This pilot trial is designed specifically to collect the preliminary safety and tolerability data necessary to conduct a future phase III clinical trial to investigate the hypothesis that deep brain stimulation of the subthalamic nucleus in subjects with early Parkinson's will slow the progression of the disease.

If there's a CHANCE that this procedure could slow the progression of PD, then I want a piece of the action! I am clearly in early Stage II (in the Four Stage Hoehn & Yahr Ratings Scale). I have a long way to go before being profoundly handicapped by this disease. What a wonderful thing it would be if this procedure slowed—or even HALTED the progression! And how wonderful it will feel to have been on the cutting edge of this thing if it turns out that deep brain stimulation someday becomes the treatment of choice for patients—earlier rather than later in the course of the disease.

There are risks. For one, I could have a stroke and die. Right there on the table. Boom. Gone. Or I could be profoundly crippled as a result. Or there could be an infection of the electrode leads or the implanted neurostimulators which would be placed in my chest. And there's a bunch of other stuff that could go wrong. And it might not work! But it probably will. The odds are in my favor. And it beats doing nothing. And for me, at least, that tips the balance.

Back home tomorrow. Back down here sometime in March for a couple days. Then April 10-18, I'm here for the 8-day drool-fest... I mean, 8 days without medication.

But the first step has been taken.

Back from Nashville

February 27, 2007

Been home about a week now. I don't think I'll be driving to and from Nashville any more. I was wiped when I got to there on the 15th, even more so when I got home on the 20th.

Depending on whether or not I'm randomized for the surgery, I may have to make the trip several more times this spring.

I'll fly, thank you.

At present, I'm waiting for Chandler to contact me with the dates for the first step in the screening—the CT/MRI, neuro and psych screening. Thank goodness they've changed the protocol to allow out-of-towners like me to bunk down in the Clinical Research Center when we're in town for these sorts of things.

After that, it's two weeks of keeping hourly symptom diaries. Then the 8-day inspection, tentatively set for April 10-18.

Actually, I'm doing well. The three Stalevo 100s per day weren't getting the job done, so my neurologist suggested taking four a day. That seems to be working quite nicely.

Did the NIH bi-weekly podcast on Friday. Talked at length about the clinical trial and why such things are important.

So... I wait. I should hear something soon I would suppose.

One thing I didn't expect was the well meaning but stupid people would say when I told them I had decided to participate in this clinical trial. Chalk it up to unawareness about Parkinson's disease.

My favorite was, "but you LOOK fine!" (I always replied—mentally—"Yes. I AM fine. I'm LYING to you about having PD! Joke's on YOU, dimwit! Ha ha ha!") Then there are the folks who think you may be faking it because you can move better today than you did yesterday.

This lack of understanding came into glaring focus when Michael J. Fox did a political ad for a Democratic candidate for Senate in Missouri in 2006. Conservative critics (like the idiot Rush Limbaugh) attacked him—first for faking the dyskinesia, then for being a shill for embryonic stem cell research. When Fox explained that the dyskinesia was caused by "too much levodopa"—he obviously meant that the "sweet spot" where the right amount of medication leaves him relatively smooth and fluid was getting smaller and smaller. Limbaugh and others took it to mean he "took an overdose" just to appear dyskinetic in the political ad.

Some people seem to prefer to be stupid.

Then there's the wearing off—when you walk into the movie theater looking just fine, and by the time the movie's done you need help getting out of the chair.

How do we educate people about this without seeming whiny about it?

OK... back to the diary/blog...

Back to Nashville for Screening

March 27, 2007

Nice place they got here at the Vanderbilt University Medical Center Clinical Research Center!

I arrived about an hour before I was expected on Sunday, but the staff was ready. They took me back to my room and got my vital signs. My BP was through the roof for some reason—I expect that part of the reason was that I had been off the Stalevo since Saturday morning. After a bit of relaxing and a couple eight-ounce cans of Sprite, I was able to register a relatively decent BP.

Slept like an innocent man on Sunday night. It's a tiny bed, but when you consider how much sleeping space I actually get at home with Gail on one side of the bed and Raven absorbing as much space as a border collie possibly can... I probably actually have MORE room here.

Yesterday morning, about a half hour before our appointment time, Dr. Charles came in and gave me the standard neurological exam. He left to get Chandler, the coordinator, and when they came back they gave me the Unified Parkinson's Disease Rating Scale—henceforth to be known as the UPDRS. I suppose I was marginally impaired after being off the meds for more than 48 hours at that point. Dr. Charles told me to take 1-1/2 of my Stalevo 100s and they'd come back in an hour.

I LIKE 1-1/2 STALEVOS!!! In about 30 minutes I was fully "on" and loving life again. Dr. Charles and Ms. Chandler returned and I breezed through the UPDRS like a person without PD. And that's one of the inclusion factors of the study... you have to have a positive reaction to your PD medications. Dr. Charles said my reaction was one of the most striking they've seen in this study.

After allowing me to interview them for the NIH podcast, they went on their way and I took a stroll down towards the location of my afternoon screening test to just get out of the room for awhile. After I located the place—the Vanderbilt Psychiatry Clinic—I ducked into a convenience store, got some sodas and chips and came back to the room all hot and sweaty.

At 3, I was back at the Psych Clinic for my neuropsychological screening with Dr. Tramontana and his assistant, who put me through the rugged paces of a cognition test. Then I visited with the doctor, he asked a few basic questions about my history with PD, my state of mind and emotion, and that was that.

Back to the room for dinner, relaxed, watched "24" and went to bed. Slept like a lord once again.

Now I'm killing time. Dr. Konrad, the neurosurgeon, is slated to drop by at 4:30 for a podcast interview and to look over the MRI's I brought down with me. Chandler just dropped by to give me a form for Dr. Konrad to sign. I just finagled a laptop from the nice folks at the nurse's station so I could enter all this fascinating information.

Tomorrow... back home after a psychiatric screening with Dr. Salomon. Then I'm back here on April 10-18.

Home Again

March 29, 2007

Why is there no such thing as a straight-line flight from somewhere to somewhere?

I got home last night at about 10:15 p.m. Plane A flew from Nashville to Memphis—which was EXACTLY the opposite direction from home. But for some reason, I had to fly THERE before I could fly to Baltimore. When I go back to Vanderbilt in April, I fly from Baltimore to Charlotte, NC, THEN to Nashville. When I come home, it will be via Chicago.

Also, as long as I'm complaining, why are airplane seats made with children in mind? There's just not enough room for a plus-sized individual like me. I had to hold my right arm over my chest to give the poor lady sitting next to me all the room she paid for with her ticket. By the time we landed, my poor ass was in agony!

Then there were the two idiot women sitting right behind me. I think it was a skank mom and her skank daughter. They both had the look of "skank" about them—the mom was nearly as old as I am, but dressed in a t-shirt and short bike pants with various piercings in her eyebrows, nose and lips. She looked like a fishing lure. She and her daughter were playing cards and SLAMMING the fold-down table as they laid down their hands, rattling my already uncomfortable seat. Must be nice to be so absolutely thoughtless as to believe you are the only two people on the friggin' airplane.

I already have plane tickets for the eight-day Droolfest in April. I may choose to drive to and from after that.

I hate flying!

HOWEVER—the overall experience at Vandy was a positive one. The staff at the Clinical Research Center was polite and professional and accommodating and pleasant beyond the call of duty. The room was small but efficient and comfortable with a little fridge for cold sodas and snacks. The bed was surprisingly comfortable. A better selection on the TV might have been an improvement, but they had all the network channels (Billy's GOT to see his "24" every Monday!) as well as CNN and ESPN—and, oddly enough, one channel that has a blue screen with white letters proclaiming "THIS IS SCREEN 2."

(So, what the hell happened to Screen 1?)

The food, by and large, plentiful and non-offensive. My only problem lies with the "Lump O' Egg" one receives with breakfast... a scoop of scrambled eggs that has something of a slight "rubber" taste—I think it gets that flavor from the container in which it's microwaved.

I mentioned my visit with Dr. Charles and Ms. Gill—on Tuesday I met for an extended and lively chat with Dr. Konrad, the neurosurgeon who will have my brain in his hands should I be randomized for the surgery. My conversations with Drs. Charles and Konrad and Ms. Gill will be included on my NIH Research Radio podcasts at a later date, as well as on my personal "What's Shakin'" podcast.

On Wednesday I met with Dr. Salomon, a psychiatrist, whose job it was to make sure I wasn't a crazy or a depressed person who was hoping to be killed by the surgery. After a spirited chat, he declared me "normal"—which was about the nicest thing anyone would say to me all day. I should have gotten it in writing.

At any rate, I'm looking forward to the eight-day Droolfest—to "Get It Over With" more than any other reason. Eight days off the Stalevo will suck in many various ways. On the final day, the flip ofthe coin and we learn if I am to be randomized to the surgical group or the control group.

But it's nice to know I'll be cared for by such great folks in a comfortable facility. That makes the small headaches—like the rubber eggs—much easier to take.

Next, the eight-day stay at the General Clinical Research Center at Vanderbilt University Medical Center – the "Droolfest." (By the way, if you are interested in seeing what "Droolfest" was really like, you should go to my You Tube channel at http://www.youtube.com/bschmalfeldt and scroll way down, you can see some delightful videos of my delightful days at several of these delightful Droolfests.)

Back to the diary/blog.

April 10, 2007

Day 0, Droolfest 1

It's Day 0: of the 8-Day Drool Fest—the first of the several visits to the Vanderbilt University Medical Center for eight days off the meds. Let us keep track of each day's events, say wot?

7:16 AM

Woke up, as usual, shortly before 4 a.m. Time for a pill. Hit the hay quite early last night—a bit after 8. Was gonna stay up to watch "24" but I was falling asleep on the recliner. Stalevo doesn't seem to have all that much impact on the "fatigue" part of PD. Added to this, the stress of my hillbilly neighbor's dog getting loose again and attacking MY chained-up dogs in MY yard. The cops are now involved. Anyhoo—we'll head to the airport in a bit more than an hour. Gonna be a lot of sitting around today—nearly a 4- hour layover in Charlotte. Why is there no "non-stop" between Baltimore and Nashville? Are they not both relatively major cities? Oh well.

12:40 PM

So far, so good. Made it to Charlotte. Oddly enough, for the first flight in MANY times, I actually had no one sitting next to me, so there was a little room to stretch out. Now I'm sitting here in the main concourse, sipping a Sam Adams, watching the folks walk by. We're about 2 hours and 20 minutes from load-up time. I'm not at all hungry, but I may go grab sumthin' anyway, cuz who the heck knows when I'm gonna get any grub tonight. Neat thing about this airport—there's a row of rocking chairs... like the kind you'd see in front of a Cracker Barrel Restaurant, for folks to sit on and relax. Very nice touch. The flight was kinda bumpy at both ends... bumpy takeoff, bumpy landing, but smooth as silk in between.

7:10 PM (CDT)

Ok... I'm in Nashville. Using the Treo to make this entry. More tomorrow when the laptop's hooked up.

Day 1, Droolfest 1

April 11, 2007

8:58 AM

Hey! The computer's working! The IT guy had to come in and add the wireless network to my network connections, but that's done and once again I'm in touch with the world. Crapped out at around 9 last night, woke up at 4 to take a pill, then slept in until about 6:45. Took a shower and laid around waiting for brekky, which showed up at 8. Sausage links, "Lump 'o Egg", French toast, cereal, orange segments, a tiny blueberry muffin, apple juice. No coffee. Then my nurse of the day, Christa, came in and took my blood pressure. 16 times. I'm not kidding. It's part of the protocol. First sitting, then standing. Then 2 minutes later while standing. Then once each 30 seconds for 6 minutes. My poor arm was purple. And we'll do this every morning. Chandler, the study coordinator, is supposed to come in sometime this morning for the 8-hour symptom diary, after which I go OFF the meds at 4 p.m. Then the fun begins.

12:54 PM

Another dandy lunch. BBQ Pork, turkey veggie soup, pineapple chunks, baked beans. Before that, Chandler came by and we went through the entire UPDRS, except for the physical exam part... Dr.

Charles is supposed to be coming by this afternoon to do that part, and get it on tape. This provides the researchers with an objective measurement of how I'm doing, and how fast I can do it. With Chandler timing me, I opened and closed each hand as fast as I could, tapped finger to thumb on each hand, and tapped each heel on the floor for 30 seconds each. Chandler produced this contraption – a long, metal thingamabob with a pair of what looked like old fashioned Royal typewriter keys about a foot apart, each connected to a counter. My job... press each key, back and forth, fast as I could, with the index finger of each hand for 30 seconds. Then we stepped out into the hallway and she measured off a set distance. I sat in a chair, and at her command stood up, walked the distance, turned around, walked back and sat down. And not once did I get a cookie, a piece of candy, or any other form of "reward" for performing these stunts.

3:09 PM

OK, so now I'm a video star. Went through the videotaped portion of the UPDRS... I'll be videotaped again on the final day. But this is supposed to show me at my most "on". With Chandler running the video camera and me sitting in a chair, Dr. Charles directed me first to open and close my right hand as fast as I could. Then the left. Then the finger tapping. Then I was told to extend my right arm with my hand positioned as if I had just picked an apple from a tree, then to invert that hand back and forth, as if I were trying to shake dew from the apple. First the right hand, then the left. Then I was directed to tap my right heel on the floor as fast as I could. Then the left. I was told to cross my arms over my chest and rise to my feet. Dr. Charles had me walk back and forth in front of the camera a couple times. Then he told me to stand still. He came up behind me, put a couple fingers on my shoulders and delivered a backwards tug to see how many steps (if any) it would take me to keep from falling. It took none. I was Steady Eddie personified! And thus ended the video session. My 8-hour symptom diary will wrap up at 4, so even though I would ordinarily take a pill right about now, there's no real reason to do so. May as well "get it on" - - as they say. I enjoyed "feeling good"... now it's time to see the other side again.

6:44 PM

More than 9 hours since my last pill. Already starting to feel the decline. Muscles starting to tighten. Feeling a little headachy. Let the good times roll.

Day 2, Droolfest 1

April 12, 2007

9:10 AM

It sucks to wake up early here. I crawled out of the sack at about 5:45 because my body still thinks we're on Eastern Time. Breakfast doesn't come around until 8 am. So there's two-plus hours with little to do. And the TV reception was crappy... it's cable/Dish TV or something like that, but it was all snowy and impossible to watch. I got cleaned up, then watched last Monday's episode of "24" online. By the time that was done, the TV situation had been remedied. At 8, brekky showed up, and it wasn't bad! No "Lump 'o Egg" today... it was a cheese omelet, and it wasn't bad. A couple bacon strips, a tiny cheese Danish, cornflakes, orange juice and coffee. At 8:30, my day nurse Christa (she's also the manager of the GCRC) came in. She's a delightful German lady of 60-some years. We did the 16-times blood pressure thing... I'm running a bit on the high side... Maybe the stress of not having my Stalevo? Then Chandler called. Dr. Charles won't make it until 1 p.m. today. Which is fine. It's a lovely day and I may head out for a stroll here in a bit. I'm feeling somewhat hindered, but not as bad as I probably will feel before I can take my next Stalevo on the 18th.

2:37 PM

I had just typed a whole bunch of stuff here, but before I saved it, the heel of my right hand touched "something" on the body of this laptop, and it decided to go back to the previous page. So I lost everything I wrote. With this laptop, for some reason, if any part of your hand is touching anything other than the keyboard when you write, it acts goofy. Anyway, Dr. Charles came by at 1:30 and we did today's UPDRS thing – basically, a reprise of the bit we had videotaped yesterday. Today my score was 4. Yesterday I was a 2. Still minimal, but progressing. Then he asked me to rate my independence, based on the Schwab and England Activities of Daily Living Scale. 100% means I can do all chores without slowness, difficulty or impairment; that is to say – normal. 90% indicates I can do all chores but with some degree of slowness, difficulty or impairment, beginning to be aware of difficulty. I decided I was at a good 90%, since I was noticing some stiffness and slowness, but not too bad at the moment. I decided to take a stroll to a little market about six blocks from here. On the way back, my upper back tightened and my legs throbbed. My brain seems to be saying, "No Stalevo, no leisurely strolls." To hell with my brain. There are little restaurants I intend to check out. Cheeseburger Charley is at the top of the list. Maybe tomorrow. We'll see.

8:22 PM

I was really wiped out from the walk. Amazing what a difference a little pill can make. Dr. Charles says it will take about 3 days to wash the Stalevo from my body... so the next couple days should be interesting. The good doctor prescribed an Ambien for sleeping, so I'm expecting a good night's sleep and a better tomorrow.

Day 3, Droolfest 1

April 13, 2007

9:51 AM

Slept through the night like a little angel. Ambien. Good stuff. Not feeling particularly hindered this morning... more "slow" than "tight". The typing is starting to slow down and get a bit difficult. But nowhere near "bad" just yet.

There was some sort of power outage early this morning. Got woke up when it came back on and the BP monitor near my bed started going "bee-DOOP! bee-DOOP!" over and over again. It's done something bad to the TV here in the room, too. I have the volume turned up all the way on the bedside remote, and you have to be lying in bed by the speaker to hear it. When you press the "volume" button on the TV... it changes the channel. But at least, you can still tell when you're watching "Screen 2." (I still wonder what happened to "Screen 1".)

Did the 16-times BP thing again.... and it's still trending kinda high. So I called and left a message with Dr. Geller's (home physician) staff asking if I should double up on my daily Lopressor script. Chandler just dropped by with some personality tests I'm supposed to fill out before seeing the neuropsych guy on Monday. And we're waiting on our daily neurology test from Dr. Charles. Such a busy, busy boy I am.

1:49 PM

Did it again! Had an entry typed and a part of my hand touched some other part of this useless laptop and it "went back to the previous page". And when I came back to THIS page, my entry was gone!!! DAMMITT!!! Anyhow, Dr. Charles and Chandler came by before lunch and we did the UPDRS thing (I swear, ossifer, I only had a coupla liddle beers!). My right hand and arm are more rigid than they were yesterday, and so is my left hand. But I still place myself at 90% because in order to be classified at 80%, I would have to take "twice as long" to do some things, and we ain't there just yet. Chandler will do the UPRDS thing tomorrow since Dr. Charles will be gone for the day. Lunch was a workable turkey breast sandwich, a cookie, a salad, some sort of soup or another, and a fruit cup. Heard back from my family doc, and now I will be taking 2 BP pills a day. Despite yesterday's discomfort, I was planning on taking a stroll, but it looks like rain is in the offing, so instead I'll eat cookies and watch TV. Yeah, it SOUNDS good...

Day 4, Droolfest 1

April 14, 2007

8:25 AM

Mmmm. "Lump o' Egg." I will miss my daily "Lump o' Egg" when I'm done here. Does that mean I'm suffering from "Stockholm Syndrome"? Watched "Law and Order" last night. The story was about a college student with PD who killed another student while attempting to assassinate an Ann Coulter type for speaking out against embryonic stem cell research. They showed the dude in court in full-blown dyskinesia, and the prosecutor said, "Hey, he had no trouble sitting still in my office." The dude's lawyer said, "That was him on medication, this is him off meds." Bullshit.

That's just the same sort of crap Limbaugh was spreading. One does not get dyskinetic from NOT taking meds. It's a small thing, I suppose, but it spreads the kind of disinformation that we had to overcome last fall with Limbaugh spreading the lies he was spreading. Grrrr.... Anyway, just had my daily 16-times blood pressure test done. Much better numbers today now that I'm taking two Lopressors a day. Now to await Chandler's visit at around 10 or so, then I'll pound out this 567-question "personality test" I'm supposed to have done for Monday. No rest for the wobbly.

3:08 PM

A crappy, miserable, doleful day here at the GCRC at Vanderbilt University Medical Center in Nashville, TN.

I'm currently on the 3rd floor. Broke out of the joint for a little while earlier today after Chandler came by to put me through the UPDRS—or, field sobriety test if you will. There was a break in the rain, so I wandered up to Cheeseburger Charley's and found the place to be aptly named. Then I staggered to the CVS store and got some chocolate milk and orange sherbet for later. Hopefully the sherbet won't be a fluid sludge when I get around to eating it—this fridge isn't the coldest in history. Pounded through the 567 questions on this Minnesota Multiphasic Personality Inventory test I'm supposed to have done before my Monday visit with Dr. Tramontana—the neuropsychiatrist. Cool true-false questions, such as, "Sometimes I'm so strongly attracted by the personal articles of others, such as shoes, gloves, etc., that I want to handle or steal them, even though I have no use for them." For the record, the answer to THAT one was "false." Other than that, just killing time, listening to music, grateful that I'm halfway through this event, looking forward to randomization and taking that next wonderful, blessed, lamented STALEVO!

Day 5, Droolfest 1

April 15, 2007

8:57 AM

How odd. "Lump o' Egg" took the morning off. Cheese omelet instead. I feel somehow... empty. It's another dreary, rainy day in Nashville... doesn't look like I'll be getting outside any time today. Even with the Ambien, I had trouble getting to sleep last night... just couldn't shut my mind off. Got up at about 7-ish. Gonna be rough getting back into the routine when I get home later this week. MAN, am I looking forward to getting home. Everyone here is perfectly lovely, especially Christa—the manager of the place. We always have a nice chat about this, that and the other when we do the 16-times blood pressure thing in the morning. Dr. Charles is supposed to come in to do my "field sobriety test" later today, but that's gonna depend on air travel. He went to Silver Spring, Maryland yesterday and is due back this evening. The weather has the entire east coast balled up. So, we shall see. Took almost a half hour to get showered this morning. The right hand is delinquent, and I'm slow and stiff. And I'm still more than 72 hours away from my next Stalevo. Bitch, bitch, bitch.

8:12 PM

I seem to be the patient that time forgot tonight. My dinner tray is still sitting here, 3 hours after the fact. And usually someone has popped in to take vitals or at least see if I'm still breathing... well... how's THAT for timing! As soon as I wrote that, my night nurse came to get my tray. She also told me that Dr. Charles probably wouldn't be in until after 9 pm. That's fine. I'll still be here. Looking forward to tomorrow, just because there will be something to DO! First the visit with Dr. Tramontana, then out to dinner with my entertainment lawyer. Three more days. Three more days. Three more days.

Day 6, Droolfest 1

April 16, 2007

7:31 AM

It's still a half-hour until brekky. I'm pretty sure "Lump o' Egg" will be back on the menu today. You can't go more than a day with no "Lump o' Egg." No doubt, there are abstracts in medical journals to that effect. I found an occasion for a little impromptu humor this morning. I had just gotten out of the shower and was shaving, when my nurse for the day—a jolly little lady named Eunice—came in to check on me. She said that if I needed anything, I should be sure to press the call button, as she would be pretty scarce today ... they have a patient who is getting her blood drawn every 15 minutes. I opened my eyes in faux shock. "A new needle every 15 minutes? Sweet Jesus! Is that a punishment? Did she press the call button once too often? I swear! I won't bother you! I promise! I'll be good! I'll be good!" She laughed nervously and retreated from my room. I wonder if this little exchange will make it into my chart? I have an appointment for cognitive testing this afternoon. (PD can affect— and WILL affect if it goes on long enough—a person's cognitive abilities.) If they greet me with one of them long-sleeved leather jackets with buckles, I'll know it DID get entered in the chart. Dr. Charles finally dropped by at about 9 last night, looking tired and unshaven. He had just flown in from Baltimore, and he's heading back up there today. Ah, the wild life of the research scientist! As for me, my right hand is so tight and stiff, it actually causes mild pain when I try to make a fist. I'm stiff and rigid and MORE than ready for a pill, thank you.

10:21 AM

I topped off the morning by dumping a full 16-oz. cup of coffee with creamer and sugar all over the floor. The nice dude from housekeeping didn't even make fun of me. Dr. Charles has come and gone for the day, and now I'm waiting for the cognitive testing—which promises to be grueling and frustrating.

12:57 PM

The world keeps turning. Horrible day at Virginia Tech... 30 dead in shootings. The story is still breaking. Back on topic, my cognitive testing for today has been cancelled. It's been reset for tomorrow at 4. Oh well. Dinner is still on for tonight.

7:51 PM

Felt great getting out of here for awhile. Had dinner at the Longhorn with my entertainment attorney. Had the 20 oz. Porterhouse and a man sized portion of mashed taters. Lifted my spirits nicely. And since I'm not taking Stalevo, didn't have to worry about the protein messing up the levodopa uptake. Now to relax and watch "24." Just one more full day, then a half day, then the coin flip, then I can take a pill and go home. Yaaay, home!

Day 7, Droolfest 1

April 17, 2007

9:17 AM

So far today, I've survived "Lump o' Egg" and the Blood Pressure Torture. Now the rest of the day is mine until about 3:30, when I will begin my shamble to the psych hospital for the cognitive testing. Hope they don't mind that one of the forms has coffee spots on it from the great Coffee Spill of yesterday. Numbers were still kinda high—but not bad—with the Arm Purpling Blood Pressure Procedure from Hell. I personally think a big part of it is that I'm not on the Stalevo and my whole body is in a state of perpetual clench. Whatever. Hopefully at or around this time tomorrow, we do the final testing, I get randomized, and I can take a Stalevo and rejoin the human race, walking erect and speaking clearly again.

6:27 PM

Went to have the cognitive testing. There was a young boy in the lobby, looked like he had Down syndrome. He walked up to me, smiling, and touched my beard. "Santa," he said, giggling. I smiled and said, "No, I'm not Santa... but I am one of his helpers." The testing was exquisite torture. And frankly, I'm too tired right now to really detail it like it deserves to be detailed. Got back to the room, had dinner, called Gail. Tomorrow... the final UPDRS, the flip of the coin, and STALEVO!!!

Day 8, Droolfest 1

April 18, 2007

7:12 AM

At last, we reach the end of the Droolfest. Sometime after brekky, Chandler will put me through the paces of the full UPDRS. Then,

I guess around 11 or so, Dr. Charles will take care of the Part III
of the UPDRS. Then the "opening of the envelope" and we'll
find out what's what. This has been a very interesting experience.
For one, I didn't know I was as impaired as I am. I must have
certainly deteriorated in the months since I went back on the
Stalevo... perception is everything, and I might have a different
perspective on it now, but I can't imagine that I lived my life
every day feeling as bad as I do now. It actually hurts to open and
close my right hand. My walk is more of a stagger—not as bad as
it WILL get if the PD progresses—but it certainly is different
from the way I walk when I'm medicated. Sitting here typing
this, my arms are aching, my upper back is aching, my neck
aches, and even my thighs are aching. As soon as we do that last
UPDRS, I will be able to take a Stalevo... so I suppose that by the
time I get to the airport I will be pretty much "ON" again. If I'm
assigned to the control group, that's fine. Over the next six
months, it will be interesting to see if I develop dyskinesia and
then again to see how far gone I am when they take me off the
meds for the NEXT 8-day Droolfest. If I were a betting man, I'd
bet that I will be in the control group. And that's just fine. Other
than the possibility of getting this surgery, the whole point of this
for me is "putting my money where my mouth is." Now, at least,
I'll have the satisfaction of having taken part—and continuing to
take part—in an important clinical research study. And that will
give me a voice of authority as I do my reports for the NIH Radio
News Service. I'll TRY to do one more entry from here at the
GCRC before I leave... otherwise, I'll hope for a WiFi access at
the airport. Once again, the folks here at the GCRC have been
great. I was kept as comfortable as person can be—in a hospital.
And everyone was delightful. Now... brekky, the Arm Purpling
Blood Pressure Procedure, then I wait for Chandler.

11:06 AM

We're almost there. Chandler just came by and we did the whole
UPDRS—save for Part III, which we'll do on tape with Dr.
Charles performing the honors. I seem to have slowed down by
about half on the right, by about a third on the left. This has
certainly been instructive as far as knowing how far along I am in

the progression of this disease. BTW—for those who might be reading this while considering taking part in this very study, if you qualify and don't at least look into participating... I have to ask you... WHY NOT? Here's my official take on it... even if you are not chosen for the surgery, it is a VERY worthwhile experience—for yourself to know where you stand in the progression of your OWN disease, and in the interest of science finding newer and better treatments for PD. I have been a bit—shall we say, "colorful" in my descriptive language regarding the bill of fare (which, as far as hospital food goes, is not really all that bad), and the Arm Purpling Blood Pressure Procedure—which isn't exactly as much fun as eating CANDY, but nor is it particularly unpleasant—but that's just the ranting of a creative writer.

6:07 PM
The last entry in CDT... and the last of the 8-Day Droolfest. Huzzah and hooray! I was randomized to the surgical group! After carrying out Part III of the UPDRS, Dr. Charles opened the little grey envelope, and it contained the initials DBS. So, sometime in June or July I will have Deep Brain Stimulation. I was 100% prepared to be told that I was going to the control group. But now I can start preparing myself—mentally, physically and spiritually—for what will, no doubt, be the greatest adventure of the latter portion of my life! I took a Stalevo at about 1:10 p.m., and by the time I got to the Nashville Airport I was almost fully "ON." It feels GREAT!!! As I type this, I'm sitting near my gate at O'Hare Airport in Chicago. My flight from here to Baltimore has been delayed about 45 minutes, so it gives me this opportunity to end today's entry on a high note. Back to work tomorrow.

The first "Droolfest" out of the way, finding myself randomized to the surgical group, all of a sudden I discovered I had some serious planning to do. And not all that much time

to do it. The first of the three surgeries was scheduled for June 5, with the implantation of the probes set for June 13. This was call for some serious considerations.

May 7, 2007

I Need A Hat!

Four weeks from today I will have my pre-op workup done at Vanderbilt University Medical Center. The next day, I'll visit the radiology clinic where I'll be put under general anesthesia. Four temporary bone markers will be inserted into my skull and I'll remain under for a CT and MRI scan. The surgeons will use these pictures to plot their course of attack in the deep brain stimulation surgery I'll have eight days later on June 13. Then, it's back to the hospital on June 25th for the installation of the IPG devices which will control the stimulation the STN region of my brain will receive.

And really, all I can do in the intervening days and weeks is wait—and prepare.

I need a hat. God, in his infinite wisdom, has decided that my scalp should be visible to friends, family, acquaintances, total strangers, and even satellite imagery. I've been bald since my mid 20s. And for everything I've heard about this surgical process being relatively painless, there will be some scarring. Pictures I've seen of folks taken shortly after their DBS surgery experiences indicate head bones that look to varying degrees as if they'd come out on the short end of a battle with a meat grinder.

I exaggerate, of course... but consider the insult my shiny bald pate must endure all in the merry month of June.

First, the installation of the bone markers. Now, thank goodness, those big "thumb tack" looking things are removed right after they get their CT and MRI pictures (a fact that my smiling, she thinks she's so funny WIFE lamented, saying that if those post were left in place she could envision a delightful macramé project that would be the talk of the DC-area craft community. Sorry, hon... the posts come out)... but the stainless steel anchors will remain embedded in the skull so the surgeons will have a place to attach the individually made platform they use at Vandy—replacing the superstructure-like stereotactic frame that gets bolted to the surgical bed, rendering the patient immobile—captive.

When I return home on June 6, it will be with four little puncture wounds in my noggin—one in front, one towards the back, one on each side, each closed with a staple. That in and of itself would make for some uncomfortable moments on the airplane ride home as fellow passengers gawk and wonder who I had angered, and why that person had used a b-b gun to perforate my scalp. Then, after the June 13th lead implants, depending on which technique the surgeon uses, the top of my big, bald head will look like it's either been bitten by a small shark with two semi-circular scars—or it will look like it's been used as a landing pad for small alien spacecraft with two parallel 4-inch scars. Either way, they'll be a stapled or stitched ugly mess and if I thought my fellow air passengers would be wondering about the four simple puncture wounds from the week before, I imagine they'll think I'm an escaped mental patient from the double-lobotomy ward of a psychiatric facility.

So I need a hat.

I have lots of hats, all of varying degree of cleanliness. Some new... like the Vanderbilt University cap I recently purchased to show my pride in the alma mater... although I've never taken a single college class at Vandy, I will have my skull opened and my brain probed there... so I get to take SOME small amount of pride in my attendance, do I not? Some hats are older—like the weather and sweat stained "ON BROADWAY" hat I still own from my days as the original program director of the show tunes channel at XM Satellite Radio.

None of these hats will do. I need a hat that will cover the wounds, keep them clean, and most of all—NOT TOUCH the wounds or allow the bodily fluids that will no doubt seep from them over the first few days to clot in the cloth, making removal of the hat uncomfortable and perhaps even dangerous.

So... my wife and I went to a place at a nearby mall that sells surgical scrubs. We bought a "scrub hat." I was hoping for something like you see doctors wearing in the OR. What I got was something that my stepson TJ said makes me look like "The Grand Mufti"—whatever the hell THAT is. I think it makes me look like an older, paler, fatter version of hall of fame NFL running back Jim Brown. But it fits the parameters. It will cover the scalp without TOUCHING the scalp and therefore STICKING to the scalp.

Oh, sure... passengers will gawk. But at least they won't be sickened. And with my wife's help, my freshly insulted scalp and I will be able to make our way on and off the airplane, into the car, and home... where no doubt my two dogs will have to be restrained from jumping onto my lap so they can get a closer sniff at the source of that strange, new aroma of recent surgery.

Thank goodness when I have the IPG devices installed under each collarbone on June 25th... that gets covered with a shirt. Although one has to wonder what fresh hell awaits the first time I strap on the shoulder belt when I next attempt to drive the car.

But that's something to worry about another time.

My co-workers at the NIH Office of Communications and Public Liaison were HUGELY supportive of my decision to take part in this clinical trial. But some co-workers are brighter than others, as I confirmed one afternoon on my way home from work.

Dealing With Morons

May 10, 2007

3 p.m. yesterday.

I'm heading out the door. I'm one of those early arrivers, early departers. I get to work at about 6:30 a.m. and I leave at about 3 p.m. For one thing, traffic between here and home isn't nearly as bad in the early mornings and early afternoons. For another thing, there's always room in the parking garage when I get here. If you wait until a more reasonable hour – say, 8 a.m. – you'll be lucky to find a spot in the parking garage. And it's a long walk to the other parking lots on the campus. So I blow this pop stand every day around 3-ish.

I'm standing at the elevator when a colleague walks up behind me. This is someone I see from time to time, we are on a first name basis but have never really been what one would call conversational acquaintances. Still, when you're waiting for an elevator, ya gotta say something.

"Makin' a break for it?" I asked. "Yeah, getting out of here early today," he replied. "This is about the time I usually leave," I said.

He nodded and the scintillating conversation was temporarily halted by the "ding" announcing the arrival of the elevator. We both stepped through the door. I pressed the button for B-3 (government logic dictates that the ground floor leading to the parking garage should be labeled the third basement level). The door "schusshed" shut.

My colleague noticed I was wearing my "Vanderbilt" ball cap. "Wearing a Vandy cap, huh?"

"Yeah," I said. "Since that's where I'm having all this stuff done, I feel a certain sense of commonality with the institution."

(See, everyone in our unit pretty much knows what's going on with me. For one thing, I've been reporting about the clinical trial in the NIH biweekly podcast. For another, when we have our monthly "all hands" meetings, during "share and care" time – as I call it – I've related to the group that I've entered the clinical trial. So my colleague instantly knew what I meant by "all this stuff".)

"So, they're gonna do it?" he asked.

"Yep," I said. "They're gonna pluck my head like a melon and see if it's ripe." (Folks who know me are used to my sense of gallows humor regarding such things.)

He squinched his face a bit. "Do you really think you're going to get any benefit from this?"

I looked at him for just a second before responding. It struck me as a profoundly stupid question.

"Uh, well... yeah. I mean, otherwise why would I be volunteering for brain surgery?"

"Mmm-hmmm," he said, turning to watch the red LED numbers count down the floors. There was silence. I felt more needed to be said.

"Besides," I said, "I make a living telling people about the benefits of clinical research. What kind of hypocrite would I be if I didn't take an opportunity to put my money where my mouth is?"

He looked at me, smiled and shook his head.

"You're a braver man than I am," he said as the doors opened on the B-3 level. We both stepped through.

"It's not a decision YOU have to MAKE," I thought but didn't say. "You're not confronting a steady decline in your motor function, the onset of dyskinesia that will have folks staring at you as you flop and twist like a fish out of water, and the certain onset of cognitive difficulties as you get older," I continued to think. "You don't lie awake at night with images of Pope John Paul II in his final days in your head – this brilliant man, stooped, trembling, hardly able to speak, his face a Parkinsonian mask. So no, I am NOT a braver man than you are. I know what WILL happen to me if I don't do this. There's a chance this might NOT happen to me if I DO take this chance. Idiot."

These words stayed safely locked between my brain and mouth. Instead, I smiled.

"Well, it's not like I'm being completely altruistic here," I said. "I do expect that this procedure will perhaps slow down the progression of the disease. At least, I should be able to get by with less medication. And if it turns out that this clinical trial leads to earlier and better treatment for folks in the early stages of PD, that's icing on the cake."

He shook his head and looked down at the floor.

"Still, you're a braver man than I am." His expression clearly indicated that he was saying the word "braver" while thinking the word "goofier". He strode towards the sliding glass door leading to the little courtyard outside the building. All of a sudden, I decided I didn't want to walk with this guy all the way to the parking garage.

"Well, have a good one," I said, as I ducked into the men's room.

Up until now, the concept of volunteering for brain surgery was just that – a concept. Now it was time to put my money where my mouth was. It was time for the first of the three surgical procedures that constitute Deep Brain Stimulation at Vanderbilt. The diary/blog tells the story.

Surgery the First

June 7, 2007

One down, two to go. My head hurts.

I look like the Peter Boyle character in "Young Frankenstein" – but not nearly so dapper or charming.

It hurts to raise my eyebrows.

The bone markers are in – the anchors that Dr. Konrad will use to attach the stereotactic platform he'll use to guide the probes and electrodes during my brain surgery June 13. And despite the bitching you might detect in the above paragraphs, the whole thing went quite smoothly... once I got through the security gate at BWI airport, anyway.

"That bag's too big," the TSA agent snapped. I looked at the small, rolling suitcase by my side. Borrowed from my stepson – this suitcase was purchased for the sole purpose of serving as carry-on luggage. I opened my mouth to inform the agent of that fact when he pointed at the plastic bag holding my toothpaste, deodorant, etc. that I removed from the bag so that the TSA could see my liquid toiletries and satisfy themselves that I was not going to concoct a toothpaste and deodorant bomb onboard the aircraft.

"It's supposed to be a QUART bag," he hissed. (I swear... he HISSED!) "That's a GALLON bag."

"I'll be damned," I said, contemplating whether or not they'd have to clear the terminal because of this breach of security. I mean, you could clearly see the toothpaste, the deodorant, the little bottle of liquid soap, the tiny bottle of mouthwash – all purchased to comply with the idiotic new security requirements designed to prevent Osama bin Laden and his legion of evildoers from blowing airplanes out of the sky with commercially-available toiletries.

"I thought the purpose was to make the items visible to the inspector," I said. "I didn't know the size of the bag was the issue."

Earning every cent of his $8 per hour salary, the TSA agent pointed at a sign. "It says right there... a quart-sized clear plastic bag. That bag is a gallon-sized bag."

I braced myself, anticipating at any moment to find myself being pushed down to the floor, my face pressed into the carpet as this diligent guardian of the airport rifled through my bag to see what other dangerous things I might be carrying in as of yet unseen clear plastic bags of unauthorized volume.

"Is there any way around this, or do you have to confiscate the bag?" I asked. The agent considered for a moment.

"Well, if that's the only size bag you have," he said, apparently deciding that my gallon-sized plastic freezer bag of toiletries was not a clear and present danger to America and its freedom. He gave me a dismissive wave and I was allowed to proceed to the x-ray conveyor belt. I pulled off my shoes, took off my hat, stripped off my belt, emptied my pockets, and placed everything into the grey plastic bin along with the freshly-pardoned plastic bag. With my suitcase and the bin on the conveyor, I showed another TSA agent my boarding pass and walked through the metal detector. No beeps. Good.

Moments later I sat in a nearby chair, put my shoes and belt back on, put the plastic bag of stuff back into the suitcase, refilled my pockets, and made my way to the gate.

Southwest Airlines has an interesting way of boarding passengers. No assigned seats. When you get your boarding pass, you are assigned a letter – A, B or C. At each Southwest gate, there are three gates marked accordingly, A, B and C. When I got to my gate, there were a few people standing in the "A" row. Most were seated in nearby chairs. I found an empty chair near the head of the "A" row – I had an "A" boarding pass, after all – and sat down.

"Do you have an 'A' boarding pass," a fellow passenger asked. I told him I did.

"The line begins back there," he said, pointing to a group of people sitting about 10 yards away. There were a bunch of empty seats in this area. But apparently this gent had appointed himself "row captain". So I shrugged and made my way towards the back of the row .

As it turned out, folks sat pretty much wherever they wanted to sit as we awaited boarding. "A's" sat with "B's" and even the otherwise untouchable "C's" were allowed to mingle among their betters without being ostracized. But once the gate personnel started loading the pre-boarding passengers... the elderly in wheelchairs, folks with tiny kids... it was every man for himself as we queued into our respective lines.

I got lucky. When I got on the plane there was a front, aisle seat. Being a fat man, I like the aisle. I can lean into the aisle and give my center-seat mate a little more breathing room. I am a humanitarian and make no bones about it.

The flight to Nashville took about 90 minutes and was without event – except for some rocky turbulence as we dropped through thunderstorms on our descent into the Music City. I was first off the plane. A short cab ride later, I was once again at the entrance to Medical Center North at Vanderbilt University Medical Center.

The door was locked.

I pondered this for a moment, recalling that my first visit to the General Clinical Research Center at Vandy also started on a Sunday, and the door was open then. I walked to the side door along 21st Street. Also locked.

Thank goodness for technology. I pulled out my trusty Treo, did a web search and found the phone number for the desk at the GCRC. A few moments a later a young nurse named Ben opened the door and let me in. I asked why the door was locked.

"It's Sunday," he said.

Ben took me to my room where I stashed my gear, turned on the TV, made myself comfortable and waited for dinner, which arrived with its usual punctuality. You can almost set your watch by the meal times at the GCRC... breakfast at 8, lunch at 12, dinner at 5.

Monday morning, I noticed something different about breakfast. "Lump o' Egg" no longer had that "rubbery" taste. In fact, it was in a different kind of container. I felt a brief, unreasonable sensation of pride believing that my blogging on the subject might have led to this improvement in the bill of fare. They're my delusions, and I cling to them fiercely.

The only official item on the agenda for Monday was the pre-op anesthesia evaluation. It was a relatively standard affair – for obvious reasons, they want to make sure the patient is likely to survive the application of anesthesia. This involves an EKG, answering questions about one's medical history, a chest x-ray and blood tests. The very nice nurse practitioner who interviewed me cleared me for the procedure, but asked that I provide her with a copy of a cardiac stress test I had in 2006 (or was it 2005) before the final procedure on June 25. This struck me as rather odd... I would be having surgery in less than 24 hours, and if I were likely to be killed by the anesthesia on the 25th, I was just as likely to die from it sooner rather than later. But I agreed to find the report and send it

At 6:45 Tuesday morning I made my way to the radiology clinic at the main hospital. After filling out more forms, I was ushered back to the preparation/recovery room. After getting into a gown and lying down on the gurney, a gent from the MRI department ran a tape measure over my mid section.

"He's right on the border line," he told one of the techs. "60 inches... that's right at the limit." This meant that I would likely not fit into the MRI tube without being stuffed into it like cream cheese into a cannoli.

"We'd have to squeeze your arms into your chest, and that would restrict your breathing... and we won't do that," the tech said.

"Well, I hope I haven't come all the way down here for nothing," I whined, wondering if this was the end of my participation in the clinical trial. I could visualize my patient file, with the word "Closed" stamped on it in bold red letters with the notation "Too Fat!" written below the stamp.

"No, Dr. Konrad says he has some old MRIs of you he can use," the tech said.

"We'll get the CT and go from there."

Bernard, the tech who checked me into the radiology department, came back and started an IV in my right hand. "This is my least favorite part of surgery," I said.

"We'd worry if it was your favorite part," he said without a smile.

Then came the procession of professionals to my little gurney. Associates of Dr. Konrad ("We've been told what a HOOT you are," one said.), members of the anesthesia department, and the folks who would drill the bone markers in my skull all dropped by to say howdy.

Then they rolled my gurney into the CT lab. I slid from the gurney onto the CT table and the professionals gathered about me. Everyone was so busy. I almost felt guilty just laying there doing nothing. The two anesthesia ladies discussed which of them would stand on my left and which would stand on my right, and I got the feeling that the younger of the two was a trainee. For a fleeting moment it occurred to me that all I had to say was "I'd like to stop now" and then everything would come to a screeching halt, I could get up off the table and go home. I decided against it.

The more senior of the anesthesia ladies told me she was just about to inject something into my IV. "This burns sometimes," she said... and it did, but just a little. Her junior put an oxygen mask over my nose and mouth.

"You're going to feel very sleepy in a second," the senior one said.

I concentrated. I focused. I wanted to actually FEEL myself drift off to anesthesia-land. I've never been able to catch the feeling before.

Nor would I this time. A moment later I was back in the recovery room. "Are they done?" I asked. "Yup," Bernard said. "What time is it?"

"About 8:30," Bernard said. The whole thing took less than an hour. I raised a hand to my forehead and gently explored the region. I was expecting a puncture mark in the middle-upper part of my forehead, since the Vanderbilt handbook on the subject indicated that the bone markers are installed in a diamond-like pattern – one in front, one in back, one on each side of the head.

I had two bumps on my forehead and two in the back... not a diamond... a rectangle.

"Don't touch those," Bernard said. "Your fingers are dirty." "I washed them this morning," I said with a pout.

I asked for – and got—three cups of coffee, and they monitored my blood pressure for the next hour before turning me loose. I felt fine! In addition to the general anesthesia, they used local anesthetic to numb the top of my head. For the first time in my life – despite taunts to the contrary over the span of my entire existence – for the moment I actually was a "numbskull."

After a wheelchair ride back to the GCRC, I called Gail and told her I had survived the procedure. She seemed glad to hear this. I took pictures of myself with the Treo and e-mailed them to her. "Oh, my!" she said as she saw the first one.

I was beautiful. But I wasn't done yet.

My nurse-of-the-day came into the room and said radiology called. They were sending someone to take me back down for an MRI.

"I thought I was too fat," I said.

"They're going to try it anyway," she said with a shrug.

Moments later, two young ladies arrived with a gurney. "Where's your hospital gown?" one asked, no doubt puzzled by the fact that I was wearing a black t-shirt, green shorts and sneakers.

"Don't have one," I said. "And this is silly. I can walk down there."

"No, this is procedure," she said.

"Fine," I said as I hopped onto the rolling bed. I pulled the sheet up over my face and said, "Let's go."

"You're gonna scare everyone," my driver said, pulling the sheet down. "Stop that."

We went back the way we came... through the tunnel separating the main hospital from the Medical Center North. There in the MRI lab was the guy from earlier – the one with the tape measure.

He rolled the gurney into the MRI room and I got on the table. He asked me to lay down with the back of my head in the coil they use to get better pictures of the brain. My head didn't fit. It's a large head. What can I say?

I sat up so they could change the coil, and noticed something trickling into my right ear.

"How did I get water on me?" I wondered as I wiped my ear. My right hand came back with my index and middle fingers soaked in blood.

"Fellas, I seem to be bleeding here," I said as calmly as a guy with a bleeding head can say." Turns out I bumped one of my new scars on the skull coil. As it was still numb from anesthesia, I didn't feel it.

They put a gauze and tape over the incision and tried another coil. This one was even smaller... it was like trying to put 10 pounds of cheddar into a box meant for five pounds. They decided to go with a larger coil. This one fit tightly, like a football helmet, but it did the trick.

"All right," the tech said, "we're going to strap your arms to your side and slide you into the tube and see if we can get you in there. Pull your arms in as tight as you can."

I did as directed and they slid me into the tube. My arms and elbows pressed into my rib cage, but they were able to get my head where they needed it. After nearly a half hour they pulled me out of the tube, injected me with a contrast agent, and stuffed me back inside. Another 12 minutes and they were done. I was treated to another gurney ride back to my room, and never was I so glad to see a hospital lunch as I was when they brought it in to me.

After lunch, I relaxed and waited for the local anesthetic in my head to begin wearing off. It did. And that's when I noticed how much the entire scalp is involved in something as routine as the movement of an eyebrow. Each motion of expression was met with pain. It wasn't so much a "headache" as it was a feeling of getting the crap beaten out of you by someone with brass knuckles. My eyes felt swollen. My sinuses ached. Tylenol took the edge off. But there was no way to lie comfortably. I was able to sleep that night, but woke up frequently – every time I moved my head.

By the next morning it felt a little better. By the time I got on the plane to come home, it was even better. I had the same seat on the flight home as I did on the flight to Nashville – but now I was paranoid about passengers swinging their carry-on luggage and smacking me on the head with it. When Gail met me at the airport, I was paranoid about banging my head on the car door as I sat down. It's amazing how much you think about and care about a previously ignored body part when it aches and throbs with each and every movement.

My sense of humor, however, was not affected. Gail and I stopped at a grocery store on the way home and I noticed an elderly woman pushing a cart towards her car. "Howzabout I take off my hat and stagger towards that lady – Frankenstein-like – and demand that she give me my brain back?" I asked. Gail shook her head.

"Yes, that's a good idea. Why don't you do that? I'll wait here."

She knows me too well.

It felt good to be home. Oddly, neither Shiloh nor Raven seemed interested enough to jump into my lap and sniff what I feared might be the enticing scent of fresh blood on my bean. Gail had purchased one of those foam wedge pillows, and that made it somewhat easier to sleep through the night.

And now, the day after, as I sit here at my desk wearing a "Thompson Cigar Company" hat to protect my co-workers from having to look at my scarred and stapled skull – unless they ask first – the pain isn't much more than a dull ache.

A week from right now will be the morning after the actual electrode implantation. With two 4-inch incisions and two dime-sized holes in my skull, I imagine that will feel a bit tender as well.

But that's another battle for another day. This one's behind me. Like I said...

One down, two to go.

Interesting thing about the MRI I had that day. Nobody ever told me the results. I had an MRI of the brain done in Feb. 2006, and it came back as a normal cranial scan. Now that I'm applying for retirement, I'm in the process of gathering medical records from all over the place. One of those records is the report from this particular MRI. It said I had "diffuse atrophy of the brain." I didn't have diffuse ANYTHING 14 months earlier. Makes one wonder what's gone on under the ol' skull cap in the three years-plus SINCE then. It also gives me a headache.

Surgery the Second

June 12-18, 2007

I have no idea why this is so hard to write about. More than once over the past few days I've found myself typing words on the blank screen, only to delete them, start over again, delete those words as well, and then just give up. It's like there's something stopping me from telling the story. I have no idea what that might be, but it's hard to get started. I'm thinking perhaps it's just a case of there being so much to write about that I just don't know where to start.

So, I guess what I'll do is just start writing and keep writing until the story is told. If I don't like it, I can change it later. Just put your head down and push. Here goes.

We parked the car in the airport's hourly parking lot – the one with the $20 daily maximum. I figured that when the plane got back on Thursday, the last thing I would want to do would be to stand around waiting for a bus to take me back to the long-term parking lot on the perimeter of the airport property. If I survived the surgery, that is...

If I survived the surgery...

Now that the deed is done, I suppose it would be all right to admit that the idea of not surviving the surgery did pop up more than just from time to time. Dying during deep brain stimulation surgery is not unheard of. It's rare, but it happens – most usually a result of a ruptured blood vessel in the brain. So the possibility is there. It's a card in the deck that you hope doesn't get turned up while you're playing. It's like the "Bankrupt" space on "Wheel of Fortune". You spin the wheel and hope against hope that you don't hit that "Bankrupt" spot and lose everything you've gained up to that point. Odds are it won't happen.

But it can. And it does. And you don't get another spin when it happens during this surgery. Instead of Pat Sajak saying, "Oh, too bad, Bill," I suspect that the last thing you would hear would be the neurosurgeon saying something like, "Oh, shit!" and then the techs would rush about in a controlled panic as everything fades to black forever.

See? These are the things a creative mind thinks about but doesn't like to write about BEFORE a procedure like this because it would be bad juju. But the possibility is there, in the shadows. The odds are in your favor, and hugely so. But that "Bankrupt" space is on the wheel. And one can never say for sure...

Not that I want YOU to worry about it if you're considering this surgery... but you will. And you will most likely do what I did... and that's go ahead with it anyway.

(Seems to me that this is the sort of thing Dr. Finder – the Vanderbilt University ethicist – wanted me to really, really think about before I signed the consent forms back in February. I thought I did give these concerns their proper consideration. Hah!)

But now that part of it is over. As I write this, I'm five-days post op. And what I really, really want to do right now is write about what happened – which I was starting to do. (Is lack of focus a side effect of DBS surgery? I'll have to check that...)

Anyway, we parked the car in the hourly lot and made our way into the airport. I toted the suitcase, and Gail trailed me like a Mama Duck following her Drake as we went inside. We checked the bag, made our way through security, and found a place to sit down for a beer.

I ordered up a Sam Adams. "Ah! Goin' to Massachusetts, are ya?" a voice to my left said.

"Beg pardon?"

"Goin' to Massachusetts?" he asked again? The stranger was wearing a cowboy hat and a shirt that was reminiscent of military fatigues. But the accent was Bostonian.

"Metaphorically speaking, I suppose," I said as the bartender handed me a tall frosty mug of the most famous non-bean Boston export. I turned away, towards Gail, hoping he would get the hint that I was not looking for a conversation partner. No such luck.

"So, you live up there or just visitin'?" he asked. He missed my metaphor.

"No, I'm from here," I said. "I was just making a little joke because you asked if I was going to Boston because I ordered a Sam Adams." I turned away again. It didn't stop him.

So, for the length of time it took me to drink a big, frosty mug of Sam Adams – which I really wanted to linger over and enjoy – the stranger to my left went on and on about the fact that he was from Boston, that he now lived in Phoenix, that he once served in the Army for six years, that he drove tanks, that his father drove tanks, that the tanks these kids have today are like luxury hotel rooms compared to the tanks he had to drive, and so on and so forth. As he would make a particularly interesting or humorous point, he would accentuate it by slapping me on the shoulder, the back, or my forearm. He did that about six times.

I pounded down my beer and looked at Gail. "Well, hon, we'd better head for the gate..."

"What time's yer plane leavin'?" he asked.

"Any minute now," I said. I told him to have a great trip and even shook his hand. As we walked away, I told Gail that if he had slapped me on the back one more time I might have knocked him off his barstool.

In fact, there was still an hour before boarding time. But folks with "A" boarding passes were already lining up in the Southwest Airlines boarding queues. I took a spot in line and invited Gail to sit and wait for the line to start moving. She decided to stand with me for a while, but as it became apparent that our plane was going to be late arriving, she sat and waited while I held our place.

We boarded, and the flight itself was pleasant and uneventful. We had good luck with baggage claim – our suitcase was one of the first offloaded – and we made our way to the taxi stand.

The taxi itself was a clean, well-maintained SUV driven by a polite young man of Middle Eastern origin. He got us to the Vanderbilt Medical Center North entrance without delay.

We were greeted by the friendly, welcoming folks in the GCRC who said that this time I would be in a special room – with wall decorations. And true it was! There was a wall painting – tropical fish, swimming in a tranquil ocean setting. Very peaceful. Nurse Ben checked me in, and Gail and I went out to get a bite to eat.

Later, Nurse Ben showed up with a rollaway bed for Gail. We watched TV until about 10 p.m. and then decided to turn in for the night.

I spent a lot of time looking at the ceiling. I was glad Gail was there with me. But at 3 a.m. on the morning before brain surgery, in a dark room, you can only be alone with your thoughts.

I checked the time frequently. Nurse Patrice said she would make sure we were up by 5 a.m. so we could check into Admissions by 6. I was ready.

After a quick shower – Gail folded up the bed, her sheets, blankets and pillows so the nursing staff wouldn't have to do it – we were ready to go. I was discharged from the GCRC and we walked the short distance to the main lobby at the Vanderbilt University Medical Center. The Admissions office was full, with only a few seats available. Gail decided to wait with the suitcase out in the main waiting area. I checked in and took a seat. As each patient was admitted, he or she would leave with a group of four or five friends or relatives. Then another would arrive with five or six relatives in tow, and they would all sit in the admissions office waiting area. When it was my turn, I gave the admissions person all my information. She punched up a wristband and a blue card with my info in raised letters and told me to take a seat in the main waiting area.

In a few minutes, a gent called my name and that of another patient. Gail and I followed into the elevator up to the pre-surgical area. Now that things were rolling, I was no longer nervous. I was just ready to get this show on the road.

Gail was asked to sit in the waiting room while I was taken to a gurney in the pre-op area. The nurse told me to strip down to my birthday suit, put on the green hospital gown, and have a seat on the gurney. I did as told and waited for the nurse, who was a cheerful, chipper middle-aged lady whose name I cannot remember. She started an IV on my left hand, and since she used a numbing agent before inserting the IV catheter, it didn't hurt much. I was visited by surgical residents who explained the procedure, anesthesia doctors who explained that I would get some sedative in the first and third phase of the operation, I signed various consents. Then it was time to be catheterized.

See, this is a long procedure. A patient cannot get up to go to the bathroom. So a tube into the bladder is a necessity. My cheerful, chipper middle-aged nurse would not be the one performing this duty. That particular chore fell to a young man named Donta.

Let me set this up properly. Donta is a very nice, very pleasant young man. He has the build and look of a middle linebacker in the NFL. He looked as if he could lift me off the bed with one hand, insert the catheter with the other, and slam me back down to the gurney – all without breaking a sweat.

Donta walked into my area with the sterile catheter kit and shook his head sadly. "You've done lots of these, right?" I asked. He nodded. He opened the package, poured out the antiseptic solution he'd use to wipe down the tip of my urethra, and applied lube to the tip of the catheter.

"Take a deep breath," he said.

Now, to be fair, I didn't scream. I didn't yell. If you had been standing outside my cubicle you would have heard sounds like "Oooof, Nnnnnngh, Unnnnnh," but no screaming. Donta showed no mercy. He got that thing where it needed to go in short order, and got the front of his scrubs doused in urine as a reward.

"Struck gold on the first try," he said. I sheepishly explained that I wanted there to be a little urine in my bladder so he'd know he had hit a bull's-eye. He smiled, then went to change his scrubs.

As the clock sneaked up on 7:30, the pre-op room got busier. Then, like the biblical Hebrews fleeing the pharaoh's Egypt, patients on gurneys were wheeled out of the staging area and into their various OR's.

As I was rolled into mine, I announced that the star of the show had arrived. The various residents and techs assured me that I was the star of this particular show, and they set about getting me ready for my performance.

I had brought my iPod along with 132 songs on a playlist I called "DBS Ditties." This included an eclectic mix of jazz, classical music, tunes from the 30s, and lounge music. The fact that I brought the iPod was communicated to Dr. Konrad, who hadn't arrived yet. I was told that the good neurosurgeon was at the moment digging through his office for his iPod player. We would have MUSIC this cheerful morning!

Dr. Konrad arrived and brandished the iPod player, he took my iPod, plugged it in, and I told him to go to the "DBS Ditties" playlist. This generated a bit of a chuckle among the crew, and the concert began with Mozart's "Concerto for Piano and Orchestra, No. 24 in C Minor, KV 491, Allegro." It set a dramatic tone as the crew scrubbed my head, set up the plastic sheeting, and generally made ready to dig in for their morning's work.

I kept up the banter, talking about things I don't recall at present. It was important for the success of the surgery that I be placed in as comfortable a position as possible. And they were able to do this quite simply. Imagine being in a large lounge chair aside a swimming pool for hours. My neck was fully supported, they put pillows under my knees, foam pads under my heels, and foam rests under the entire length of each arm. Then Dr. Konrad said it was time to numb up my skull. I had been expecting to be sedated for this portion, but wasn't feeling the effects yet. "This is going to feel like giant hornet's stinging," Dr. K said. And he wasn't far off. After a few very painful injections, I began to feel the sedation... don't know what caused the delay. But it didn't seem to hurt quite as badly after the sedation started running in.

I didn't feel it at all when they pulled out the staples over the bone markers, nor did I feel it when they cut two four inch lateral incisions into the top of my head. I was good and groggy when they drilled holes into my skull. Dr. K made a point of explaining that the driver on the drill was set to cut off instantly when there was no further resistance from skull – thereby avoiding the damage that could have been done to the covering of my brain. And darned if it didn't cut off the instant it was supposed to. I felt the vibration through my entire skull, and smelled the kind of "burned bone" smell one might recall from drilling at a dentist's.

I felt myself being roused from my groggy reverie, and asked if this was being done intentionally. I was assured that this was the case, because they needed me awake and alert for the next phase. I felt somewhat nauseous from the sedative and my entire body had broken into something of a light sweat. Everyone was so busy fastening the frame to my bone markers, installing the probe drivers, and getting everything else ready to go, I didn't want to bother them with such a petty complaint. Eventually, someone noticed I was glistening and asked if I was warm. They covered me with one of those air-cooled blankets and it was like heaven.

As I lay there, fully awake and listening, they began inserting the probes. First, the "listening" probes. Now keep in mind that for the last eight days, they had a good map to go by – my CT and MRI scans. And based on previous experience and using data from other patients they had a pretty good idea of where their "target" would lie. The subthalamic nucleus isn't highlighted on the scans. And every brain is slightly different. But you go with the averages, and you have a general idea of where this tiny, football-shaped piece of brain will be found. So, since my right side is the most profoundly affected, they advanced the "listening" probe into my left brain.

(And here, I will mention that once they had my head opened, one of the doctors called down to the waiting room and left a message for my wife, saying that they had dug two holes in my head and found brain in both of them. Knowing my sense of humor, they felt my wife would appreciate the joke. She did. She also appreciated Dr. K sending her a photo of me on the table, taken with his Treo cell phone. I showed him how to shoot it to my phone number. He also took a photo of what was going on there on the other side of the plastic sheeting. He sent that to Gail, too. I wondered how much she would appreciate that.)

As the probe advanced, we could hear what sounded like an AM radio that wasn't set on a station, picking up faint static. As the probe approached the target, the static started to pick up in intensity, like there was a thunderstorm in the distance. They attempted a few different approaches, and each time in the area of the STN, there were the crackly sounds of misfiring neurons... and they were able to increase the intensity even further by manipulating my right shoulder, elbow, wrist, and foot, demonstrating that these were movement neurons that were misfiring. Dr. K remarked how easy it had been to find the area.

"And to think, not a year ago, I was seeing a neurologist who stated that I did not have Parkinson's," I said.

"We'll send him a copy of the paper we're writing," Dr. K joked.

It was necessary for me to be quiet during this portion of the operation. If I spoke, there was a problem with bone conduction artifact... meaning that the test probe would pick up the sound of my voice as it was heard in the depths of my skull. But being quiet came with some challenges.

For one, my neurologist, Dr. Charles arrived around this time and took part in the limb manipulation efforts. He stood at the foot of the OR gurney and waved. "Hi, Bill! David Charles here."

"Hi, Dr. Cha..."

I could hear my words coming out of the speakers, distorted but recognizable. "So, this is how my brain hears sound," I thought. I smiled and waved.

Other times, if something was said that I wanted to agree with, I found myself nodding my head. Not a good idea when you have probes in your brain. I adopted a "thumbs up" signal to indicate my agreement with something being said.

Now that they had secured the target area, it was time for the stimulation test.

This was, in a word, freaky. I had no idea what to expect, save for some possible pulling, numbness, tingling and the like. But they needed to find that "sweet spot" between "no effect" and "side effect" and this was the only way to do it.

(Now, keep in mind that what follows isn't exact, that for the sake of narrative I am playing fast and loose with the numbers being called out, but that this is generally how it went.)

They started with the left brain and advanced the probe to an area close to the target they had identified. Dr. Charles held my right arm and began to manipulate it. "One. No efficacy," he said, meaning that set at 1, the stimulation had no effect. He called for it to be raised to 1.5.

"There it is," he said. And he continued manipulation. He asked me to open and close my fist, and to rotate my hand. Even though I had been off the medication since the previous Sunday, my hand was loose and free.

"You can really feel it," he said about the stimulation. "The cogwheeling (that ratcheting stiffness in a limb that comes with Parkinson's) just melts away. Raise it to 2."

He asked me how I felt, and I replied "fine."

"OK, 2.5 then."

I felt something... even now, it's still almost impossible to describe the feeling. It was something like nausea, but not quite. But "nausea" was the only word I could think of for it. Dr. Charles told me to take a few deep breaths and we'd try one more.

"Up to 3," he said. "How's this? Any different."

"It's... It's... It's..." "Yes?" "...hard ... to ... talk..."

And besides, I noticed I couldn't move my eyes. He held a fist up for me to look at, and I was able to follow it on one direction, but not the other.

"Turn it off," he said. And as if a magnet that had been holding my eyes and tongue had been turned off, I was able to at least try to explain what had happened. But words still failed me, and I was more than just a little freaked out by the experience.

But now that I knew this was likely to happen with each successive testing of the electrodes, I was ready for it and felt I could make a good effort to define and describe what was going on with me.

Bit by bit, the electrode in my left brain made its way towards, into, and through the target area in my STN. We found that with therapeutic stimulation, the symptoms on my right side were eliminated. With too much stimulation, I had varying degrees of dysarthria (difficulty in speech) and eye-freeze. The speech difficulty ranged from speaking in a slow, slurred voice, to being completely unable to think of the proper word, or even to think of a word to say.

Testing my right brain followed a similar course. The only difference was when they reached the high end of stimulation on the last few passes, my mouth pulled to the left with a half-grimace as I tried to speak, and my gaze was averted in that direction as well. But the instant the stimulation was turned off, I would return to normal.

Dr. Charles seemed a bit frustrated that I wasn't able to be a bit more specific with what I was feeling and experiencing, but Dr. Konrad seemed more than satisfied with the electrode placements and they agreed to lock them in place and close me up.

By this time, the cooling blanket had left me feeling cold. A heated blanket placed over my chest and shoulders warmed me up nicely as Dr. K and his team began the process of locking everything down, securing the electrodes, and closing the wounds. They put me back into sedation and I listened as the doctors chatted amongst themselves as they applied the absorbable sutures and covered the incisions with derma bond liquid sutures – like Crazy Glue, but more expensive. They created pockets in the skin under my scalp for the wire leads from the electrodes that will be attached to the IPG devices when they are implanted on July 3rd – that date was changed from June 25th due to Dr. K being called out of the country to take part in some other seminar or something... I'm still kinda foggy on the details.

At about 1:30 – six hours after they started, they rolled me into the post-op recovery room, and Dr. K went down to the waiting room to tell Gail the operation was over and I had done well.

In the recovery room, I was assigned to Nurse Tom. A great guy, with a soft, southern drawl, he was easy to like. I asked for water and he brought me ice chips. Never in the history of the world had ice chips been so delicious. Our next step was for me to be taken to radiology for a CT scan, which we did about an hour after I rolled into the recovery room. They let my wife come up to see me briefly, and told her that the CT would determine whether or not I went to a regular room or neuro-ICU. "If there's no bleeding, he'll get a regular room," the doctor said. Shortly before 3 we headed down to radiology.

There was a Tennessee Highway Patrolman in the elevator when we got on. "Afternoon, Officer," I said. He wished me a good afternoon as well.

"I understand I have the right to remain silent, everything I say can and will be used against me in a court of law..." I said. I was recovering from surgery, but my sense of humor was intact.

"Don't ask him any questions, Officer," Nurse Tom said. "He's already had his brain picked today."

I gave Tom a high five for the zinger.

Still woozy, I crawled onto the CT table. I could still feel the catheter, a very annoying sensation. But they were quick about the CT and I was in and out of there in just a few minutes. We rolled back to the recovery room and waited.

And waited. And waited. And waited.

A couple hours later, Dr. K's intern came by and asked how I was doing. "You tell ME," I said. "I've had my CT taken." He went to a nearby computer monitor screen and took a look. He came back smiling."

"We do good work here," he said. "No bleeding, just some air, but you expect that in this surgery." He assured me that it was just a matter of waiting for a room to open up and I'd be on my way to a regular room on 6 North.

While we waited, Donta came back and pulled out the catheter. I won't say it was like he was trying to start a lawnmower, but it sure felt that way. "It's gonna burn when you pee at first," he said. I asked for a urinal. He was correct.

Nurse Tom was my constant companion for the next few hours. We chatted about everything under the sun. In the meantime, he kept me hydrated with Sprite, brought me a tub of Jello, and when it was clear I would keep the Jello down – a sandwich.

And we waited, and waited and waited for a room.

Around 6 p.m., Tom rolled me into a larger room with chairs and TVs and said he would bring my wife up to sit with me. Poor Gail had been waiting since being told that the CT scan would determine whether I spent the night in ICU or a regular room. No one had told her the CT was OK. So she was relieved when she showed up to sit with me.

When we were alone, she offered me a Milky Way candy bar. She bought me a candy bar, thinking I might want it. I love her with all my heart.

At 6:30 Nurse Tom went to dinner. Shortly after, the charge nurse for the post-op recovery room told me that they found a room for me, but that we'd have to wait for Tom to get back. When Tom got back, he said we'd have to wait until after shift change, but by 7:30 or so, we'd be in our room. And we were.

For the first time, I got a look at my gruesome surgical scars. I look like I was bitten on the head by a shark. My face was swollen, my head hurt. Gail took pictures to preserve the moment.

There was no rollaway bed for Gail in this room. But they were able to get a pull-out chair for her to sleep on, which she did with varying degrees of success. I know, because I was awake most of the night. For one thing, I was nauseous from the Lortab pill I had taken for pain. The ache wasn't so severe that I wanted morphine, but I had hoped the Lortab would cut it back a little. All it did was make me sick. And I felt constipated. And my head was crackling like a bowl of Rice Krispies.

Seriously. As I lay there, trying to sleep, my head kept up a steady "snap, crackle, pop" as the air that got into my skull was reabsorbed. If I opened my mouth, you could actually hear it. All night long. Snap. Crackle. Pop!

I had no appetite at all the next morning. I was able to eat some of my breakfast, but the eggs, bacon, etc., went uneaten. They were very nice to sneak some brekky in for Gail. Same thing for lunch... just a bite here and there. Dr. K popped in to check me out and said I was free to go home. My nurse for the morning arranged for me to be transported to the Admitting Office in time to catch a cab to the airport. Gail and I spent the better part of the morning dozing and watching TV.

It wasn't quite as nice of a cab that took us to the airport. A chatty young Arab in a run-down, rattletrap cab drove like a madman and hummed Arabic songs to himself when he wasn't grilling me on my medical condition. But we got to the airport alive, and I was able to secure a pre-boarding pass to make sure we got on the plane ahead of everyone else.

I've been home now for four days. In that time, my appetite has returned, my bowels have started working again, my head is still swollen, and I'm sleeping very well. I'm glad I was warned about this, but now my eyes are swollen almost shut because of the downward migration of all the fluid that accumulated under my scalp during and after the surgery. I look like I've done 12 rounds with Mike Tyson – bite marks and all.

Gail has been taking wonderful care of me. She is my healing angel.

TJ has been great, too! Yesterday was Father's Day. He smoked up a bunch of brisket and ribs. I got a pewter Homer Simpson statue to take to work with me. Life is good. I got an e-mail from my daughter Kendra, and Peter called from St. Louis – we talked for nearly a half hour.

Just one more surgery to go. Dr. K. says this one's a two-hour, in- and-out breeze – compared to what I've just gone through.

He's been right so far.

The third surgery was originally set for June 25. Then it got pushed back to July 3. So I had some time to sit and heal and contemplate what had been done to me and consider what the future had in store.

A Week Later

June 20, 2007

God, has it only been a week? Or... has it been a week already?

Either one of those would describe how I feel at the moment. Or both. Take your pick.

It would be a lie to say that I feel bad at the moment. In fact, it would be a lie to say I feel much of anything. I'm just kinda flat at the moment, like root beer that's been left to sit for too long.

I've made the airline reservations for the trip on the 3rd and 9th. Turns out I had to swap out the reservations for Gail and myself on the 24th... since we're not going. But it's all good – the new reservations for the 2nd thru the 4th actually saved me $94, which at this instant, carrier pigeons with arthritic wings are carrying in lead-lined wallets from the SWA headquarters in wherever the hell their headquarters are towards my bank in Maryland.

To be fair, I just checked the bank balance again. I swapped out the flight on Monday, asked SWA to put the $94 into my account – and here it is Wednesday – TWO DAYS LATER (I can hear those words in my mind as if they were being spoken by my grandmother, who watched each and every penny as if it were a little copper- covered grandchild) and the money is still not in my account. "It's HIGHWAY ROBBERY!" (Another of Granny's favorite sayings when the price of pork chops went up a penny or two a pound.)

Maybe they're waiting to see if I'm actually going to try to fly on the 24th... which I can't, because they cancelled the reservation when I made the new one. Or else they're just screwing me.

I will be going back down on the 9th to get the units programmed. This will be a day trip – down and back, same day. No need to... ooops. Hang on a sec.

That was the phone. It was Ida from Doctor Konrad's office. My appointment's been changed yet again. It's still on the 3rd... just not as early in the morning. Now it will be at 11 a.m. on the 3rd, instead of 10 a.m. which means I don't have to get to admitting until 9 a.m., which means a longer period NPO during that special time of day when I really, really DO want a cup of coffee.

Oh well... Like I was saying...

No need to linger about and take up a room at the GCRC when I go down for the programming.

Shit. I should have asked Ida about the "No Driving" rule. She wouldn't have known, but she might have checked with someone.

See, I have "No Driving" restrictions. I've been taking the train to and from work last couple days.

Work. Cute name for it. Not busy at all. Folks coming by to gawk, to tell me how "good" I look. And I suppose that considering that I had brain surgery a week ago today, I do look pretty good. The swelling around the eyes is going down – not gone yet, but going.

The Derma Bond on my head scars is starting to flake off. Feels like rubber cement. The staples over my little frame holes will be coming out soon. Gonna do it myself... ordered a stainless steel surgical staple remover over Amazon. I'll do the front two (4 staples total) then show TJ how to do the back two (another 4). No sense paying someone else to do that which I am perfectly capable of doing myself. And TJ's been ITCHING to do something to my head... back when I had the bone markers put in, he volunteered to take them out for me using tools from his garage at work. When I said I was going to buy a surgical staple remover, he said a friend of his at work has a staple remover, so I should save my money. It's a staple remover, a regular one. Such a good son to his doddering old dad.

Anyhoo... I'm just a little flat. The writing is coming along nicely (and if you don't think so, who the hell asked you?) but the speech is still a little rough and stilted. I'm not quick with a comeback like I was pre-op. In a few different conversations today, I found myself struggling to keep up the banter. Oh, I'm sure that I still seem like Noel Coward to some of the folks around here, but to my own mind I sound more like Barney Rubble. The timing just isn't there. No snap. No zing.

But I feel good. I feel strong, considering. I am tired and fatigue easily. But I knew what to expect. And I know it gets better with time.

Just don't anyone ask me to do any "stand up" in the meantime...

Do Not Peel the Derma Bond!

June 29, 2007

The head scars are coming along nicely. Most of the "Derma Bond" has flaked off. Nah, that's not accurate. After each shower, the edges of the "Derma Bond" on each scar would sort of pull away from the skin, like dried rubber cement. Although the post- op instructions said, "Do not peel the Derma Bond" – I dare you NOT to. It's like peeling skin from a sunburn. There's this little edge there, taunting you from the mirror.

"Come on, fat boy," it says. "Just give us a little tug. One little tug. That's all. We'll come loose REAL easy! And that's a PROMISE!" So, with the dexterity of a surgeon, I would grasp a small portion of the edge where it was most noticeable and give it a slight tug. And then a little harder tug. Finally enough would come loose to make it worth my while – satisfying, like the aforementioned sunburn peel and not nearly so painful.

I think the people who write things like "Do not peel the Derma Bond" are the same people who advise against scratching mosquito bites.

The scars look much better for my efforts. For one thing, when the doc applied the Derma Bond, in some places he did so over leaking blood. So the stuff dried over the blood, creating instant clots. Ghastly looking things. Now, my head scars are all shiny and clean. No infection (one of the biggest dangers mentioned in the "things that could kill you about DBS" portion of the handbook). The absorbable sutures are still in there, but that's because they haven't absorbed yet. Let's face it... we're not talking about deep, rich turf here. We're talking about thin skin stretched over bone.

I still have the staples in the bone anchor holes. They will come out tonight. I'm doing it myself.

I was a hospital corpsman in the Navy for a number of years. And that number would be 5-1/2. I have both put in and taken out surgical skin staples. There's no trick to it. The only thing you need is a surgical staple remover, which I ordered 8 days ago over Amazon.com – which means they will be here tonight.

Supposedly.

I placed the order and the clippers were immediately shipped from the company that sells them to a Fed Ex warehouse in Keasbey, NJ. That's about 187 miles from my front door in Elkridge, MD. Then, for some reason (I suspect President Bush had something to do with it... no reason, I just tend to blame him for everything) the remover was shipped to the Fed Ex location in North Salt Lake, UT. That's more than 2,000 miles from Elkridge. I know this, because I got the tracking number and checked. "How odd," I thought, "that in the process of delivering this surgical staple remover they would ship it from New Jersey – which is NEAR to Maryland – all the way to Utah – which is FAR from Maryland.

Several e-mails to Fed Ex later, I now can happily say the surgical staple remover and I are in the same state. A nice customer service person at Fed Ex said he (or she, I forget which) would get to the bottom of the problem and fix it... if such problem could be fixed.

I'm guessing the staple remover was just stuck to something else. Perhaps, even stapled. At any rate, it's on its way to me and should be here tonight.

Supposedly.

We'll have those staples – all eight of them – out of there by the time I go to bed tonight. Then my head will be clean and metal-free for the trip to Nashville on Monday.

Finally, it was off to Nashville for the third and final surgical event of the DBS trilogy. The one that was supposed to be a "cinch." The one that, frankly, caused more pain than the other two put together.

July 5, 2007

Surgery the Third

I was in the shower when I heard a knock at the door.

"I'M IN THE SHOWER," I hollered. My wife was going about the business of getting dressed and folding up the little cot the GCRC staff had given her for the night.

"They want you over there right now," the nurse said through the door. It was not quite 7:30 a.m.

"I was told I wasn't supposed to even check into the Admissions Office until 9," I replied through the shower door.

"That's what we were told, too," the nurse said. "But they just called. Someone cancelled and they're ready for you now."

"All righty, then," I said. It was good news. I was originally supposed to have this third and final phase of DBS surgery on June 25th. Then it was rescheduled for July 3rd at 10 a.m., meaning I was due in Admissions at 8 a.m. Then it was rescheduled for an hour later. Now, here it was, just about 7:30 a.m. and I was dripping wet in the shower and they were waiting for me in the operating room.

It would be wrong to say I had been "dreading" this operation. All along I had been told that this was the "piece of cake" portion of DBS surgery. Just two hours, in and out. Two cuts into the side of the noggin to locate the ends of the electrode leads left coiled like little wings on the side of my head since June 13. Two cuts into the area below my collarbone to make little pockets for the little Medtronics "Soletra" neurogenerators that would provide the electrical stimulation to the subthalamic nucleus. They run the wires up along the side of the neck from the neurogenerators, connect them to the leads, stitch everything up, badda bing, badda boom! Done! No more surgery!

So I was certainly not dreading this surgery. Perhaps I should have been. Of the three procedures I've gone through thus far, this was the most painful.

We arrived at the GCRC at Vanderbilt University Medical Center the night before after flying in yet again on Southwest – henceforth to be known as "Squealing Baby Airlines." (If anyone is reading this and wants to make a little money, come up with a line of "Thank You for Sharing Your Delightful Screaming Child with the Rest of Us" greeting cards that you can hand out to parents on these kind of flights.) This time, they were clear on the fact that Gail was going to stay with me and they were ready for her with the fold-out cot. The room was smaller than the one from my previous visit, and Gail didn't think there'd be room for the bed, so she at first said she'd be happy to sleep in the little recliner in the room. "I just don't want to put anyone out," she said. But as night came, she was happy to have the bed.

I slept moderately well, but – as one might imagine – I was somewhat apprehensive. In and out, two hours, piece of cake aside... it was surgery, and it required general anesthesia. I had that feeling one has at the beginning of what one knows will be a long, trying day – I'll be glad when this is all behind me.

So now this news that they were ready for me hours earlier than expected came as excellent tidings. All the sooner, all the better to get this whole thing over with once and for all.

This time Gail didn't have to drag the suitcase along with her since we were going to be returning to the GCRC following surgery. We headed out through the front door at Medical Center North and made our way to the Main Hospital Lobby. After going through the Admitting Office, Gail and I sat in the lobby waiting for someone to come take us to the pre-op room.

Eventually a lady called my name and that of five other folks. (I can always tell when someone is about to call my name in a medical office. The nurse – or whoever – will look at the piece of paper with my name on it and say, "William...." and then her expression will become one of confusion as she grapples with my utterly unpronounceable last name. "Schmalfeldt," I will generally interject. On the rare occasion that the person gets it right, I will be profuse in my congratulations. It's not a hard name to pronounce – think of a small hat made out of felt. Then say it as if you had a German accent, and you will have a "schmal felt hat". Leave off the "hat" and you have pronounced my last name correctly. Thank you.) We crowded onto an elevator and made our way to the pre- op room. A smiling young lady named Bonnie showed me which bed was mine, and told me to strip down to my birthday suit, put on the hospital gown, and wait on the bed.

Then came the traditional parade of experts – a representative from Medtronics was first. They apparently like to meet the people who will be walking around with their devices implanted.

Then the anesthesiologist who told me much more than I needed to know about what he would be doing with me before, during and after putting me to sleep. Maybe I'm wrong, but if I'm not going to be awake for it, or if you're going to give me a medication that will cause me to not remember you did it, then I don't really need to know about it in advance. But that's just me.

Whenever I have surgery, I always seem to present the anesthesiologist with a bit of worry. For one thing, I have a huge neck. That sometimes makes for difficult intubation. Then there's my overall size. Although I've never had a heart problem (knock on wood!) my bulk makes anesthesiologists wonder if they're going to be able to give me enough "nite nite gas" to put me to sleep – without killing me. So far so good. After we got the IV started, the anesthesiologist told me he was giving me a little "calmative". It made me nice and calm. I may have even been singing when we rolled to the OR.

They got me to climb onto the operating table, and I was very happy and very calm and very relaxed when the anesthesiologist said he was going to give me MORE medicine and I don't remember much of anything that happened in the next two hours. In fact, the next thing I can clearly recall is wondering why in the hell my neck hurt as badly as it did. Was I hard to intubate? Did they have to twist my neck into unusual contortions? Did someone put me into a headlock while I was out? What the hell did these people DO to me???

I opened my eyes and realized I was back in the post-op recovery room. My nurse, in a gentle and reassuring way, told me the operation was over with and I was fine. I asked if they could lift the back of the gurney so I could sit up a bit, and she complied. I took mental stock of my condition. I noticed my two new wounds on my chest and I gently felt the sides of my head for the two new incisions that were there. But I was still wondering about my neck.

Eventually it dawned on me that they had to run the wire from the neurostimulators up through the lateral sides of my neck to where they were connected to the electrode leads... and that since there was no natural passage for these wires to traverse, they had to make one. And that would likely cause a bit of trauma. It all started to make sense as I sat there, blinking, taking deep breaths, trying to wake up. After about an hour they brought Gail in to see me. She walked up to my gurney and gave me a look that reminded me of the way Jackie Kennedy looked at JFK in Frame #317 of the famous Zapruder film. She waited outside the curtains as I got dressed and sat on the wheelchair they brought to roll me back to the GCRC. When I was done, Gail gave me the same look. "There's a huge blood clot on the back of your head," she said. I felt, and sure enough there was a large area of dried and matted blood and hair. "There's a huge blood clot on the back of his head," she told my nurse. Between the two of them they got the blood cleaned off and I was soon on my way back to my room at the GCRC.

The surrealism continued on the following day. I woke up early and trudged out into the hallway to find a cup of coffee.

"Where are you heading," the overnight nurse asked.

"Going to the patient kitchen to get a cup of coffee," I said.

"There isn't any," she said. And it dawned on me. It was the 4th of July. I was the only patient in the joint. The kitchen staff was NOT going to come in and make coffee for just one patient. The nurse said she'd try to find some instant coffee. I told her that would not be necessary.

They brought a heated-up breakfast at 8 a.m. At 9 a.m. we were in a cab heading for the airport. We checked our bag and got into the security line. Gail went through the metal detectors. I got to the head of the line and showed my temporary Medtronics ID card to the TSA agent. (I'll get my permanent one in a couple weeks.) It notifies the agent, "The bearer of this card has an implanted medical device prescribed by his or her doctor." The squat, swarthy TSA agent asked what kind of device.

"Deep brain stimulation," I said.

"What?"

"Like a pacemaker... for the brain," I said.

"If it's safe for you to go through the metal detector, go right ahead," he said.

"I don't think it is," I said. "I just had it put in yesterday." See, the metal detector can turn the neurostimulator on. It can turn it off. It can mess with the stimulation parameters.

Realizing that this meant he'd have to get off his chair for a moment, the agent rolled his eyes and told me to put all my stuff in a bin and run it through the x-ray machine. Then he escorted me through a gate and directed me to take a seat. He pointed to a small row of chairs, in front of each was a small mat with the white outline of two footprints upon it. That way, I would know where to put my feet for the upcoming search. How convenient.

The agent WAS very thorough and after he was done, I realized he knew as much about my physical anatomy as my wife does. As he approached the newly implanted neurostimulators in my chest area, I asked him to be gentle. He was. Thank you.

The flight home was a surreal mixture of comedy and drama as a hyperkinetic flight attendant insisted on playing "Are You Smarter Than a 5th Grader" with the passengers for small door prizes, and various people got sick. One young man staggered to the front of the plane. The flight attendant gave him a large plastic bag and directed him to the lavoratory. Then she had the teenager sit down on the aisle seat, right across from me. I began to wonder how quickly my new wounds would take to infection should this kid puke all over me, but thankfully it didn't happen.

Eighty or so minutes in the air, and we were on the ground in Baltimore. Then home.

Then we had to bail for a tornado warning. We had been home all of 15 minutes when the Weather Channel said there was a tornado heading directly for our trailer park. We piled the dogs into the car and took a drive to an open spot where we could watch the weather and dive into a ditch for cover should the need arise.

It didn't. A rather scary wall cloud rolled past as the dogs heaved and whined in the back seat. Raven, especially, is an auto coward. She drools and weeps and rolls her eyes in terror thinking that each trip in the car means she's going to be spayed again. Shiloh seemed to be upset by Raven's mental anguish, but otherwise took the emergency in stride.

Thirty minutes later we were back in the trailer. Now it was Shiloh's turn to be afraid as the local idiots with their fireworks were out in the driving rain making noise. The thunder competed with the firecrackers and for awhile it seemed as if God and my hillbilly neighbors were having a contest to see who could be loudest and most destructive.

I stayed home from work on the 5th. But I was back at my desk on the 6th, regaling friends with much the same details I've just shared here.

Back to Nashville for programming on Monday. Then, hopefully, I'm done for awhile.

Now that the surgeries had been completed, it was time to schedule programming sessions. It's a trial and error sort of thing. They know they've got it "just right" by checking your reactions to the stimulation.

Day Trip for Programming

July 10, 2007

I overslept this morning. Got home from Nashville at around 8:15, went to bed shortly after 9, got up at 4:45 a.m. I'm usually up by 4. It's an occupational hazard. Now that I'm taking the train every day, I gotta be at the train station by 5:51 in order to get to work at or near 7 a.m. No time for coffee this morning, and that probably has more to do with my sense of ennui than does the fact that my Deep Brain Stimulation is turned on, programmed and functioning.

The flight to Nashville was uneventful, except for the young father and his two darling, precocious little treasures who sat in the seats in front of me. I'm guessing they were around 2 and 4 respectively and neither child has yet developed an "inside voice." They weren't crying or fussy. But they SQUEALED the entire flight.

"Oooooh, Daddy! Lookit this PICTURE, Daddy! Lookit the PICTURE of the KITTEN, Daddy! Lookit! Lookit! Awwwwww! Lookit the KITTEN, Daddy!"

Daddy was reading a magazine and only nodded the most perfunctory acknowledgement to his daughters and the picture of the kitten.

Grabbed a cab at the airport with a garrulous country boy driver named "Steve" and we chatted like chums all the way to Vanderbilt's Medical Center North. I made my way to the 3rd floor neurology department, checked in, took a seat, and waited.

I resolved that I would try to be a better, more communicative patient during this session than I was during the initial brain surgery. For instance, as I think back, when I told Dr. Charles that I was feeling, "nausea, but that's not the right word for it" during the test stimulation, I felt like I wasn't really communicating the effect the stimulation was having.

Chandler called my name and led me back to an examining room, where Dr. Charles was waiting. I brought along my Access Review Model 7438 Therapy Controller (It looks like a garage door opener, and it will be my faithful friend and constant companion for my remaining days) and hopped onto the table at Dr. Charles behest.

"Remember when I said during the test stimulation that one of the side effects was nausea, but that wasn't really the word for it," I said without waiting to be asked. "I've been thinking about it, and in retrospect I think the best way to describe that feeling would be just a general feeling that something 'wasn't quite right.'"

Dr. Charles frowned and looked at Chandler.

"Scratch that paper we were writing on DBS and Nausea," he said grimly. Then he smiled.

Dr. Charles produced a controller that made my little garage door opener look puny by comparison. He explained the programming process and said that his gadget would be able to tell him if the leads were situated correctly, and if there were any problems with the hardware. They were, and there weren't.

Each lead has four electrodes. It's necessary to test each of the electrodes for efficacy and side effects. That's what we did. First with the left brain, since my right side is the one most affected by PD symptoms. The first electrode was able to reduce my symptoms somewhat. Then the side effects kicked in with a buzzing feeling in my right hand and foot, and double vision as my right eye went off its axis. The second electrode eliminated my PD symptoms completely and the worst side effects consisted of a buzzing in my fingers, foot and lips and tongue. Electrode three didn't score as well, neither did electrode four. He put the control magnet on my right-sided neurostimulator and repeated the procedure. The side effects weren't as pronounced, and it seemed as if the second electrode was the "money" electrode on that side as well.

When we were finished, Dr. Charles said the session was a great success. He turned on both neurostimulators and put them at a low setting, directing me to continue taking my Stalevo as before. I'll go back in two months for another programming session to get the voltage kicked up a little and that is when we'll start drawing back on my PD medications.

Dr. Charles had a flight out of Nashville International as well that afternoon and offered me a lift to the airport, which I gladly accepted. We talked of many things, including his idea for a web forum of some sort for those of us in this study to use to stay in touch with each other, to touch base on therapies, and to share the latest news on the study. I said I'd be glad to spearhead such a thing.

On the subject of "other people in the trial," Dr. Charles shared an experience that happened during a recent surgery with another of the DBS-randomized participants. Actually, it's something that didn't happen, but might have had not "better sense" ruled the day. One of the patients – he didn't say who, since we all (technically) don't know each other as we maintain our anonymity – mentioned to him during a subsequent programming session that he had entertained the idea of playing a bit of a joke on the good doctor during his DBS surgery – specifically during the electrode programming session.

"He said, 'I was gonna pretend to be paralyzed on one side,'" Dr. Charles said.

"Well THAT would have been a good idea," I said. "Very clever! Very funny! And frankly, I entertained the same idea once... for about a half-second. Then I thought that you guys might have a syringe full of 'something' that you would immediately inject into the IV line that might save my life if I were REALLY having a stroke, but might otherwise kill me if I were not. And knowing that my self-satisfied chuckling might be the last sound I ever heard, I decided against playing that particular joke on you."

"What is it with you guys?" Dr. Charles said, shaking his head. "You're laying there, on the table, your skulls open, having brain surgery, and you're thinking of jokes to play."

"Gotta do something," I said with a shrug.

He dropped me off at the door leading to the Southwest Airlines portion of the terminal, I thanked him for the ride and went in.

The flight home was uneventful, save for a young girl traveling by herself, taking her first plane trip to see her grandmother in Albany. She kept up a steady litany of questions to her seat mate and harried flight attendants.

"How can you tell if a plane is going to crash?" "Does lightning strike airplanes?" "Is there a ramp at the end of the runway?"

I was grateful when the flight attendant said we could use approved portable electronic devices. My iPod drowned out the nervous child for the remainder of the flight. So did a double scotch on the rocks.

I was celebrating. I made it through the DBS procedure and was sailing down the downhill slope. No more procedures until September.

Life is very, very good.

Getting On with the Healing

August 7, 2007

I'm feeling pretty good. Having a bit of minor discomfort from time to time in the area of my scalp... feels like worms are crawling under the skin between the two incisions sometimes. And there's still some minor pain in the neurostimulators... more on the right than the left. Sometimes it feels like the wire between the head and chest on the right is a bit too tight, like there just isn't enough slack there. But it's nothing horrible. The incisions behind each ear are still a bit tender to the touch.

And it's no big deal, but it seems like I have two dents on the top of my head.

Since the healing of the surgical scars from my DBS surgery on June 13, I've noticed that there's a bit of a dent towards the front of the scar on the right side of my scalp, and another one just posterior of the burr hole cap that fills the hole the doctor drilled in my skull. It's nothing terribly serious... they look like what you might expect from a large hailstone hitting the hood of your car. My son the auto mechanic has offered to get his hands on a dent-puller at work to fix these dents, but somehow I don't think that is a good idea. Nor do I like his suggestion of filling in the dents with spackle and then sanding them down. But his heart is in the right place.

Now that the old bean is healing up, I will actually walk around in the presence of people without covering my disfigurement with a hat. When everything was still all scabby, I felt the least I could do was keep 'em covered. But now, and especially in these warm, muggy DC-area summer days, I enjoy the feel of air conditioning blowing on my still somewhat-sensitive scalp.

And nobody asks why I'm sitting in the "handicapped" seat on the subway.

On that note, there's this one guy who I think of as a "handicapped bully." I see him from time to time on the MARC train from Union Station to BWI that I ride every afternoon.

The handicapped seats on the MARC train are well-marked, but not reserved. That is to say, if a handicapped person comes on the train, and you are sitting there, you are supposed to rise and allow the handicapped person to sit there. I generally get on the train early enough and can therefore sit wherever I choose.

But every few days or so, this one guy shows up about 10 minutes before the train departs and will walk up to someone sitting in the handicapped seat, point to the sign, and say he wants to sit there. And I have no problem with that. But then, this same guy—this same, I can't tell WHAT his handicap is guy—will save the seat with a box or a briefcase, and then STEP OUT ONTO THE TRAIN PLATFORM, STAND THERE IN THE MUGGY August HEAT, WITH THE HUMIDITY MAKING IT FEEL LIKE 105-degrees, with the SWEAT DRIPPING DOWN HIS FACE... this HANDICAPPED GUY will STAND there and SMOKE until they tell him to get onto the train so they can leave! And maybe this is just me, but if this guy is able to STAND on the PLATFORM and CHAIN SMOKE in the hot, muggy, miserable DC summer afternoon, he can bloody well take whatever other available seats there are on the train and not bother other people to move so he can park his not-all-that-handicapped ass there.

Stuff like that makes me mad. And I think it leads to bad karma.

Add to the mix the fact that I am bored out of my skull at work. It's summer, this is the government, and nobody seems to be in the mood to do anything. The run of press releases has been slow, so there's not a whole lot to write about for the radio news service or podcasts. We did shoot an interesting video podcast the other day with Dr. Joe Pancrazio at the NINDS... it was on the subject of DBS, focusing on my surgery. It was interesting to see – to actually HOLD – an example of the electrode leads that currently reside as a pair in my dented, scarred noggin. It was also interesting to get a look at some of the prototypes of the new technology currently being tested for future DBS... although that is some time away. I imagine at some point, decades from now, we will look at DBS the way it is currently performed and marvel at how barbaric and clumsy it was. But for now, it's state of the art.

Not that it makes my itchy scalp feel any better knowing that...

The Second Programming Trip

August 21, 2007

A crazy Elvis lady, a pain in the butt New York lady, a fellow traveler in the clinical trial, and – dyskinesia? These are the things I want to write about in connection with my second DBS programming trip to Nashville yesterday.

Let's take up that last one first.

At first I wasn't quite ready to declare this dyskinesia. And it certainly was not caused by the hiking up of the wattage in the old fuse boxes yesterday, and here's how I know. I felt this way yesterday morning, in the Baltimore airport, while waiting for the plane to Nashville. I attributed it to nerves and the two candy bars and bottle of tea I had just consumed. But it got to the point where I had to get up and walk around a little because sitting still just was not an option.

Then, after the adjustment yesterday, I took a Stalevo 150 at about 4pm. An hour later I was sitting in a restaurant at the airport and the feeling came over me again. This time, I was less successful at forcing myself to hold still. It lasted for about 15 or 20 minutes, and for the first time I began to wonder if this was the dreaded onset of that bastard side effect of levodopa therapy.

How to describe it... are you familiar with what they call "restless leg syndrome", where it feels like your legs want to just jiggle and dance, and you wanna get up and walk because it's driving you nuts just sitting there with your legs NOT moving? Imagine that feeling in the entire body. Right now, it's 8:51 in the morning. I took a 150 mg. Stalevo at 3:30 when I got up. It's almost time for another pill. And about a half hour ago, I started getting that "higgledy- jiggledy" feeling where I just... could... not... hold... still!

OK. I took a few minutes there to call Gail. She says she's noticed in my sleep (I take a Stalevo 150 right before bed) that I've been unusually restless lately, with a lot of fidgeting and such in my sleep.

It's subsided somewhat now. At this point, I'm just sorta rocking in my chair, sliding back and forth in my seat, readjusting my position, and missing the keys on the keyboard which calls for much backspacing and correcting as I go along.

I don't think it's noticeable yet. If someone were to see me right now, they might think I was acting a little – antsy? But I don't think they would notice anything really out of the ordinary.

So... the race is on. And the stakes have just increased. As we kick up the stimulation, we'll decrease the Stalevo pills. And that will take care of the dyskinesia. Now, instead of four Stalevo 150s each day, I'm directed to take three Stalevo 150s and one Stalevo 100 for the late morning dose.

I just shot an e-mail to Chandler down at Vanderbilt asking her to pass this info on to Dr. Charles. We'll see what they have to say.

OK. It's 9:15 a.m. and the feeling is almost gone. My typing is better, and I don't feel like I want to jump out of my skin and run around in my skeleton anymore. Now, what were we talking about?

Oh yeah, the trip to Nashville.

Possible dyskinesia aside? It went well. The flight down was jammed – what flight isn't during the summer months? There was one squealing child on the plane, and I was jammed up against the bulkhead in a seat that is far too small for the immense likes of me. But that's air travel.

On arrival at Nashville I had a bit of time to kill, so I dined on some boneless chicken wings at a little restaurant at the airport. A three person combo destroyed some of the American standards for my entertainment. It made me a little sad to think that this group harbored any misconceptions about being talented. I figure if you're playing for tips at a public area in an airport – especially in "The Music City" – then I think it's safe to say you're not fated to "make it big" in the music business.

Got a cab to the Vanderbilt Clinic and made my way to the Neurology Clinic where I found myself chatting with an older guy with PD. The topic? Gun control, and how the only reason cops don't want us to have guns is because they know we'll use them. On cops. Sometimes, I find myself limited in conversation to just nodding and smiling. This was one of those times. I smiled and nodded and smiled, all the while my mind crying, "Chandler? It's my appointment time. Come and get me, Chandler! Rescue me, Chandler!"

Sure enough, Chandler stuck her head through the door and invited me back into the exam room. She asked the usual questions... still taking the same meds? Any adverse events lately? (I didn't mention the "thing" at the airport, as I was still convincing myself that it wasn't dyskinesia.)

A few minutes later Dr. Charles came into the room and asked if I had any objections to meeting another patient in the clinical trial. I said I would love to, and in walked a gentleman wearing a white t- shirt with the name of some company or other on the front and "Job Well Done!" on the back. His name is Ronnie, and he had his surgery back in November 2006. In fact, he was featured on the TV show about DBS that was aired on a Nashville station last spring. We had a nice, spirited chat – compared scars and stories – and he left. He'll be there for the eight-day Droolfest same time as me, so that should be fun.

Dr. Charles came back and pulled out the neurotransmitter programmer, which looks like a big, old fashioned hand held electronic game. He put a transponder over my left neurostimulator and began taking readings.

I mentioned how I had set off a theft protection device at a liquor store last week. "Yeah, I see that on here," he said.

"No you don't," I said. "That thing tells you if the unit has been turned off and back on, but it can't tell you whether or not it set off an anti-theft device," I said.

"You're right," he said. "I like telling people that I can tell where they shop, what they buy, what movies they've seen."

"Santa Claus is watching you," I said. He smiled.

A few minutes later, we were all done. He had upped the wattage, but just a little. We agreed to change my medication as I described earlier. Soon thereafter, I was in a cab on the way back to the airport.

After my second episode of suspected dyskinesia – while eating a cheeseburger at O'Charley's (as Dr. Charles will no doubt see on the programmer during our next visit in September) – I started getting that "can't hold still" feeling again. I found myself shifting in my seat, moving my arms and head, and generally acting like a person with ants in his pants, so to speak. Like I said, it lasted about 15 to 20 minutes, then subsided.

This time, I had a "B" boarding pass... my first one ever for a Southwest flight. Passengers can print out their boarding passes online 24 hours before takeoff. I didn't print mine out until 23 hours and 50 minutes before flight time. So, instead of the "A" line, I found myself waiting among the second class citizens in the "B" line. Not as bad as the "untouchables" in the C line, however, one of which was a woman carrying bags of Elvis paraphernalia. She and her granddaughter had been celebrating the anniversary of Elvis Presley's death by swinging through Memphis and Nashville. She struck up a conversation with the lady at the head of the "B" line about her adventures, including following a tour of Elvis impersonators and sleeping in the $600-per-night "Elvis" room at the "Heartbreak Hotel." I mentioned that if I was ever going to pay $600 for a hotel room, I would expect room service... served by Elvis, himself. That made the Elvis lady look sad, so I decided to keep my yap shut about the late King of Rock and Roll. The woman in front of me, heading to Albany, New York, covered for me – talking about how if someone got $600 worth of happiness by sleeping in a hotel room that Elvis once slept in then it was money well spent.

Then the Elvis lady mentioned downloading the new album in which, through electronic means, Lisa Marie Presley sings with her late father. The New York woman asked how much it cost. The Elvis lady said, "Nuthin'. I knows a place whar you can git songs fer free."

That set something off in the New York woman, who began what, I'm sure she felt, was a very polite lecture about how downloading free music was cheating the artists, and in this case, the homeless – as Lisa Marie had promised a certain portion of the proceeds from this new album would be going to feed the homeless or to house the hungry, or something like that, and for just a minute I feared this small but rotund and powerful little Elvis grandmother would launch herself over the retractable strap that separated the "B" line from the "C" line and all hell would break loose with hair pulling, screeching, punching and cries of "ELVIS WOULDA WANTED ME TO HAVE THAT THERE ALBUM...".

Thank goodness they started loading the plane and hostilities were soon forgotten.

Once again, I was crammed into a window seat. The flight home was delayed as we sat on the runway for about 30 minutes – first, waiting out a "hold" on takeoffs because of congestion in the northeast, then waiting for planes to land so we could get on the main runway without getting killed.

90 minutes, two old-time radio shows on the iPod, and a double scotch on the rocks later, the plane landed at BWI. Gail picked me up at the departing flights area (yep, departing flights! That time of night, the arriving flights area is jammed with vehicles. So I generally have Gail pick me up at the departing flights area. Less hassle that way.)

In four weeks, I'll do it all again.

And now it's 10:50 in the morning. The "higgledy-jiggledys" (a much nicer way to describe it than dyskinesia, don't you think) are just a memory. No response to my e-mail to Chandler yet, but they're an hour behind us. I don't know what they can really say, anyway, other than, "Yeah, sounds like dyskinesia. See you on the 17th."

But I do want them to know about it.

The Third Trip for Programming

September 18, 2007

And now, a new feature—

Parky Bill's Helpful Tips to Get You Through the Day.

First a travel tip. Want to ensure an empty center seat on the airplane, giving you a little bit of elbow room? Try this. Oh, a disclaimer. For this to work, you will need to be overweight, bald, and have recently undergone Deep Brain Stimulation surgery or some other procedure that leaves multiple, visible scars.

1.   When you get on the plane, do a quick scan for OTHER fat passengers. Look for one in a window seat. Then sit in the aisle seat on the same row, leaving a space between you and the other chubby flyer that only a circus rubber man could possibly squeeze into. This works even better if the other passenger also has visible scars or some other noticeable disability.
2.   Take off your hat. They're YOUR head scars! Show 'em off! Few people will willingly sit down next to someone with visible head scars. They don't know how you got them, or what you're likely to DO on the flight as a result.
3.   As people make their way down the aisle, shooting evil glances at you for daring to be overweight, smile at them. In a slurred voice, say "you can sit here if you wanna." Rub your scarred, bald scalp when you say it. I'm not saying you should go so far as to drool on yourself... but it works. And you're probably never going to see these people again, so what the heck?

And now... a tip about how to cover up that pesky dyskinesia. Get an iPod. They've just lowered the price, so now's the time. When the twisting and writhing come over you and everyone in the subway car is staring at you, put an expression on your face that indicates you are merely grooving to the music. If you want to, say something to the person next to you like, "there's an audition for one of them iPod commercials where they show them silhouetted morons hoppin' around like savages as they's listenin' to them iPods. I'm just gettin' my MOVES down." And the side benefit will be that you'll have pretty much that whole section of the subway car to yourself after that! So enjoy!

So... there you go. I came up with both of those ideas yesterday during my trip to and from the Vanderbilt Clinic in Nashville to get my DBS unit adjusted. And here's where I helped myself to a heapin' helpin' of hubris.

Doctor Charles, the lead investigator for this clinical trial, is one of my favorite people in the world. While I was holding the little transponder over the neurostimulator buried in my left chest, he turned the screen of his programmer so I could see what he was doing and he explained everything about it.

"Can you play Tetris?" I asked.

"No, and for what this thing costs, you SHOULD be able to," he replied.

Both stimulators were previously set at 1.0 watt. I watched as he set the left one to 1.3 watts. As this was the third and final adjustment according to the study protocol, I asked if that's where we would leave it.

"I'd like to go to 1.5, but that represents a pretty big jump for someone without advanced PD," he said.

"What the heck," I said, "let's give it a try."

So, he jumped 'em both up to 1.5 watts. Then he asked me to hang around the clinic for about a half hour so we could make sure he hadn't bounced them up TOO much. He told me what to expect and what to do if I should run into trouble with the adjustment after getting home. He said it would feel like I'm overmedicated, and it it's something I can't deal with – turn them off. Simple enough.

So, I went to the cafeteria and sat until about 3:10. I felt a little "antsy in the pantsy" but not particularly dyskinetic. And, as we will recall, I had dyskinesia LAST time after an adjustment. After balancing out the meds, the dyskinesia went away. So, I called a cab and went to the airport. I swallowed a Stalevo 100 and went to the gate.

And then they hit.

Not horribly so, maybe only slightly noticeably so... but there I was, with a case of the flibberty gibbets while waiting for an airplane.

And they lasted all the way home, despite my attempt to drown them in a double scotch on the rocks. And then, as I tried to fall asleep, my flibberty, jibberty legs would NOT let me drop off.

So, at about 10:30, I got up and walked out to the kitchen where the remote control was... and for the first time since Dr. Charles turned on the neurostimulators in July, switched 'em off.

I slept like a LORD! But when I got up this morning, I was really off. So, back to the kitchen, and on with the neurostimulators.

Good morning, flibberty gibbets!

So that's where we are now. I took a Stalevo 100 at 4 this morning. Nothing since. I'm still bouncing around a little, but not nearly as bad as earlier today or last night. It seems like my legs are the most affected... I can't remember them ever feeling so... loose! No stiffness at all. Arm swing? I've got THAT! Don't stand next to me while I'm walking.

I'm gonna just let the whole thing sit and stew awhile. If it's still doing this tomorrow, I'll shoot Dr. Charles an e-mail asking for advice. I really don't want to turn the whole thing off for four weeks. And it's not THAT bad. We'll just hope that things eventually wind down. I'll let you know what happens next time.

Remember what I said about how programming of the DBS devices is a trial and error process? Sometimes it takes awhile to get everything just right.

What Ho! A Mystery

September 24, 2007

Well. Darned if THIS isn't turning into something of a mystery!

As I mentioned in my previous entry, I had planned to just let this thing sit and stew awhile in the hopes that the dyskinesia and other side effects would just calm down. Then, on Wednesday, I had a revelation. An incorrect one as it turned out... But still...

As I stood on the train platform waiting for the Maryland Amateur Railroad Club to arrive, collect its passengers and whisk us all to DC, I realized that I could NOT get my left knee to lock and allow me to put my weight on my left leg, stiff-legged.

That's when the light went on. Left side. Controlled by right brain. Both sides of the brain getting the same, new setting of 1.5 watts from the adjustment on the 17th. As I am primarily RIGHT sided with my symptoms, this MUST mean the RIGHT brain (which controls the LEFT side, which is NOT as badly affected by my PD) is getting—TOO MUCH STIMULATION and that HAD to be causing loose muscle tone in my left side!!!

Right?

So, I turned off the stimulation in my right brain. Badda bing! My right side felt fine, and my left side no longer felt loosey-goosey!

I got to work and fired off an e-mail to Chandler and Dr. Charles informing them of this great discovery and, no doubt history-making revelation.

That night, Gail almost had to get up and sleep in another room. My right side, all stimulated and such, was trying REAL HARD to flip over in bed, while my unstimulated left side was having none of it.

Thursday I got an e-mail from Chandler. She and Dr. Charles had been discussing my situation and suggested that I TURN THE STIMULATOR BACK ON! My little "loose muscle tone" theory was something the good doctor had never even HEARD of in connection with DBS.

So, as directed, I turned the stimulator back on. And within minutes, I experienced the worst case of dyskinesia I have ever had, before or since. It hit as I was walking down the hallway towards the elevator to go down to the little snack bar we have on the first floor. All of a sudden – and bear with me, because it is difficult to describe – my legs didn't want to do what my brain was telling them to do, and my upper body began to twist and bend at the waist. I had to quickly place by back against the wall to keep from falling. Once I felt secure enough to try walking again, I could only take small, halting steps. And just then, the elevator door opened and several people I knew stepped into the hallway. Now, everyone here who knows me, knows I had the operation in June. And for the most part, I haven't given folks much to gawk at. On Thursday, we made up for lost time in the gawking department. Other than the usual greetings, no one said anything as once again I flattened by back against the wall to try to stop the bouncing and twisting, so I could let these folks walk past without having to see my twisting, turning and writhing efforts to get back to my office where I could sit down without being looked at. It took some doing and some real concentration, but I made it back to my office and plunked down on the chair behind my desk. My head and neck were bobbing and twisting as if I were some sort of curious chicken trying to see everything around me, and my arms... especially the left one ... were not at all interested in holding still.

I managed to punch the correct buttons on the phone to call my wife. I told her what Dr. Charles said, and what was happening, and she suggested that perhaps, until the dyskinesia settled down a bit, I should use a cane when I walk. I laughed out loud at the thought, as I explained to her how my arms were flailing in the hallway, and how a cane at that time would do nothing more than help me to cut a swath through the onlookers.

I shot an e-mail to my boss and begged off of a meeting we had scheduled and was soon on my way home. Folks on the Metro subway and the MARC train, especially as we stood and waited to be let onto the train, looked at me and looked away quickly when they noticed I was checking them out. Their expressions said it all – "kinda early on a Thursday to be quite so shit faced, ain't it, fat boy"?

I stayed home from work on Friday. Dr. Charles called me at home that evening. He said the fact that I'm having dyskinesia is, in a way, a good sign. It means the electrodes are where they're supposed to be. Now it's just a matter of finding the right balance between medication and stimulation.

He suggested I try half a Stalevo 150 when I get up, then half a Stalevo 100 at 9, half a Stalevo 150 at 3, then half a Stalevo 100 at bedtime. I tried that on Saturday with minimal success. By

Sunday, the dyskinesia was bad in the morning, not quite so bad in the afternoon, and almost gone in the evening, except for when I went to bed and my left leg developed the worst ever case of "restless leg syndrome."

Now it's Monday, and I'm taking even less medicine. I took half a Stalevo 100 at 4 this morning. In a few minutes I'll take another. Then another at 3 before I go home. Then another at bedtime. I will, by this evening, be taking about a third of the Stalevo I had been taking before the surgery.

As I write this, my upper body isn't quite so affected. An occasional twitch in the trunk causes me to rock back in my chair. While seated, my legs are just dandy. But as soon as I get up to walk, the dyskinesia kicks in – but not as badly as before. My right leg feels just fine. My left leg feels like a spaghetti noodle.

On the way in this morning, another co-worker asked why I was limping. I winked and said, "Interesting weekend." So now, no doubt, the nice lady thinks I hurt myself having sex. Let her think that.

So... What have we learned?

I am not a neurologist. I don't even play one on television.

And... since I have been spending a great deal of money for travel to and from Nashville to take part in a clinical research study with a top notch neurologist... Therefore, I should DO what the neurologist SAYS!!!

Which I will do from now on. With one caveat. When I go to bed at night, and I cannot sleep because my left leg wants to get up and run up and down the hallway by itself, and no relaxation technique I know of will FORCE it to just lie there and go to sleep with the rest of the body, I will turn OFF the stimulator. I'm sorry, I love my wife and do not want her to get used to being kicked. And, I need my sleep. I'm assuming as we go through the "getting used to it" process, the leg will eventually come to terms with the rest of the body and stop acting like the renegade puppy that wants to keep the rest of the litter awake all night – bouncing and flipping and jiggling—when all the other puppies want to do is get some shuteye.

At least, that's what I hope will happen. You can always give away a naughty puppy. Not so, a naughty leg.

Oh, and since you're no doubt wondering? I'll put this as delicately as I can.

Dyskinesia sex? It's not... good. That may come as a surprise to you. Sure did to me. But it is not... good. And that's all I'm going to say about that.

Dr. Charles Makes a House Call... Almost

October 9, 2007

Yesterday was Columbus Day. That being one of those phony baloney government holidays, it meant I had the day off as I am a phony baloney government employee. As we are in the midst of the most ungodly hot and humid October on record here on the Eastern Seaboard, I was lounging about in my summer "at home" uniform. Underpants.

Shortly after noon, the phone rang. It was Dr. Charles. He was in Washington. He had brought the DBS programmer along with him. And he offered to fix the problem I was having with the stimulation in the right brain if I could get to his hotel at 6 that evening.

Now here I had been expecting to just leave the right brain electrode turned off until the end of the upcoming 8-Day Droolfest. But the good doctor said he preferred that I have the thing turned on and set at a comfortable level, even though in a week we will be shutting the whole thing down for eight days.

So, I put on some clothes (after a nap), got into my non-air conditioned car, and headed DC-ward. I drove to the Grosvenor Metro station, just north of where I work, parked the car there, and took the Metro to the Woodley Park station. The doc's hotel was right across the street.

The hotel lobby resembled nothing less than one of Saddam's presidential pleasure palaces—marble floors, wide-screen TVs, plush furnishings, and pleasant perky uniformed folks. OK, that part was different than what you would see in one of Saddam's palaces, but you get the idea.

Dr. Charles greeted me and we walked to sit in adjoining chairs in a discreet part of the lobby where a neurologist could adjust a fella's DBS units without making a scene.

I described what had been happening to that point, what my current Stalevo intake is, and Dr. Charles did the rest. He reset the right brain electrode to 1.0 watts—right where it was before I went to Nashville last time. And I was good as new. He watched me walk a bit, and we decided I was good to go.

As I was leaving, Dr. Charles introduced me to the young lady who was coordinating the neurology event he was in DC attending. The lady smiled, shook my hand, then she said to Dr. Charles that he would be seated at Dr. Howser's table at that evening's dinner.

"Doogie? He's here??" I asked. They both managed a quick smile at my idiotic comment. I sure do think I'm funny sometimes.

There were a total of five "Droolfests" – those eight day stays at the General Clinical Research Center at Vanderbilt University in Nashville. After the second one, the other three were remarkably similar. So to save a few trees in the rain forest, I'll revert to the blog/diary to tell you about Droolfest 2, then I will leave the other three to your imagination.

Day 0, Droolfest 2

October 15, 2007

Well, here I am — same room as last time I was here for an 8-day stint. I'm all checked in. Nurse Eunice has strapped the wrist band on. I have officially begun the 8-Day Droolfest II.

I'll write more in a bit. Dinner just got here. And it's meatloaf. Mmmmmm. Meatloaf.

———

Well, I made quick work of that. Wasn't really hungry... pigged out at McDonalds at BWI before getting on the plane.

Ah, the plane. There's usually at least one major annoyance per plane trip. This time it was the yammering, nattering old lady in the seat behind me. This easily offset the bonus of having an empty middle seat next to me. I employed one of the "How to Get an Empty Seat" techniques I defined in a recent blog entry — find a fat guy sitting by a window, grab the aisle seat, leave an impossibly thin space between you and the other fat guy. It worked again. But the yammering, nattering, high-pitched old lady behind me who talked and talked and yammered and nattered and WOULD NOT SHUT HER MOUTH THE ENTIRE TRIP ruined it for me. That, and the fact that it seemed for a moment that the plane might crash on landing here in Nashville.... The pilot seemed to be riding the controls pretty hard, but we got all the wheels down at roughly the same time and... well, here I am.

It's warmer here in Nashville than it has been in Maryland. Mid 80s today. A bit on the muggy side. It matches he weather I understand will be coming to Maryland in a few days. Gail is keeping busy by painting the bathroom and our bedroom. Girlfriend knows how to PARTY!!!

Anyway, Eunice reminded me that I can continue to take my meds until tomorrow, when Dr. Charles tells me to stop. OK. That's why I'm here.

Oh, another DBS-buddy dropped by. Donnie's bald, too, but his head looks like it healed without dents. You could use the divots in my skull as ashtrays. But please, don't.

Now to sit and chill and watch TV and... I guess... chill some more.

Day 1, Droolfest 2

October 16, 2007

7:40 am

Got up about an hour ago. Felt a keen desire to take a Stalevo. May as well take them while I still can, right?

We're about 20 minutes away from the first appearance of our old friend, "Lump o' Egg." That is, if they don't cross me up and put an OMELET on there today. That could happen. I won't know until it gets here.

Met the other three DBS dudes here for their own 8-day assessment. Two have had the surgery, one is in the control group. Those guys are the real heroes, I think. They devote themselves to coming here and taking part in the study, even though they haven't had the surgery. But without them to compare the surgery patients to, this whole thing is a waste of time from a research point of view.

Oooooh. The CNN weather guy says we might be in for severe weather here. Cool. But I do need to dash out to a convenience store today to get some basic staples... soap, shampoo. I forgot. This ain't a hotel.

Having my first cup of the pale brown water they call coffee. It's not horrible... it's like what you might expect at a Denny's. Of course, when I make coffee, one generally has to cut off a chunk... but that's me.

Eunice dropped by. My first "Arm Purpling Blood Pressure Torture" will be at about 9:30. That's the thing where they have to take my BP 16 times, once every 30 seconds, etc.

Then at some point, Dr. Charles comes in, does my Hoehn and Yahr scaling, turns off the DBS device, and let the fun begin.

12:20 pm

Lunch was just here. Country Fried Steak, mashed taters, green beans, cornbread, pecan pie, orange jello. Not bad. Tonight? Grilled chicken breast.

Eunice came in and performed the "Arm Purpling Blood Pressure Torture." Gee. Just seven more days of that! My next door neighbor, Don, dropped by. Nice fella. Nice head of hair to hide the DBS scars. He and Wayne are probably gonna head to the golf course this afternoon. I think I'll pass. Supposed to rain this afternoon.

Had my Day 1 videotaping done. Wore a hat to disguise my readily apparent head scar from the independent analyst who will review the tape. With my meds and current settings, my PD is virtually non-noticeable. That will change over the next few days. After 4 pm, no more pills, no more neurostimulation. Whee.

I'm waiting for Chandler who said there was something she needed to go over with me, then I'm gonna dash across the street to the drug store to get some stuff I need.

3:25 pm

Chandler came and went. We did the test with the finger tapping on the counters. Both hands had the same score... 42/41. Then she asked several UPDRS questions and timed my walking and sitting.

And that's all for now!

Went to the CVS across the street and got some snacks and shampoo and such.

Took my last Stalevo 150 at about 12:30. That makes 300 mg for the day.

And now, since I don't suppose a half hour will make that much difference in the scheme of things, I'm going to turn the stimulators off. Let's get it on!

First the one in my right brain... off.

Now the one in my left brain... off. Okee doke. Let's rock and roll!

Day 2, Droolfest 2

October 17, 2007

9:19 am

What I want to know is, whose brilliant idea was it to conduct overnight construction projects here in the Medical Center North area? Since about 10 pm last night, someone (it sounds like he's one floor below me) has been running what sounds like a pneumatic paint chipper. Forget getting any sleep. The grinding, grinding, grinding and grinding have put an end to all hopes of that!

I have to wonder... did whoever authorized this overnight work realize that there is a Clinical Research Center here on the third floor, with PATIENTS, some of whom might want to actually get some SLEEP at some point during the night?

I'm sure it seemed like a great idea to someone. We'll chip paint, or remove plaster, or grind up drywall or whatever the bloody @($#! they're doing down there at almost 2:30 in the morning while all the offices are empty.

I know we PD patients are not the only ones here in the Research Center tonight. Sorta makes you wonder what sort of shape we're all going to be in during the day. It also makes you wonder — is this just the first night of some ongoing project and we can look forward to six more nights of this?

It's too late to ask for an Ambien now... but I'm damn sure gonna ask for one tonight!

9:42 am

The drilling or grinding or whatever the hell they were doing went on until just after 3 am. All the while I lay there, fantasizing about going down there and showing the operator a new use for his equipment — mostly involving his ass. But it would have been too much work to walk the hallways looking for him, and besides — I'd be in jail right now.

Got up at around 7, got coffee, took a shower, got dressed just in time for the arrival of breakfast. Sausage, French toast, and the ever-present "Lump o' Egg," which no longer has that "burned rubber" taste I remember from my first 8-day assessment.

Just had a nice visit with Nurse Sheila, who administered the "Arm Purpling Blood Pressure Torture."

I feel somewhat crappy — lack of sleep, tightening muscles, bit of a headache... I'll live.

12:50 pm

Just had lunch. BBQ pork sammich, beans, pineapple chunks. Not bad.

I miss my Stalevo and how it makes me feel.

Ahhhhh.... Stalevo! Click here to see how I feel when my stimulation is on and my Stalevo is working!

(Yes, I do have too much time on my hands this afternoon...)

6:19 pm

Well, looks like dinner with my DBS chums is going to be the order of the day. That's great. These are some nice fellas — I hope I have the names right... Dwayne and Ronnie, both of which have had the surgery, and Wayne who is in the control group.

They hipped me to the fact that they like to gather in the patient dining room for the evening repast last night. Everyone looked a little more ragged than they did last night. Dwayne wasn't there — he was out golfing still. Wayne and Ronnie had their wives with them... delightful ladies. We had a nice dinner and a very nice chat.

Symptom-wise, I'm not feeling it too much in my hands as of yet. My legs, however, feel slow and stiff. And my right arm isn't swinging when I walk.

So, on to tomorrow then. Hopefully the demolition on the second floor is put on hold.

Day 3, Droolfest 2

October 18, 2007

8:47 am

Slept like a lord last night. Two Ambien before bed did the trick. I don't think there was any construction going on, but really they could have torn down the hospital and built a new one around me and I probably wouldn't have noticed.

Just had brekky... bacon, omelet, a tiny Danish, cereal and coffee.

Typing is beginning to get challenging. Perhaps it would be instructive in one of these posts to just leave up what I originally type without going back to correct it. Maybe by Sunday or Monday I'll give that a try.

Other than my morning visit with Dr. Charles and the "Arm Purpling Blood Pressure Torture," really not much on the agenda today.

7:30 pm

Man, I really have been out of it today.

Really nothing to write about today. I took a 45-minute stroll around the campus this afternoon and have been wiped out since. My legs ache, my arms weigh a ton, and even my FACE feels tired.

Talked to Gail for awhile this afternoon, and she noticed that I'm slurring my speech a little. Right now, I feel like I could just sit motionless in my chair for hours.

Maybe tomorrow will be better. Sorry, just don't feel much like sharing today.

Day 4, Droolfest 2

October 19, 2007

8:34 am

We're halfway through. Huzzah!

Actually feeling slightly peppier this morning than I did yesterday. Maybe that was the low point and it gets better from here. We shall see.

Slept great, thanks again to Mr. Ambien. I understand there were severe storms that rolled through Nashville last night. Couldn't tell by me. Closed my eyes at around 10:30 and didn't open them until about 7.

Just had a shower, followed by breakfast. Not quite feeling "energetic" or anything like that, but I do feel like I'm in a better mental place today than I was yesterday.

So... we await the "Arm Purpling Blood Pressure Torture," the visit from Dr. C, and then a visit with my little brother tonight.

8:18 pm

I think I've figured out why my BP has been trending high during the "Arm Purpling Blood Pressure Torture."

When we do the sitting part, I generally sit on the edge of the bed, which presses into the back of my thighs, cutting down on the flow of blood in my femoral arteries. It finally dawned on me that's what was happening, so I moved and my diastolic pressure dropped about 15 points in subsequent measurements. Then tonight, I had my BP taken sitting in the chair here, and the diastolic was in the 70s.

Anyhoo...

Just got back from dinner with my little brother Joe. He's the chair of the Phys. Ed. Department at Lane College in Jackson, TN. We went to the Long Horn restaurant and enjoyed tasty porterhouses. Good stuff.

Now I'm back in the room... time to wind down for the night, then the fellas and I will hike over to the PD Symposium here at Vandy tomorrow .

Day 5, Droolfest 2

October 20, 2007

7:39 am

It sure is hard live blogging ANYTHING when you just don't feel like writing...

I passed on taking the Ambien last night because I had a drink with dinner. So the night was spent flipping and tossing and having wild dreams about driving a tanker truck and getting it stuck in sand and having minor accidents banging the trailer into things and getting dispatched to far off odd locations...

I think I'll have the Ambien tonight.

In about 20 minutes, the lads and I will toddle over to the PD Symposium being put on by the VUMC Neurology Department today. Should be interesting. Maybe I'll feel like writing something about it.

4:40 pm

Well, right now the lads are off enjoying themselves with one of the original DBS guys... and I'm sitting here in the room waiting for a phone call from my little brother cuz I dropped my Blackberry in his car last night.

I noticed it was gone when I put my jacket on. Then I recalled how I heard a "clunk" when I sat down in Joe's car as we left the restaurant. I felt around, but only found the seat belt thingie. But the "clunk" had to be the Blackberry.

I eventually got hold of Gail who got Joe's number from Mom and left a message. Now we wait for him to call. Hopefully he can swing by on his way home tomorrow and drop it off.

It was an excellent symposium. About 250 PD patients and their families were gathered to hear from four neurologists, including Dr. Charles. We DBS dudes got a round of applause as we were introduced.

Ever want to be in a really slow buffet line? Do so with a bunch of PD patients with bradykinesia as they slowly and stiffly pick through the bacon, eggs, etc. If I didn't have PD myself, I would think it cruel to smile at the thought.

Met Dale, the first guy to get the surgery in the clinical trial. He's the guy the other fellas are out with now as I wait for Joe to call. And wait. And wait.

I did find time to stagger to the convenience store and get some provisions. I'm exhausted.

Day 6, Droolfest 2

October 21, 2007

7:43 am

Whew! That's a load off of my mind. Joe got in touch with me last night and will be here with the Blackberry around 9-ish. I'll take him out to breakfast for his trouble. I knew that the blackberry was in his car, but still there's that little bit of uncertainty...what if it isn't?

Yes, I am typing wihtout correcting my mistakes this morning. Just want to see how far the hand coordination has gone. Not too bac, actually.

Dr. Charles will be in around 8:30-ish to do the daily UPDRS thing, then my breakfast with Joe. The other fellas are heading off to church and then for lumnch over at Wayne;'s place. I'd go alonmg, but I really, really meed my Blackberry back — it's government- issue, and hey don't look kindly on little boys who lose their Blackberriues!

Ten, an afternoon of waching football. Thjey actually have a Redskins game on down here today. Now that the Packers have beaten the Skins... go Skins! (Tbhe Pack has a bye week...)

More later...

7:47 pm

Had my morning visit with Dr. Charles and my daily Arm Purpling Blood Pressure torture. Then Joe got here around 9:15

and we went to breakfast. Thank God he did have my Blackberry. That would have been a real embarrassment, losing it so soon after getting it.

Spent the afternoon lounging around, watching TV. One more full day, then I get to go home. Yay!

Day 7, Droolfest 2

October 22, 2007

10:29 am

It occurs to me that this would be far more interesting to "live blog" if there were more interesting things HAPPENING!

Sadly, it's just another day at the GCRC. Had my breakfast (spilled my cup of coffee all over the floor, thanks), had my visit with Dr. C, had my Arm Purpling Blood Pressure Torture, and now I'm sitting in my bedside chair, getting caught up on some work, and deciding to write something in the blog about how there's really nothing interesting going on.

Let's face it. This has been like watching paint dry.

I'm entirely washed out. I feel slow and stiff, my typing sucks (I'm correcting it as I go, because otherwise you wouldn't be able to understand it...) but I don't know how this compares to the LAST Droolfest in April. I guess we'll see tomorrow when I take the final UPDRS tests before turning the devices back on and taking a Stalevo.

So, it's about 90 minutes until lunch. It's Fried Catfish today. Uh, yay? Then we wind up back where we started with our meat loaf dinner... just like a week ago tonight when I first got here.

This afternoon at 5:30, I gotta get a computer with a printer so I can check in to tomorrow's flight and get the "A" boarding pass. Gotta get that "A".

7:20 pm It doesn't get any more exciting than THIS!!! Spent the day lounging around, watching TV, feeling crappy.

Had my final meal with the rest of the Gang of Four. They're all splendid fellows and I will look forward to seeing them again in April.

Got my boarding pass. It's an "A".

I'll get my final UPDRS tomorrow, get videotaped, and be on my way!

Day 8, Droolfest 2

October 23, 2007

7:56 a.m.

I get to go home today. Yaaay! This has been a long week. But in a way, I think it's a good thing — not just for the fact that the researchers need this week to measure our progress. I think it's good for each of us to know how bad the disease is, unmedicated or unstimulated. It can't help but make us appreciate how good we have it when the devices are turned on and the meds are working.

Dwayne, Wayne, Ronnie and I will go our separate ways today after we each get our final UPDRS check on videotape. Then we can take our pills and (except for Wayne, who's in the control group, God love 'im) turn our devices back on. I wonder how long it will take to get back to "where I was" symptom-wise.

Brekky will be here in a minute. Then the final "Arm Purpling Blood Pressure Torture." Then we wait for Dr. Charles and Chandler.

Oooh! It's HERE!!! With RAISIN BRAN!!!

8:55 am

OK. Odessa (Chandler's helper) came in and had me drink from a cup of coffee and button my coat. I did both to perfection. She asked how I felt, and "mildly impaired" seemed to fit best. But I do feel better, if memory serves, than I felt on Day 8 of the last Droolfest.

Then Chandler came in and we did the finger tappy test... On Day 1 I scored 42/43 on both hands. Today, it was 25/25 on the right (a 40% decrease) and 35/35 on the left (a 19% decrease). Last time, I was reduced by half on the right and a third on the left. So there's a measurable improvement right there!

I also did the stand and walk test, but I have no idea how I did or how it compares to last time.

Now I'm just waiting for Dr. C and the videotape. But first? THE ARM PURPLING BLOOD PRESSURE TORTURE!!! That's next!

9:49 am

ALL DONE!!!

I'm turned back on and I've taken a Stalevo 150. I changed my flight (at a cost of $63) and will be in Baltimore an hour before I was supposed to leave Nashville.

Gonna pack, have the ladies call a cab for me, and be on my way. And this endeth the Droolfest II.

CHAPTER 3

The Decline

**After this entry, I blogged at length about further
"Droolfests" and other events in my life. I left NIH and went
to work at the US Department of Agriculture, only to return
to NIH in September 2008. I took a prolonged break from the
blogosphere when my older brother, Jack, died from lung
cancer in January 2008, and I realized I was likely to be the
first male member of my family to reach the age of 55. It was
another "psychic shock" to the system. The first was when
my twin brother, Bob, died in 2004. I noticed my PD
symptoms picked up considerably later that year, but I had
no health insurance and could do nothing about it. Then Jack
died on my birthday in 2008, and it's been downhill since
then. I started blogging again one November morning when I
fell and broke the shower curtain.**

Faw Down! Break Shower!

November 28, 2008

It was Monday morning, Nov. 24. Shower time. Time to scrape
off the scuzz of the weekend and make myself dainty for the first
day of the work week.

I woke up that morning feeling particularly unfocused. It's one of
the symptoms of Parkinson's disease. It's called bradyphrenia.
Loosely defined, it means "slowness of thought."

I get that a lot. My limbs move slowly before the first pill of the
day. The deep brain stimulation (DBS) devices are always turned
on, but they're not sufficient in and of themselves to control all
the symptoms. And, usually, I take that first hit of
levodopa/carbidopa an hour BEFORE getting into the shower.
But I woke up late that morning.

The shower proceeded with no problems. It's a small shower, so I am able to keep one hand on the wall and stay steady.

I turned off the water, opened the curtain and grabbed the towel from the nearby table. Slowly and carefully, I dried myself. Making sure my pins were under me, I gingerly stepped over the rim of the tub. Right leg first. Then the left. So far, so good. I slipped on my underwear and shaved the undergrowth from my neck and lower lip. I picked up the towel from the toilet seat and — much as I've done at the conclusion of a shower for DECADES — flipped it over the shower curtain bar.

My wife, God love her, slept through the crash. I didn't even know what had happened, but somehow I was plastered against the far wall of the shower, the towel — and most of the shower curtain bar, in my hands. The brackets that were supposed to keep the shower curtain bar fastened to the wall? In pieces on the floor and in the tub.

"Gail's gonna notice this," I thought. "Better leave a note."

I stepped out of the bathroom into the hallway — a passage that, at this time of the morning, is generally strewn with dogs. Our two beauties — Raven and Shiloh — tend to present themselves as obstacles to my progress at this point of the morning. I've long since learned not to try to step over them, as they tend to wait until I have one leg over their prone bodies before leaping to their feet in their daily attempt to kill me.

Now I stand there and growl a single word.

"Move!"

And they do. Grudgingly. They get up, stretch, shoot me an evil glare, and make their way either to the couch or the recliner. Now I can just kick the dog toys out of my way and step safely — first into the living room, then into the kitchen.

Coffee's ready by this point. So I pour a cup, dispense my morning pills, and sit down at the laptop at the kitchen table to check the morning headlines and e-mail.

After about 10 minutes, it was time to get back into the bathroom, brush my teeth, then finish getting dressed for the day. I felt foggy, cloudy-headed, unconnected, and apathetic. I thought about leaving the empty coffee cup on the table, but decided against it. I stood up and turned on my left foot to put the cup on the counter top near the sink.

I meant to just turn around and take a step. Instead, with my left foot stuck to the floor — a condition Parkies know as "freezing" — I found myself wheeling around nearly 360-degrees. I grabbed the back of the chair and steadied myself, preventing a fall.

Twice now. In the span of a morning. This was going to be a FUN day. I just KNEW it.

I've been aware for awhile now that I am not the steadiest fellow in town anymore. I've nearly fallen quite a few times... getting into the car, getting out of the car, walking up stairs, walking DOWN stairs, and almost always when I least expect it. There's no sense of dizziness. There's no sense that something isn't quite right. There's just that sense that the top half of my body is just about to go over the lower half to a tipping point past the center of gravity and if I don't GRAB SOMETHING, I'll go ass-over-teakettle into somebody's lunch at the cafeteria.

That's what the cane is for. I figure I actually only need it once out of every several thousand steps I take. But I'd rather have it and not need it than need it and not have it.

So... where were we?

Right. My balance issues.

I sent an e-mail to the very nice lady at Vanderbilt University Medical Center — where I'm taking part in a clinical trial testing the safety and tolerability of Deep Brain Stimulation in early Parkinson 's disease. I told her what happened that morning. I also explained the fogginess I had been experiencing. How I sometimes lose track of a TV show because I zoned out for a few minutes and missed a plot point, or how I can watch a football game and not remember why the score had changed. I explained how my speech had been more slurred than usual, and how Gail was noticing my face wasn't showing its usual range of expressions.

That evening I went to bed shortly after 8. I was practically incapable of holding a conversation and just wanted to let my brain reboot.

On Tuesday, I was slightly better. Still feeling foggy, still wobbly. But I didn't fall. Gail had replaced the shower curtain with a nice new one.

When the neurologist called me back on Wednesday, I was actually feeling better. Not as foggy, not quite as wobbly. But still stiffer than I would like to be. Still slower. And still having moments where, if I weren't hanging on to something, I would probably fall.

He explained it clearly. Parkinson's is a progressive disease. Mine is progressing. We noticed during my last 8-day stay at Vanderbilt as part of the clinical trial that my balance was becoming an issue. Postural instability is one of the cardinal symptoms of the disease. Like bradykinesia (slow movement), rigidity and resting tremor. (I have three of the four... although tremor is the symptom most people associate with PD, it is not the most disabling... and I don't have much. Which is why, when I tell folks I have PD, they invariably respond, "but you don't LOOK like you do!")

We decided against changing my meds for the time being, and I said I would keep a daily track of "how I'm doing" and we'd discuss it when I go back down to Vandy in April for my last 8-day stay in the clinical trial.

Then, shortly after Thanksgiving, we learned that my older sister had been diagnosed with a terminal case of esophageal cancer. That's the day I wrote this next entry.

Hairy Thunderer or Feckless Thug?

December 12, 2008

I recall an episode of "The West Wing" where, after the death of an assistant and long-time family friend, President Bartlett walks into a church and curses at God.

President Bartlet (Martin Sheen): You're a son of a bitch you know that? She bought her first new car and you hit her with a drunk driver. What, is that supposed to be funny? "You can't conceive nor can I the strangeness of the mercy of God," says Graham Green. I think I know who's ass he was kissing there, 'cause I think you're just vindictive. What was Josh Lyman, the warning shot? That was my son, what did I ever do to yours but praise his glory and praise his name? There's a tropical storm that's gaining speed and power. They say we haven't had a storm this bad since you took out that Tender ship of mine in the North Atlantic last year, sixty-eight crew. You know what a Tender ship does? It fixes the other ships, and, delivers the mail, that's all it can do. Gracias Tibiago Domine. Yes, I lied. It was a sin, I've committed many sins. Have I displeased you, you feckless thug? Three point eight billion new jobs that wasn't good? Bailed out Mexico, Increased foreign trade, 30 million new acres of land for conservation, put Mendoza on the bench, we're not fighting a war, I've raised 3 children. That's not enough to buy me out of the doghouse?

Hace credam a deo pio? A deo iusto, a deo scico? Cruciatus in crucem. Tuus in terra sertvus, nuntius fui. Officium perfecti. Cruciatus in crucem. Eas in crucem.

(Translation: Am I really to believe that these are the acts of a loving God? A just God? A wise God? To hell with your punishments. I was your servant here on Earth. And I spread your word and I did your work. To hell with your punishments. To hell with you.)

A nice piece of writing, and it really goes to show the anger and frustration and powerlessness we confront when faced with bad news... when things happen that are beyond our control... when bad things happen to good people.

We wonder why God permits evil to exist while the righteous suffer. Is that fair?

We wonder why God allows decent people — children, adults — to suffer from dreadful diseases while those who prey on others enjoy long, healthy lives.

We wonder, sometimes... "God? What the fuck are you doing up there?"

If you're of the Judeo-Christian tradition, your mind turns to the book of Job, where God visits his good and faithful servant with death and disease and poverty to win a bet with Satan. And when Job finally turns his eyes skyward and asks the Almighty to explain, "Why me?" God answers — "Because! That's why! And by the way, where were you when I created the universe? Huh? So, which one of us is God and which one of us is YOU? Ah ha! I thought so! Piss off." Of course, God does replace everything He took from Job, but still...

If you're a Steven Sondheim fan, you think of the lyrics to "Epiphany" from "Sweeney Todd."

We all deserve to die. Tell you why, Mrs. Lovett, tell you why. Because in all of the whole human race, Mrs. Lovett, there are two kinds of men and only two. There's the one staying put in his proper place, And the one with his foot in the other one's face. Look at me, Mrs. Lovett, look at you!

So, I have to wonder. Are we to blame for the bad things that happen by virtue of the fact that we are mortal? Does God cluck His almighty tongue in contempt for humanity when we plead for mercy, for forgiveness, for special treatment, for a cure to disease? Does He flip us the Eternal Bird when we ask him to protect the airplane we're riding, when we beg him not to wipe out the city we live in as the hurricane approaches, when we pray for the Queen to come up as we draw to an inside straight?

Or is the problem merely the way we think of God?

Could it be that God is NOT a cosmic "Daddy Warbucks" — to be called on for rescue when we're in trouble?

Why would God divert a hurricane from New Orleans to have it strike in Houston? Are the people of Houston less righteous? Why would God answer YOUR prayers to cure YOUR cancer and not answer my father's prayers to cure HIS cancer?   Why would God allow a plane carrying good and decent people to crash into a mountain when planes carrying wicked people fly cross continent unharmed? And why would God kill the GOOD people on that plane at any rate, even to get at the Mafia Don who happens to be sitting in first class on his way to commit wicked deeds?

Could it be that God created a universe that is random in nature... that things sometimes "happen" for no good reason?

Could it be that we are as capable of understanding eternity or the rationale of an omnipotent being as my dogs are of understanding why water is falling from the sky and why their fur is getting wet and why I — as their master — can't STOP this nonsense?

I don't know what lessons are meant to be learned when we or our loved ones are dealt shitty hands in the card game of life. Actually, I wonder IF there is a lesson to be learned. I wonder if we're not supposed to just pick ourselves up, dust ourselves off, and get back to work with a smile on our faces and a pound of lead in our hearts.

I do know that there are times when I've found I can handle things better when I ask God to just give me a bit of strength to DEAL with misfortune.

And frankly, as a finite being keenly aware of his own mortality, I think that's all we really have any right to ask for.

So, in the words of the National Lampoon parody — Deteriorata... Therefore, make peace with your god Whatever you conceive him to be— Hairy thunderer, or cosmic muffin.

With all its hopes, dreams, promises and urban renewal The world continues to deteriorate. Now pick yourself up, dust yourself off, and get your ass to work.

My sister Cindi, ever graceful, ever optimistic, had surgery for her condition. She did everything she was supposed to do, with the help of her loving husband and her devoted kids. She died on November 4, 2009.

The year of 2009 brought about some real changes in my life. Parkinson's disease had morphed from an "exquisite little inconvenience" into an everyday hindrance. It caused me to quit driving. It caused me to eventually need to work from home. And it eventually led me to make the decision to seek disability retirements.

These blog/diary entries detail the process of decline, as it happened.

Me So Happy!

January 28, 2009

Wanna know how happy I am right now? I had almost a full entry typed when, all of a sudden, my right pinky finger hits a key that highlights everything on the screen, and before I can recognize that this has happened, I hit another key — ALL GONE!

Vanished.

Into that black computer hole from which nothing emerges.

But I'm too pissed off to just say "fuck it" and quit at this point. I feel like bitching, and goddamn it straight to HELL if I'm not gonna do it, if for no other reason than to indulge myself!

(He hits the "save and continue" button.)

Felt relatively decent when I got up this morning. Then Raven showed me a puddle of pee on the carpet. Shiloh saw me looking at it and ran behind the couch. She's been "demonstrating" lately... when Gail leaves to go to the store... Shiloh pees on the carpet. When we go to bed at night and leave them alone, Shiloh pees on the carpet. Sometimes, when she's really upset with us, she poops.

Gail just shampooed the carpet yesterday.

I waited for Shiloh to peek out from behind the carpet and called her over. I put her collar on and attached her leash. She figured this meant she was going outside. Which she was but not quite yet.

I started walking toward the puddle. She realized where she was being led and put on the brakes. I am stronger than she is, so I dragged her to the spot, laid her on her side, and — just like the Dog Whisperer says to do — I assumed the position of a dominant dog correcting the behavior of a subordinate. I put my face over hers and growled. I rubbed her little snout in the pee. Then I smacked the palm of my hand on the carpet like a referee pounding out a three count at Wrestlemania, accentuating each slap with a "NO! NO! NO!" Then I dragged her little canine ass to the door, hooked her up to the outside leash and tossed her out into the cold, dark yard to consider her crime.

I will do this every morning from now on if there is pee on the carpet. SHE will get tired of it looooong before I do.

So now, it's almost time to go to work. Gail notices I am limping. I tell her that it's because my right Achilles tendon hurts, which is true. But walking out to the car, I notice that the leg is having trouble obeying simple commands, like "step". (Great, something ELSE that won't listen to me. At least it hasn't peed on the carpet. Yet.)

(He hits the "save and continue" button.)

No problem driving to work, except my head feels like it's stuffed with lead. So do my bowels. Every morning for the past week or so, I manage to crap out a hunk of granite — after struggling like Hercules for 10 minutes or so. I ate a bowl of Cream of Wheat last night. That USUALLY results in a steady, flowing stream of poo right away in the morning — followed by a sense of "gotta go and I mean right NOW" urgency when I'm in the car, stuck on the Beltway, 10 miles from the office. Not so this time. If I were to die today, I would feel very, very sorry for whoever has to do my autopsy. I must have four or five days of backed up crap in there.

I get to work, get out of the car, and my leg is still acting stupid. We get to the office, I get inside, take off my coat, take a seat, and chat with some co-workers. This is when I discover that my mouth is set on "stumblebum."

(He hits the "save and continue" button.)

I wonder what my co-workers think about the normally well-spoken and eloquent Bill as he stammers through simple conversation.

(And suddenly, my right hand hits SOMETHING that causes the blog program to close. He begins again with this paragraph.)

9:45 — I have a 10 o'clock appointment to discuss podcasting with a potential interviewee. I throw on my coat and drag myself to the Clinical Center... a 10-minute walk that takes 20 on days like today.

I get there, meet the person I'm supposed to chat with, and stammer and stumble my way through a description of the podcast, what I'm looking for in a subject interview, etc. The person I'm talking to is a nurse. She looks concerned. Or worried that this babbling idiot sitting before her thinks he can INTERVIEW someone. For a PODCAST???

(He hits the "save and continue" button.)

I drag myself back to the office, And this is a problem. Most days, it's tiring to walk from Bldg. 61 to Bldg. 10 and back again. Today? I feel like I'm ready for bed. My head feels heavy. My thoughts feel like they're being strained through thick layers of gauze. My fingers are practically mashing the keyboard — especially on my right hand.

I notice I'm leaning to the right as I type, and mayhaps that's why my back hurts.

To sum it up... I rarely despair. Parkinson's isn't a death sentence, it's a life sentence.

There are far worse things. But still... if I may be allowed a brief, profane explosion of anger? (He hits the "save and continue" button.)

A Lovely Weekend, Except for When I Fell

February 16, 2009

It was a wonderful day! We stayed at a 4-star hotel in DC, I yelled at a protestor, had our picture taken with "The President", fell down while walking, helped a kid get his football back, and somehow bled all over the sheet on our bed and the hotel bathroom floor.

It really was a great idea! Who needs to drive long distances to "get away" for a night when you have a world-class city like Washington, DC, just 30 miles away. Saturday morning, I went on to Priceline and Bill Shatner got me a great deal on a 4-star hotel... the Renaissance Mayflower Hotel.

We checked into our room and took a stroll. The White House was about two blocks south.

After walking for awhile, I was getting pretty tired by this point, so we had to stop and sit from time to time on our way back to the hotel. We got back to the room and rested awhile. Then we went out to see if we could find a restaurant that was open. We couldn't find a thing! Even the sandwich shops closed at 6! As we walked, I fell. Just, WHOOP! Straight down to the ground. It's like I put weight on my leg and it just wouldn't hold me. Skinned the hell out of my knee.

Gail was ticked at me for "pushing myself too hard," but we both know that the day will come soon enough that we won't be able to take long walks together. We went back to the room and ordered room service.

Then we hit the hay for a much-needed night's rest.

I got up once at 5 or so to go potty. Gail got up at 6:30 and came right back out of the bathroom.

"Do you have any idea how blood got all over the bathroom floor?"

I got out of bed, almost lost my balance, and staggered into the bathroom. It didn't QUITE look like OJ Simpson's driveway, but there were blood smears all over the tile floor. I looked at the scab on my knee, and there was no leakage. Gail asked to look at my feet... and there it was. Somehow, during my sleep, I had gouged out a small hunk of the back of my right heel, probably by kicking myself with a toenail during the night. There were streaks and smears of blood on the bed sheets as well.

We made coffee, Gail slept for about another hour, we got dressed, checked out went home.

Best Valentine's Ever! Except for falling down, that is...

Zoloft and a Handi-Capable Placard!

April 14, 2009

Had a visit with a nurse practitioner this morning. Talked about the depression (apathy, etc.) symptoms and got a prescription for Zoloft, which I will start taking tonight. Also got my Maryland MVA request for a handicap placard signed.

I'm not really bummed out about any of this... more of a sad resignation that things aren't ever really going to be any better, physically, from this point on. And they will get worse.

Meeting My New-Rologist

April 20, 2009

After originally being told that he didn't have any openings until the summer, I managed to get on the cancellation list and — viola! Dr. Stephen Grill of the Parkinson's and Movement Disorders Center of Maryland had an opening this morning. Excellent!

We had a very nice visit, and I'm looking forward to an excellent doctor/patient relationship.

We did all the standard tests and he seemed pretty encouraged about the condition my condition was in. Balance problems, yeah. A very minor tremor... but with the DBS and my meds, no sign of rigidity.

We did some speed tests... walking a certain distance, putting blocks on pegs, putting dots in squares and the like. I was thrilled to hear that I'm either as fast or faster than I was when I saw Dr. Goldstein in Feb. 2007 — until I realized that I wasn't on meds when I last did these tests for Dr. Goldstein. That was the visit where I went back ON the meds after being off for several years.

But still — for someone who has had this thing for more than 9 years now — not too shabby!

He stressed getting more exercise, so I think Gail and I will get a treadmill — provided I can find one of those "fold-up" models so it's not out in the open all the time.

We'll get together twice a year unless I need additional attention.

Balance Becomes an Issue

May 20, 2009

Last night, right before bed, I had a drink of water from an onion-shaped cocktail glass. As I tilted back my head to drink the water, I lost my balance. I didn't fall — but it was a close one. During the night, about 11 pm, I woke myself up violently shaking in bed. It stopped right after I woke up. This happened either Saturday or Sunday night, too. This morning, I'm wobbly, wiggly and altogether unsteady on my feet. I almost fell over one of my dogs. I don't feel safe driving or walking. So, this is a good day to just sit at home.

DAMN you, Parkinson! AND your disease!!!

LATER THAT DAY

I got my first driver's license when I was 17 and living in North Dakota. For awhile, I had a CDL and drove a tanker truck. Until today, I spent nearly 4 hours each day commuting to and from work. It ends today. After getting up this morning feeling wobbly and unsteady, after discussing the situation with Gail, after doing some reading up on the subject of driving with Parkinson's disease, I've decided it is in everyone's best interest to hang up the keys and rely on Gail and public transportation from now on.

The worst part (so far) is making the decision and realizing it's necessary. I haven't noticed any real difference in reaction times, but I have noticed that I sometimes step on the gas and the brake at the same time and my foot will — from time to time — slip off the gas pedal. Better to make this decision now on my own than to wait until after an accident.

So, starting tomorrow, it's the MARC train to DC, then the Metro Red Line to Bethesda.

Yay!

Training Days

May 26, 2009

Tomorrow makes one week since the day I gave up driving. So far, so good.

Gail has been wonderful about taking me wherever I need to go. She drops me off at the train station in the morning and picks me up in the evening. We went clothes shopping on Saturday (needed new pants because of the weight loss) and grocery shopping on Sunday. On those occasions I choose not to go into the store with her (like Sunday when she went into the Wal-Mart to get a new BBQ grill grate), she refuses to park in the handicapped spots, since she can walk just fine... a less moral person would use the placard. I admire the woman.

As far as the train ride goes... again, so far, so good. I get the 6:45 am train to DC at BWI, jump onto the Red Line Metro as soon as I get to Union Station, and ride it back out to the Medical Center station in Bethesda. It's out of the way to have to go all the way down to DC and then slingshot back out to Bethesda, but until they put in that new Purple Line Metro — sometime in the next century — my choices are limited.

Once I'm at the Medical Center station, it's up the longest escalator in the world, about a 150-yard walk to the NIH Campus Shuttle, and they bring me to within about 300 yards of my office.

The only problem so far... my stability. I almost tumbled out of the shuttle bus this morning, and the walk to and from the shuttle bus stop is over a small hill... and I don't have a low gear these days, it would seem.

But all in all, compared to the very real chance of a car accident if I kept driving — it's been a fair tradeoff.

For now.

Whining About Declining

May 29, 2009

The last thing I want to do on a blog like this is come off as "whiny." When I came up with the idea for a manuscript about my experience with deep brain stimulation (and that manuscript turned into this blog), the intent was to describe in as non-maudlin fashion as possible what it's like to experience the gradual loss-of-control that accompanies a progressive neurological disorder like Parkinson's. The idea is to bring folks in on — and, hopefully, help them understand — the experience. Sometimes, however, I'm not sure I understand it myself.

Since having the operation nearly two years ago, I've noticed that my "slowness of movement" in my hands and arms is almost gone. I can do finger taps with the best of them when the devices are turned on and my meds are working. But my walking, my balance, my coordination? All seem to have suffered over the past year. And from what I've seen in a VA/NIH study on DBS, that's pretty much par for the course.

According to the study, "The authors caution that the benefits need to be weighed against the risk of complications related to DBS surgery. "As with many effective therapies, there may be a price to pay in terms of increased risk of adverse events," said Dr. Moy. The total number of adverse events was 3.8 times higher in the DBS than the BMT group. The most frequent adverse events in both groups were gait disturbance, falls, motor dysfunction, balance disorder, depression, and dyskinesia and dystonia, which cause involuntary movements. There were more falls in the DBS group, often resulting in injuries (fractures, dislocations, head trauma) requiring surgery and other interventions. It is not clear whether DBS increases fall risk directly or patients are at higher risk of falling due to their improved overall function and greater activity level. "

For myself, I think it's the former and not the latter. My activity level is about the same as it was before the surgery. But before I had this done, I was able to stand at the toilet in the morning and not be in danger of resurfacing the wall with wee-wee because I can't seem to hold still at times when I need to. I'm probably walking LESS than I did before the surgery because I didn't suddenly feel my upper body shifting to the left or right when I walked before — and even if it did, it was easier to keep my balance than it is now. Before I had the surgery, I could stand on an escalator stair without bouncing and shifting from one foot to another. Before I had the surgery, I could reach for a coffee cup with my left hand and not feel the need to kick with my left leg. Before I had the surgery, I could lie in bed without my entire body jumping and twitching as if someone were touching me with a live wire every few minutes.

Now, is this a result of the surgery? Or is it just that SOME of my motor functions have been improved by the DBS, while others have declined at the same rate they would have if I never HAD the operation? I guess there's no way to tell.

I'm not complaining. I'm glad I had the surgery, especially since it was an experiment to see if DBS can be safe and tolerable for those of us in the earlier stages of PD. Hopefully, if the clinical trial bears out that this thing has benefits that exceed the risks, then folks will have it offered to them sooner while they can still preserve some motor function.

All I can say for sure is that 2009, so far, has seen this thing really picking up steam in my life. And it puts a little bit of the fear of the future in me as I wonder if this is just a momentary acceleration in the downspin and things will eventually level off for awhile — or is this just the beginning of a slide towards total infirmity.

Time will tell. And I'll talk about it — here and elsewhere.

It was in 2009 that we really started to notice – and treat – some of the NON-motor symptoms of Parkinson's – my REM Sleep Disorder, for instance...

Yelling in My Sleep

May 30, 2009

Every night, it's the weird dreams with me. Last night, for instance, I had a very realistic dream in which Gail and I were living back in Iowa back in the 90s and she decided she didn't love me anymore. She wasn't mean about it, it was more of a "matter-of-fact" realization that we could keep living together, but there'd be no more hugging, kissing or any kind of affection between us. At one point, she unplugged the TV and said that she had just finished HER three hours of TV watching and now it was MY turn. She handed me the electric cord and I knocked it away, saying, "What the hell! We're not doing THAT!!!"

Only, I didn't just say that in my dream. I shouted it for real. Woke up Gail (who actually DOES still love me) and knocked my blankets out of the bed. If Gail and I hadn't have gone the twin bed route several months ago, I certainly would have smacked her when I lashed out. She went back to sleep. So did I.

Gail. I honest to God have no idea how I would have gotten this far without her. She refuses to allow me to feel sorry for

myself. She is there to help me every step of the way. She is my constant friend, companion and caregiver. And her sense of humor can really take a tense moment and make it light. Like this example.

Miserable Morning

June 1, 2009

I'm having a miserable morning. My arms feel like lead weights. My fingers are missing the keys when I type. When I try to walk, my feet freeze to the ground and for a few seconds I'm motionless and frustrated. Freezing of gait is another delightful part of Parkinson's. Fortunately, at this point when it happens to me it's generally for just a second or two and most of the time it happens when I'm trying to start walking, or when I try to navigate a turn, or when I find myself going from an open space to a narrow space (or vice versa), or when I go from a smooth surface to a rough surface (or vice versa). It's hard to describe — think of walking up to the edge of a diving board and your legs just don't want to take that next step. That's really about as close as I can get to describing it.

Experts on the subject say that when freezing gets to be a major problem, a person could find himself frozen to the spot for as much as 30 second. They say that visual or audio cues may help a person get un-stuck. There are special canes and walkers with lasers that give the Parky a visual cue to "step over" something. Even just telling your foot "one, two, three, MOVE!" can help.

My wife, Gail, however, has a "better" idea.

I stayed home from work this morning because I'm having real difficulty with walking — and other motor activities. A little while ago, I started walking down the hallway to the bathroom. As I got from the wide-open living room to the narrow hallway, I froze. "THIS IS SO FUCKING FRUSTRATING!" I yelled.

Gail came up behind me. "Maybe I should follow you with a cattle prod, and when you freeze up, I could just give you a little jolt and then you could get going again," she said in a sweet, caring tone of voice. I started laughing and continued towards the potty.

My wife. She always knows just what to say. I sure do love her.

As my condition continued to worsen, especially after my decision to hang up the car keys, getting to and from work (and getting around when I was there) was becoming more and more problematic.

To Go In, or NOT To Go In

June 2, 2009

It's a little after 5 am as I sit in our little home office. I have a black border collie curled up behind me in the corner and cup of coffee on the desk to my left as I try to figure out what the hell I'm going to do about today. It was a much easier decision yesterday — not only was I wobbly and "freezy", but I felt like crap — like my stomach was still full of food from the night before, headachy and just plain "bleh." Not quite so clear cut this morning. I'm wavering back and forth in the seat as I type, my fingers are hitting the wrong keys, and I am not so much "walking" as "stutter stepping" when I maneuver around the house.

But I slept pretty good last night — weird dreams about buying an old clunker car and witnessing a shootout between cops and armed citizens and then reporting about that shootout for a radio news station... but when I woke up I still had my covers on the bed, so I'm guessing I managed to stay more-or-less still during the night for once.

So, as I see it, the question is — do I go to work on days when my main difficulty is in the area of walking? Ordinarily, I would say yes, even though it's getting tougher for me to get from where the shuttle bus drops me off to my office about 300 yards away. Then there's the matter of having to walk to and from the Clinical Center for lunch. Today, that's complicated by the fact that I have to add two extra trips to and from the CC to escort a filmmaker doing a project on the early days of AIDS research.

Am I up to that today? And if I am not, am I admitting to myself that I may be getting closer to the day where I just can't work anymore? It would be an entirely different matter if I were able to take a train/subway to work, get to my desk and just sit without having to walk around so much. But that's the job.

No answers. So, I guess I'll probably just go in today and see how it goes.

UPDATE: It's 9:45, I'm here at work. So far, so good despite almost falling on the train and shuttle bus again. Such is my life. May as well just get used to it, cuz it ain't gonna get any better — physically speaking. Mentally, mood-wise, I feel just fine. So... up and at 'em.

Being a Slacker is NOT a Handicap
June 3, 2009

Got to Union Station in D.C. a little earlier than usual yesterday, so I had an opportunity to ride an express train on the Penn Line to the BWI station. As the conductor came by and checked tickets, he told me that BWI-bound passengers needed to be at least three cars up from where I was sitting, as the entire train would not fit at the platform at BWI.

So, cane in one hand and the seat hand-grips in the other, I made my wobbly way three cars up. The train was full, but there are seats that are clearly identified as being reserved for the elderly and handicapped. Surely someone would see the wobbly guy with the cane and twin scars on his bald noggin and, at the very least, be shamed into giving up a seat.

The handicapped-reserved seats were all taken. The oldest passenger appeared to be in his mid-40s. Now, I don't know if they had heart conditions or any other sort of disability that would render them as officially "handicapped," so I can't really judge. But one thing stood out to me. You never saw people try so hard NOT to see someone. After giving me a quick glance as I hung on to a hand grip — wobbling and trying to keep from falling as the train jostled on the tracks, you could almost hear the neck bones snap as heads turned away as faces suddenly found something interesting out the window to look at, or something on their cell phone that caught their eye, or a scuff on a shoe tip that needed immediate buffing.

I stood there, wobbling, clutching my cane, clearing my throat, hoping that common decency might kick in. No such luck. As the train continued to roll north, all I could do was sit on the stairs.

I'm not going to be so nice about it next time.

I'm Scaring my Friends!

June 10, 2009

I'm finding that when I walk with people who aren't used to walking with me, I scare the hell out of them. When motivating by myself from point A to point B, I generally do OK, slow and clumsy, but OK. However, walking and carrying on a conversation is becoming very difficult. So when I'm walking with someone and a foot sticks to the floor, or digs into the tile and I almost trip, it invariably elicits a shriek from my companion. I've told everyone that it's all part of my ordinary day-to-day existence now, I've grown quite used to it, and unless I fall — in which case, they should at least offer to try to help me get back on my feet — it's nothing to worry about.

One such occasion was Monday. A young colleague and I were walking back from a podcast interview when my left foot dug into the floor and I stumbled. A few minutes later as we made our way down a long hallway, another gent with a cane approached from the opposite direction. He notice me and my cane (and the young lady I was walking with, no doubt), and brandished his cane as if it were a sword. I stopped and did likewise. "YOU WANT SOME OF THIS?" I said with a smile. He smiled, too, and continued on his way. "Manchild," my wife would say. Nice to know I'm not alone in that respect, either.

Yesterday was particularly difficult. I needed to get from our building to the one next door and as I opened our door and pivoted to exit, I lost balance and slammed my right shoulder into the light switch. "God dammit," I said. The ladies in the office thought someone had opened the door in my face... but it was just Willy the Weeble crashing his bulk against the wall.

I believe I'll try to make it through the day with a modicum of grace. That is, get to work, get in my chair and stay there until it's time to come home.

UPDATE: After writing this entry, I went into the kitchen to load up the "man bag" for the day with lunch, Gatorade and a Mountain Dew. Bending over to get the Gatorade, I misjudged how far I was away from the wall and busted my skull on the corner next to the fridge. It left a bump. Just what I needed.

GET OUT OF THE HANDICAPPED SPACES!
June 11, 2009

Gotta say, this new way of commuting since I gave up driving last month is really wearing me out. By the time I get to my office, I'm exhausted — and generally in need of a shower, given the recent spate of warm, muggy weather. But I don't trust myself behind the wheel and just don't want to risk it.

Of course, it would be extremely helpful if folks on the MARC train and Metro subway could READ the freakin' SIGNS! Like these two jolly fellows featured in the photo. I got on at Union Station and stood there, staring at them — cane in hand, as they both looked for other things to look at. Just when I was about to say something, a gentleman behind me (in a seat NOT reserved for the elderly or disabled) stood up and offered me the seat. But I thought I'd just go ahead and immortalize these two assholes for you.

Anyway, like I said, it's a wearying experience.

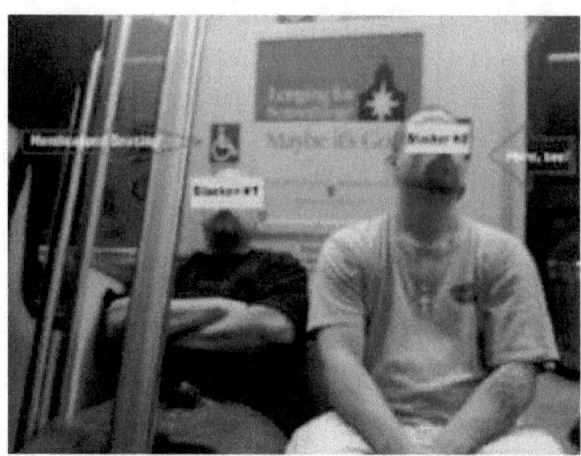

Yesterday afternoon, after walking 15 minutes to get to the shuttle that would take me to the Metro, then a half hour on the subway, then a long walk (up a broken escalator) at Union Station to the MARC train, I finally had a minute to relax. With my iPhone cranking tunes through the headphones, my mind started to wander. I thought about my nephew, Matthew, who is in the Navy in the Middle East and how he invited me to take part in a "Tiger Cruise" when his ship comes back to the states. And I wondered to myself "how many other folks can say they've been in the Navy three separate times?"

I pondered that thought for a moment — and then snapped out of my reverie. I wasn't IN the Navy three separate times. It was TWICE. Once from 1973 to 1977, then again from 1981 to 1985. This is a clear warning sign that I need to try to stay focused — and ask Gail to let me know if I ever babble on about anything that she knows did NOT happen. With my "acting out" at night and vivid dreaming, this is one of the symptoms of incipient Parkinson's psychosis. So far, it's just the one episode. But for the last few nights, I've woken up and have not been clear as to where I was or if I was awake or asleep... eventually, I realize I'm awake and look at the clock to see if it's time to get up yet. It generally is around 1 am or so when this sort of thing happens.

Walking at Work is Wearisome!

June 12, 2009

Yesterday was a bit more strenuous than I generally like 'em. Since hanging up the car keys, I'm doing considerably more walking than I used to, and that's a good thing. My neurologist stressed that the last thing I need to do is sit around and grow sluglike — or MORE sluglike, as the case may be. But yesterday, I'm pretty sure I overdid it.

It used to be I would walk out the front door to the car, then from the car in the parking lot about 20 steps to the office. Then I would repeat the process coming home.

Now, I walk from the car when Gail drops me off at the train station, to the elevator at the BWI Amtrak Station, across the catwalk over the tracks, down the other elevator, then to the train. When we get to Union Station in DC, I walk from the train into the station, down to the Metro station. When the Metro gets me to the Medical Center station in Bethesda, I walk from the train to the escalator (the longest such contraption I'VE ever seen...) and up to the front gate, after which I step onto the campus to await a shuttle bus. The shuttle drops me at the bottom of a hill, about 300 yards from where I work, and I walk the rest of the way.

Considerably more walking than I used to accomplish.

Add to that, yesterday, an additional walk from my office the quarter-mile or so to and from Bldg. 1 to take part in a Communications Director meeting, and I was POOPED when I got home yesterday.

Got up at 4 this morning and decided I just didn't have the steam to go in today. I need to fill out that "work from home" paperwork so I can stay home on days like this and not have it charged against my leave balance.

Eventually, my wonderful boss at the NIH Clinical Center Office of Communications helped me devise a plan by which I could work from home. I was able to do podcasts, answer phone calls, and do everything I was required to do from my home computer with a broadband connection. At first, it worked out very well!

Working from Home

June 19, 2009

Did my first unofficial "work from home" dealie yesterday. (I still have to get it officially approved, but since it was my boss's idea, that shouldn't be a problem.) It went pretty well. Wrote a story for the CC News, wrote some podcast scripts, checked the media line about once an hour. All in all, a successful day.

My "interns" however? Less than helpful. Shiloh came in from the yard yesterday morning (freshly de-pooped and feeling sassy) and stood at the office door barking at me. I told her she was interfering with the work of the Federal Government and was subject to disciplinary action. She gave me a look that seemed to say, "Federal, Schmederal. Throw the friggin' ball!" I reminded her again that this was WORK time, not PLAY time. She would not relent.

"President Obama called, fat boy! He said throw the friggin' ball!"

She gave up after awhile. This morning she just sat and stared for awhile... before barking at me.

She did come to my rescue this morning, however. I got out of the shower and was talking to Gail in the living room before going in to get dressed. As I turned, my foot stuck to the floor and I wobbled towards the wall. Gail, who is very quickly becoming VERY GOOD at telling when I'm gonna topple, reached out and grabbed my right hand. That steadied me for a moment, so I let go and started falling again. Gail grabbed my right hand again, I threw out my left hand... which Shiloh jumped up and grabbed! She wrapped my hand in her front paws and held on. So I had Gail holding my right hand and Shiloh holding on to my left as I regained my footing and kept vertical! Good dog!

Next time, it will be Raven's turn. Today, she's sitting here barking at every little sound she hears outside.

On the "new symptom" front, I had a little trouble swallowing yesterday. We were having some chicken for lunch and a hunk went most of the way down my esophagus... and stayed there. This has happened once before, and it's very uncomfortable. I just had my food tube scoped recently, so I know for a fact there's no obstruction in there. Trouble swallowing — or, "dysphagia" as the docs call it — IS a symptom of Parkinson's disease. Most of the time, it leads to choking or aspiration of food into the windpipe. But it can cause problems with the valve allowing food to leave the esophagus and enter the stomach. We'll hope this doesn't become a regular thing.

Stayed home again today. Got up at 4:30 to let the dogs out, took a few steps, foot froze to the floor and I decided, "Screw it. Not gonna chance a fall." So, I'm taking a break and then it's back to work.

My Mind's in a Good Place

June 26, 2009

As I drifted off to sleep last night, my mind was in a pretty good place. (I don't suppose the three glasses of port had anything to do with that...) As I contemplated the sad news about Michael Jackson and Farrah Fawcett, it dawned on me — again — I have it pretty easy.

I think the thing about sudden and unexpected celebrity death that hits us so hard is, if it can happen to THEM, it can happen to US! If someone with Michael Jackson's fame and wealth can keel over and die at age 50, then what sort of guarantees do WE have that we won't be sitting in the front car of the DC Metro the next time they have an accident? How do we know that there isn't a clot in a cardiac artery or a tumor in the colon or a weak blood vessel in the brain, or some clown on his way home from the bar who will get to the intersection the same time as us?

There are no guarantees. Like my Dad used to say, "you pays yer dime, you takes yer chance!"

I lay there for awhile contemplating this truth, which first occurred to me back in 1977 when Elvis died (and I'm pretty sure with each passing day, the similarities between the King of Pop and the King of Rock and Roll — at least in their manner of "check out" — will become even clearer). We never know what we're gonna get smacked with. A speeding car while crossing the street? Cancer? A stay bullet?

Unless you're suicidal, you don't get to choose. The wheel spins and lands where it lands. That's why otherwise healthy folks drop dead while jogging, while others — my grandmother, for instance — live into their 90s on a diet of pork chops and creamery butter.

When you wake up in the morning, you agree to spin the wheel again. If you're lucky, you'll make it home that night. If not, you could be in that Metro car I mentioned earlier. For my father, the wheel stopped on Pancreatic Cancer in 1983. He was 54. Same age I am now. Same age my older brother was when the wheel stopped on Lung Cancer. The wheel stopped for my twin brother in 2004 when he was 49. Stroke.

I may live to be 100. I might die on my way home from work today. We never know. And when things like this happen to famous people, even when it was clear that MJ was FAR from the healthiest person in the world — mentally OR physically — many of us take a little inventory of ourselves.

For me, the wheel stopped on Parkinson's disease. But I got a free spin. I don't think I will die from PD. Unless cancer or that aforementioned Metro car gets me, I probably WILL die from a complication of it... pneumonia, choking on my food, falling and breaking a hip — something. Whatever. No idea.

But, as I said about seven paragraphs ago, I have it pretty easy.

I have a wife who loves me and who I trust to take care of me as my condition gets worse. I have a supportive family. My boss is incredible. The feds have a great "work-at-home" policy that I will use on an as-needed basis until the time comes when I can't work at all... and then, early disability retirement at 60 percent of my pay awaits.

At this point of my dance with the disease, Parkinson's doesn't hurt. It doesn't make me feel ill. Sitting in a chair with my meds working and my deep brain stimulation devices turned on, you wouldn't know there was anything the matter with me — until I stand up and start walking. (I carry a card in my wallet in case I ever get stopped by a cop wanting to know why I'm weaving and walking — it's not P.I. [public intoxication], officer! It's P.D.!)

My biggest day-to-day worries now tend to center on questions like will there be a seat available on the Metro or will the "reserved for the disabled and elderly" seats be filled with 20-year old slackers again?

I'm doing OK. I'm a "Weeble." Remember them? "Weebles Wobble but They Don't Fall Down." Except for now and then. But not often.

Every night when we go to bed, my wife gives me a kiss on the lips, then a kiss on the forehead. She says she's trying to make my brain "better." I love her so very much and I know I couldn't manage without her.

I think of the folks with PD and other diseases who don't have that kind of support or assurance. The folks who lose their jobs when employers can fabricate a "reason" that has nothing to do with the disease. The broken marriages when a spouse just can't handle the PD symptoms or the stress of being a "caregiver." The folks in nursing homes who are left to "go it alone".

Taking stock of what I have and what I haven't, what do I find?

Not only do I have the Sun in the Morning and the Moon at Night...

I have Parkinson's. I've had it for almost 10 years. And I'm a lucky, lucky man!

Some Useful Suggestions

June 29, 2009

OK, let me start this essay with a comment on the title. For most of us, this list will be MUCH different than it would have been if I were writing this 20 years ago. In fact, that list would probably only have one entry... depending on how mad my wife was at being woken up.

Um... on second thought... she would ALWAYS be mad about being woken up. So maybe this list won't be so different after all...

If you're anything like me (and God help you if you are), then you know that one thing we Parkies have a LOT of time to do at night is think about stuff. The challenge is to find things to do that divert the brain from contemplating the negative and to occupy the intellect with something positive.

Or, at the very least, something shiny.

Here are some suggestions for things you can do as the hours tick away and the Sandman is caught in traffic.

1. Lay there very quietly and see if you can hear your hair growing.
2. See if you can think of a tune that is in the same tempo as your spouse's snoring.
3. Consider your toes. Wonder about how they're doing down there.
4. Run various scenarios through your mind about what you would do if a tornado were approaching or what you would do if a burglar tried climbing through your bedroom window. Bravely discard the ones that have you screaming like a little girl.
5. See if you can imagine what President Obama is doing — RIGHT NOW!
6. Run your favorite album in your mind. I like Gilbert and Sullivan's "the Mikado." If I'm in the mood for rock, Pink Floyd's "Dark Side of the Moon" works well. (For extra fun, try to sync it with "the Wizard of Oz" in your mind as you play it.)
7. Get out of bed, stagger into the living room, see if you can stare down the fish in your aquarium.
8. Wake up the dogs. Wait for them to fall back asleep. Wake them again.
9. Get back in bed. Stare at the digital clock. Start counting the seconds when the minute changes. See if you hit "60″

just as the minute changes again.

10. Lay there very quietly and see if you can hear your toenails growing. (This can be done in conjunction with #3.)

11. Try to come up with a list of things to do when you should be sleeping but aren't, and write a funny blog post about it.

No Wonder I'm Always Tired!

July 1, 2009

Let's get this out of the way — I feel like crap this morning. I feel better than I did when I got up at 4:30 to take out the dogs and then get ready for work. But I had a headache, I was wobblier and slower than usual, and my brain felt like it was wrapped in gauze like a mummy. So I wrote a quick e-mail to the office — mashing the keyboard with my barely-responsive hands — telling my boss that I was taking a sick leave day.

After a couple more hours of sleep and a shower, then some coffee, I feel marginally better. But no way able to navigate the trains, subways and shuttle busses that I would need to get to my office.

This is one of the rare days where PD makes me feel "sick." On days like this, usually by early afternoon I feel much better. But even now at nearly 9:30 in the morning, I'm mashing the keyboard with thick, fat fingers, misspelling words, and deleting whole lines and paragraphs after typing them, making me have to retype them.

It seems like the dreams I have before days like this are even weirder than normal. Before I got up, I dreamed that I was sharing a large house with an old guy with long hair (who may have been Ben Franklin) who was having sex with an old, chubby woman in the room next to mine. Then I noticed that a sheet in my bed, a mattress on the hardwood floor, was a sheet he had used before — stains and all.

Two weird dreams after I went back to bed. In one, Gail and I were on Main Avenue in my little hometown in Iowa. We were sitting on a park bench near a tree, and a little female sparrow was sitting on a branch very close to my face, holding a dandelion seed in her beak. I held out my finger for her, and she perched on it. I brought her close to my lips to give her a little birdie kiss, and she put the seed in my mouth. She flew away, and I turned to talk to Gail about the whole thing. But I felt the birdie land on my shoulder. We started walking up 3rd Street towards the house I grew up in (we were living there in the dream) and the birdie flew away again. It came back just as we made a right turn onto 26th Avenue North, and we noticed a bunch of costumed kids heading up the alley towards "our" house. Gail said, "Oh no! It's Halloween, and we don't have any candy."

Then, the dream shifted to me sitting with a bunch of friends (very few of whom I recognized) at a party. They were apologizing for what happened earlier that night when another guest at the party was making fun of me. This guest was apparently using a candy dish — which looked like a white Mexican wrestler mask — and pretending it was me, making fun of my weight and my Parkinson's. I told the guests not to worry about it, that I wasn't sensitive about my weight, and if someone were so crass as to make fun of a guy because he had Parkinson's disease — well — what does that tell you about HIS character.

A former co-worker asked me when I was going to bring Gail down to SW Florida to live — so I guess this dream was centered in Naples, Florida, where I once worked at a radio station. I told her that Gail couldn't live there because the heat wasn't good for her scleroderma. And I had to drive home, but suddenly I wasn't in Florida but in California, and that meant I would have to drive across country.

Then, I woke up.

Staggered out to the living room. Gail had the coffee already made and a cup poured. I sat in my recliner, and a bright-eyed German shepherd dropped a ball in my lap. The look said it all — "OK, fat boy, if you're gonna hang out here with us, you gotta pick up the slack in the ball-throwing duties."

CHAPTER 4

Coming to Terms

As the condition continued to worsen, it became clear I could do one of two things. I could sit around and be miserable, or I could find a way to laugh at it and make others laugh at it. I chose the latter, and frankly I think it unleashed a wave of creativity that has helped me keep my brain about as active as it can be.

From the diary/blog...

"ODE TO A FROZEN FOOT"

July 24, 2009

As I sit down to write this, I am feeling pretty good.

Having had PD for 10 years, I feel better than I should.

The stiffness and the slowness are well handled I confess

All thanks to Levodopa and that thing called DBS.

I don't have dyskinesia and I have no trouble dressing.

I'm grateful every day and thank God for every blessing.

I work at home more oft than not, in that way I'm in luck!

There's just one thing to gripe about — the way my feet get sstuck!

At lunchtime Gail and I go to the store to browse the deli

To get some ribs or chicken or something else to fill my belly.

She parks the car and we get out and I hobble towards the store.

My feet freeze to the ground as I get close to the door.

I look down at my shoes and they're stuck there on the floor.

"What are you sissies scared about, it's just a stupid door?"

My brain sends down a signal to my hesitating feet.

"Come on, you lazy tootsies, let's go get something to eat!"

I think they are embarrassed as they turn loose of the floor

And they make their cautious way and proceed right through the door.

And now our goal's is nearer as I hobble down the aisle

"I hope they have some meatloaf," I say with a hungry smile.

We're making decent progress as we get close to the food.

I can almost taste the mac and cheese when... BAM! My feet are glued.

"So what's the problem NOW?" I ask the feet I walk upon.

"The pattern on the floor has changed. It scares us," they respond.

I roll my eyes and start to rock to free my frozen feet.

My wife holds out her hand to help. (She loves me, ain't she sweet?)

My feet, at last, break free from their invisible detention.

I hobble to the counter and make clear my lunch intention.

With food in hand we make our way to the checkout for to pay.

I'd like to take our food and go, my feet decide to stay.

"I've really had it with you guys," I say through gritted teeth.

"But there's a RUG there on the floor," they whisper from beneath.

With mental calculations that would make an Einstein strain

My legs receive commands from my confused, beleaguered brain.

"YOU'VE NEVER SEEN A RUG BEFORE?" My brain begins to shout.

"IT'S JUST A STUPID RUG, YOU DOLTS! STEP OVER, AND GET OUT!"

My feet may be reluctant, but they know my brain's the boss.

They free themselves and step into the street so we can cross.

Gail, she walks behind me ever ready to assist

To gently jab me in the butt if my feet again resist.

We're almost to the car when the rain begins to fall.

It's not a gentle shower, it's a sudden summer squall.

I'm getting soaked, I cannot move, I'm frozen to the spot.

I look down at my soggy feet, I whisper "thanks a lot!"

Gail runs on ahead so she can bring the car around.

She opens up the door and I get in without a sound.

I'm wet, I'm miffed, my shirt is soaked, my feet squish in my shoes.

I'll say this about Parkinson's. It always does amuse.

Freezing by the Frozen Foods

July 29, 2009

Yesterday around lunch time, as we usually do, Gail drove me up to the supermarket so we could get some eggs. We had all the ingredients for ham, egg and cheese sammiches... except for the eggs. So, off we went. I love going to the store these days. Since I work at home almost every day, it's a rare opportunity to get out of the house and test my feet and legs to see how well they're working that day.

As usual, I was slow and freezy. There really is no way to explain what that's like to someone who hasn't experienced it — it's easy to describe losing your balance because it has happened to almost everyone. But how to make somebody understand what it's like when you're walking and your feet stick to the floor?

Anyhoo...

We got the eggs and started making our way to the checkout. There were obstacles ahead — a shopper at the service desk, a clerk stocking a shelf, and a guy with some sort of pushcart filling most of the aisle. Gail weaved her way through and kept going. I got as far as the ice cream freezer and stopped.

My feet... would... not... MOVE!!!

Gail was getting further and further away. I tried rocking loose. No go. Gail was getting smaller and smaller and I was stuck FAST to the floor.

"Um, Gail?"

She's a little hard of hearing, but I didn't want to cause a scene, which I surely WOULD have if I did what I WANTED to do, which was...

"GAAAAAAAIIIIILLLLLLLLLL!!!!! Don't LEEEEEEEEEEAVE MEEEEEEEE!!!! GAAAAAAAIIIIIILLLLLLLL!!!!!!!"

So, I repeated — a little louder.

"Um, Gail?"

She turned around and saw me standing there, smiling sheepishly, trying to work my feet loose and she came back for me. A touch of her hand and I was free.

I guess I shouldn't panic about stuff like that. She SURELY would have missed me at some point... hopefully before bedtime.

Step on a Dog, Fall on your Butt!

August 2, 2009

It's been quite awhile since I've taken a spill. I'd have to do the research to see what day it was the last time I actually fell, but it's been awhile.

Until...

Gail and I were playing with the pooches last night, and we were looking for a particular toy — a rubber bowling pin that gives off a peculiar sound when it's squeezed. I thought it might be under the recliner, so I stood up and tipped the chair forward. I took a step back and...

YIPE!!!

...stepped on Raven's paw.

Startled, I immediately lost my balance. Rather than try to stumble my way towards regaining it and getting hurt even worse in the process, as soon as I realized I was gonna fall no matter what I did, I just did a quick tuck and let my upper back take the brunt of it. See, last time I fell I was in the yard and I ended up staggering several feet trying to get my feet under me before finally toppling. If I did that in my house, I might have gone through a wall or creased my head on the exercise bike or an end table.

I'm fine. My butt was a little sore last night, but it's OK now. Raven, who is remarkably perceptive about such things, felt very bad about what had happened and spent the rest of the evening looking at me very sadly.

Gail said, "I guess we can't call you a 'weeble' anymore." Weebles wobble, but they don't fall down. I — it would seem — am no weeble.

Explaining What FOG Feels Like

August 7, 2009

I've been experiencing the phenomenon known as "freezing of gait" or "FOG" for a couple months now. For the longest time, I've found it difficult to explain what it feels like when you're walking along and — all of a sudden — you can't take that next step.

I finally hit on it. Do a little test with me. Stand up. Lift your left foot off the ground. Now... without lowering your left foot, lift your RIGHT foot. Can't? Ofcoursenot.

Imagine BOTH feet feeling like that when you come to a small incline or go from tile to a rug or there's a pattern on the floor or someone suddenly cuts in front of you in a crowd or for whatever reason your brain and legs lose contact with each other.

Now you know.

"Be Careful, Dimwit!"

August 17, 2009

This feels like one of those days where I am going to have to be especially careful.

(And right now, in my mind, I can hear Gail saying, "You should be especially careful EVERY day." Let's pretend we can't hear her.)

("Typical male thing," Gail says. We'll pretend we didn't hear that, either.)

What was I writing about? Oh. Yeah.

Got up this morning at about 6:20 a.m. Took the dogs out. (It dawns on me the first words I speak out loud on a given day will likely be, "Raven, go potty." This is because Raven — our nearly 5 year old border collie whose birthday is tomorrow... same as Gail's, but Gail is a little older than Raven is... just sayin' is all — will tend to dilly dally around first thing in the morning, smelling grass, looking around, doing her "fierce dog" pose in case anyone is watching...)

Walked into the kitchen to check e-mails and make coffee. Looked to see if there were any new comments on the blog from the previous day.

Went into the bathroom to go potty. (No one has to say a thing to me to make ME go potty. I'm all BUSINESS as far as that daily chore goes...)

Finished my business. Stood up. Turned around. Lost my balance. Fell against the wall.

Boom.

Gail says she heard something, but as it wasn't followed by cursing or screaming — she went back to sleep. Good. Save the emergency reactions for actual emergencies, says I.

Still... I feel exceptionally wobbly today. And these are my choices.

1. Turn off the DBS devices, be immobile, withdrawn, unresponsive and feel like crap.
2. Suck it up. Leave the devices on. Take the L-dopa. Be wobbly, but alert, responsive and mobile. Rub some dirt on it, as my father and Peyton Manning would say.

Great choices. Am I done whining yet?

Yeah, I guess.

The Situation Hits Home

August 20, 2009

Not a great day for me yesterday. Other than being my usual bumbly, stumbly self, the enormity of this whole situation kinda came crashing down on me yesterday afternoon.

It started, as these things generally do, stupidly. Gail was getting irritated with the dogs. Shiloh, in particular. Our 3-year old German shepherd has been very annoying as of late... making you think she HAS to go OUTSIDE and go POTTY and RIGHT NOW! And then, when you take her out, she pokes around, chases bugs, sniffs the air, stares off into the distance, does everything but go potty and that would be FINE if it weren't so bleeding HOT and MISERABLE! Gail's scleroderma causes her to have difficulty with heat. My Parkinson's does the same.

So, she hooked Shiloh and Raven — our 5-year old border collie — on their leashes and set them out in the yard... which would be FINE except for the fact that Raven thinks everyone is Osama bin Laden and will bark her foolish head off if someone walks down the street. And if you bring RAVEN in and leave SHILOH out in the yard, then SHILOH will stand on the porch and bark because she doesn't want to be ALONE in the big, scary yard where somebody — perhaps that bin Laden fellow Raven is scared of, might come STEAL her.

So, I decided to slip on my shoes and sit outside with the doggies so I could be there to bring Raven back into the house if she started barking.

Gail, annoyed with Shiloh, objected. She told me it was just too hot for me to sit out there, baking my brains in the sun, just to keep an eye on our neurotic dogs.

She was right, of course. But as I sat on the recliner, I felt this wave of sadness come over me. The realization that, at THIS MOM- ENT, I am as "able" as I'm ever going to be. Parkinson's is, of course, a progressive disease. It doesn't ever get better. And it's going to get worse. Much worse. And if I'm too frail, too "feeble" to help Gail with the mundane crap NOW, what's it gonna be like when the day comes when I can no longer do the mundane stuff — shower, shave, brush my teeth — for myself?

I know Gail will take excellent care of me when that time comes. That's not the issue. The issue is — I guess — I have this lingering "machismo" about "taking care of my wife, like a man should." And Parkinson's is stealing that from me, bit by bit.

After a considerable bit of feeling sorry for myself, I got up, went into the kitchen, and did something I knew I could do and it made me feel marginally better. I whipped up a tuna-noodle casserole. Got cooked noodles all over the floor, but that's what dogs are for, right? To clean up the spills of a Parky cook?

I'll be OK.

This Time, a CONTROLLED Fall!

September 2, 2009

Inasmuch as I generally need an excuse to get out of the house at least once a day, as we generally do on weekdays, Gail and I took a drive up to the grocery store to get a bite of lunch. I'm not having the best of days today — my leg and hand and foot muscles have been cramping (as has my right butt muscle — but try not to think about that too much).

Some days are worse than others with Parkinson's disease. Today, I'm freezing more than usual, and I almost toppled over walking into the store when I tried to get my left foot unstuck from the pavement by rocking back and forth. Then, getting back into the car, I turned to sit on the passenger seat. I can't just raise a leg and climb in like I used to... I need to turn so my back is facing the inside of the car, bend my knees, sit, and then rotate and bring my feet into the car. This time, my knees would just not bend to allow me to sit. I stood there, wobbling, trying not to fall forwards or backwards. Gail came around and took my hand. I unfroze and sat.

Anyway, on a wobbly day, a few close calls, but no falls.

Until...

The car pulled into our driveway. I rotated my body, put my feet on the pavement and stood up. I started leaning to my right. Ordinarily I would just thrust out my cane to stop the lean, but my right arm didn't answer the signal and I began to slide to the ground. I leaned back onto the body of the car so I could slide rather than just drop to the rough pavement and I grabbed the car's frame through the open door and held on. I looked to see if Gail was watching. She was walking around towards the back of the car and hadn't seen me yet.

"Uh, Gail?"

She turned and saw me through the car's windows. My right hip plastered against the car's body, my left hand clutching onto the door frame for dear life, my cane having skittered uselessly under the car.

She came to help, and I realized it would be easier to just use the car's body to control my descent the rest of the way to the pavement, then I could roll over onto my knees and get up without my wife of nearly 20 years having to tear every muscle in her lower back trying to lift me from where I was currently dangling.

I assured her it was a "controlled descent" and that I was fine. She gave me her arm to hold onto, and eventually — slowly — haltingly — I made it back into the house.

Then I ate some chicken and had a chocolate milk. How's YOUR day been so far?

In my entry about the first surgical procedure in the DBS surgical trilogy, I included a note about something I learned more than three years later that MAYBE I should have been told about before now. Here's another little surprise I learned after the fact in 2009.

"Whachoo Talkin' About, Vanderbilt?"

September 10, 2009

I got this mailing from my friends at the Neurology Department at Vanderbilt University Medical Center a couple weeks ago. It was another revision in the standard consent form they keep on file for the clinical trial in which I'm involved — a Phase I trial of deep brain stimulation in early Parkinson's disease.

If I remember correctly, there have been a couple of these since I joined the trial in 2007. Pretty routine stuff — look it over, sign it if you agree, mail it back. So I didn't really rush to deal with the one I got a couple weeks ago.

Today, Gail is having a house dusting extravaganza. Anything not moving WILL be dusted! Anything not where it is supposed to be WILL be put WHERE it is supposed to be. One such item was the large manila envelope with the consent form update. So, I decided to take a look at it — finally.

Here's the update: (emphasis added)

"The following sentence was added: 'It is also possible that the use of DBS in early stage PD *may speed up progression of the disease* and may make you ineligible in the future for the FDA-approved DBS for advanced PD."

Um... OK.

I'm thinking that there must be a reason at this late date for adding that to the consent form. I'm wondering if I am not the only one of the 15 out of 30 people who had the surgery who is having a sudden downturn in symptoms. No way to know for sure until the study is published, since it would violate patient confidentiality to share that info.

The logical question is, would I have consented to taking part in the clinical trial if that part had been in the original consent.

Yes. I would have. And here's why.

If it turns out that doing DBS in early stage PD doesn't slow the progression of the disease (as was and is hoped), and — instead — speeds UP the progress of the disease... there's only one way to KNOW that... and that's to DO THE SURGERY!

And the only way to know whether or not DBS surgery is safe or effective in early stage PD is to have DONE the surgery on a few willing volunteers and then measuring their progress.

I'm only in sporadic contact with a couple fellas who are in the clinical trial. One was in the control group, meaning he did not HAVE the surgery. The other one, who DID have the surgery — last I heard he was doing very well.

So. This is just something else to think about, something to discuss with my neurologist when I see him next month

Having the surgery did NOT give me Parkinson's. If the DBS surgery DID speed up my disease progression, which no one is saying it did, then what the hell... I would have eventually reached this point ANYWAY.

You gotta break a few eggs to make an omelet. And I am still very happy to have been part of this clinical trial, no matter how it turns out.

LEG CRAAAAAAAMP!!!!

September 12, 2009

Right before 2 am this morning, I woke up to "the leg cramp from hell."

I've been troubled with these things on and off since earlier this year. At first, I thought I just needed more potassium in my diet. But now it's clear what's going on.

There is a demon in my right calf. It wakes up at night and torments me.

I think the demon (which I shall name "Chtulu the Cramper") dwells mostly in the peroneus longus muscle. During the day, he fidgets and twitches. But during the night, he comes alive in a hellish torrent of ouchiness.

Generally, the demon attacks when I mindlessly extend my right leg when rolling over in bed or while trying to reposition my top sheet and blanket. He comes on like gangbusters, creating a golf ball- sized lump on the lateral side of my shin. Usually he attacks once or twice a night. Recently he came and went six or seven times over the course of the night.

Last night he manifested himself for nearly a half hour.

I tried everything I could think of to drive the demon into submission. Pulling my toes toward my shin. Rotating my ankle. Bending my knee. Sitting up on the edge of the bed. All to no avail!

Oh, the DOGS were happy about it, having daddy sitting up on the edge of the bed at 2 in the morning could only mean GOOD things as far as THEY were concerned. Gail had just gotten back into bed after taking them out for their middle of the night lawn watering, and they were awake and ready to PLAY. But I was in no mood.

Raven jumped onto my mattress in the mistaken belief that having a warm dog lie next to the cramping muscle would help somehow. (Maybe it would, if she weren't inclined to lay there and PANT for a half hour before going to sleep, making my bed jostle and bounce like a sleeper car on a railroad train...) I appreciated her effort, but it was up to ME to silence the demon.

I rubbed. I flexed. I twisted. I got up and walked around a little.

And that quieted the demon. For awhile.

He's asleep now. Every few moments I can feel a twitch in the painful muscle as Chtulu the Cramper dreams of causing me further pain later tonight.

I wonder if self-amputation is an option.

Damn you, Parkinson! AND your disease!

(During the intervening time between the prior entry and the next one, my sister Cindi's condition worsened. It was hard to blog about my emotions at the thought of losing the third of my seven siblings – my twin brother died of a stroke in 2004, my older brother died from cancer in 2008, and now Cindi was fading. She died on November 4, 2009. I spent a week with my mom and my two remaining sisters in Milwaukee while my little brother Joe represented our family at the memorial in New Mexico.)

It Helps with the Screaming, But Not with the Dreaming

November 19, 2009

Before we begin, I should note that I use the generic version of Klonopin, but it's easier to fit the brand name into a headline than writing clonezapam.

That being said...

My nights have vastly improved since my neurologist prescribed clonezapam for my REM sleep behavior problem. No more shouting at night. No more punching or kicking the walls. And I generally feel more rested when I get up in the morning.

It hasn't done anything about the vivid dreaming that comes with Parkinson's disease, but at least I'm not acting them out any more.

Had a doozy this morning right before I got up.

My dead twin brother and I were in Japan together. It was his first visit, and I was showing him all the high points of Yokosuka — the town I lived in for 18 months back in the 80s. We hit all the bars, browsed all the stores, dined at a restaurant and went walking down the streets. At one point, I recognized that we were in my old neighborhood, near the house that my ex-wife Janina and I rented in 1984-85. I wanted to show it to Bob and get a photo of it. (Side note — I once DID actually find the house using Google Earth, which is a neat program, but has nothing to do with this dream, although I did mention to Bob in the dream that I had found the house once on Google Earth...)

But as we looked for it, I saw that we were actually on the EAST side of the Kanagawa peninsula, and our old house was on the west side, so we gave up looking for it. Bob saw some birds down on the beach and went down to give them some bird seed. Some ate the seed, others made a big deal of spitting it out in disgust.

We went back to our walking and Bob mentioned that he had tickets to fly home that evening. I mentioned that I did, too, although we were both flying United Airlines, we had different flights. We found ourselves in a residential neighborhood as it grew dark, and Bob was afraid to walk into it until I told him that street crime is practically unheard of in Japan.

Then I woke up.

Shiloh, being bored, had barked and that got Gail up. So I went out and sent her back to bed. Now I'm making coffee, sipping cappuccino, and writing this.

See how my life is? :)

Falling in the Bedroom

November 21, 2009

I fell in the bedroom when I was getting up this morning.

Actually, it was more like I slid from the bed to the floor.

I woke up after a particularly crampy night and noticed Gail and Raven were already up. So I figgered I'd get up and get the cappuccino going. So, with some difficulty, I managed to swing my legs over to the left side of the bed and sit up. I put my hands by my side, grabbed the mattress to use them to push myself to a standing position, when...

Whoopsie Daisy!

My arms wouldn't support my weight and I slid to the floor.

For a few seconds, I laid there, my hiney on the floor, my upper back and neck braced against the mattress. I thought about calling Gail, but after realizing that I wasn't hurt, I figgered I could just slide the rest of the way to the floor, roll over, get on my hands and knees and get to my feet. Which I did.

Maybe it's time to start thinking about bed rails?

PD is a Disgusting Disease

December 7, 2009

Taking a sick day. Here's why. (And be warned... this post makes reference to bodily functions. If that kind of thing repels you, stop after the next paragraph.)

First thing, I've been getting kinda sloppy with "putting the caps back on things." The other day, a whole bottle of rum flavoring extract. It spilled. This morning, I made Gail's coffee and didn't put down the cap on her creamer. When she went for her second cup and shook the container of creamer—the dogs had a delightful mess on the floor to lick up.

Then... (and here's where you should stop as forewarned).

I went to take my shower. As usual before a shower, I decided to go potty. It was a great success. I did the "post potty paperwork" and stood up to take some ibuprofen, cuz I woke up feeling headachey and head-cloudy today. I looked at my right hand and wondered, "Are those coffee grounds?" A quick sniff showed that they were NOT coffee grounds. So I washed my hands thoroughly and got the shower water running.

I sat down on my shower seat. Then I realized I had forgotten to take down the shower nozzle (we have one of those shower nozzle on a hose kind of things). It was impossible to reach from my seated position, so I stood up—and instantly realized there was something amiss.

I turned around and looked at the shower seat. And there it was. A small dookie! Sitting there, mocking me... like a profane Hershey's Kiss.

So, I hosed down the shower seat, I hosed down myself, I finished off the rest of my shower, I shaved my cheeks and neck taking special care not to slash my own throat in the process. I got dressed, and sent my boss a note saying I'm taking the day off.

The only thing I feel capable of doing right now is staring at the wall. Maybe the TV, if there's something not-too-involved that requires a lot of thinking I can watch.

And now, we first begin to notice the onset of executive dysfunction, a harbinger of Parkinson's Disease Dementia.

My Brain is Soft and Chocolatey!

December 9, 2009

I swear, my brain is turning into a soft pudding.

Some time ago, I set my iPhone to alert me when it's time to take a pill. Now, unless I get up right away and take the pill when the alarm goes off, I forget.

Yesterday, I blew off two pills. I was sitting here at my keyboard, my iPhone alarm went off, I turned it off and instantly forgot. I've been doing that a lot lately.

I remember to take my pills when I get up in the morning cuz it's part of the routine. Check e-mails, take pills, make coffee. I remember to take my nite-nite pill, cuz it's nite-nite time. But my 11 and 4 pills? There isn't any other action associated with taking them, so I have to jump up from what I'm doing and take them, or I forget until I either start wondering why I'm so stiff, or it dawns on me that an hour or so has passed and I didn't take them.

This is one of the reasons why I got one of those daily pill compartment things. I load it up with the number of pills I need to take each day. That way, if I think I may have forgotten to take one, all I have to do is count. Like right now, I should have no levodopa/carbidopa pills in the Wednesday bin. Which I don't cuz I just took the last one... an hour late.

I think it's my brain...

One thing I've certainly learned in my decade-long dance with Parkinson's disease is that it becomes easier to tell who the nice people are – and who the jerks are. There certainly are a LOT of the latter.

Sucks Being Slow When it's Cold

January 6, 2010

One of the more charming things about having Parkinson's disease at this stage is how SLOW I am. Being a large individual, I imagine watching me walk from Point A to Point B is something like watching a huge, lumbering ship make its slow way through the Panama Canal. Whether I'm using my walker or my cane, I'm a slow and unsteady traveler.

Gail and I have joked about this very thing. She's suggested that I get one of those "slow moving vehicle" symbols and hang it from the back of my belt. I countered with a suggestion that I should put a "This Vehicle Makes Frequent and Sudden Stops" sticker over the back of my pants.

Gail is a godsend. She walks—slowly—by my side. When I use my walker, she's there to steady me if I begin to list to the port or starboard. When I'm using my cane, she gives me her right arm as we walk to steady me. I've lost count of how many times I would have fallen if Gail weren't there to grab me before reaching the tipping point.

Still, I can't expect the REST of the world to slow down to my pace.

On my birthday Monday, Gail and I went to a nice restaurant. The hostess greeted us and showed us to our table. Off she went, at what I believe was probably a normal rate of speed. I was using my cane, Gail had my left arm as I took slow, careful steps—freezing once when I came to a downward slope in the floor, regaining my slow, unsteady pace as the hostess reached our table, turned around and wondered where the hell WE were. This happens a lot at restaurants.

Yesterday at my doctor's office, the medical assistant called my name and held the door as I ambled toward it. I cautioned her that I was a bit on the slow side (which is like saying Bill Gates is sort of "well to do") and she assured me that was fine. She got my height and weight and scooted down the hallway towards the doctor's office. I froze up once trying to get through the door to the hallway, almost lost my balance in the hall, and eventually made it to where the assistant was standing, by an open door—bless her heart—she smiled at the poor old man and his slow, slow gait!

These are both benign incidents. They are perfectly understandable. I certainly do not expect the world to slow down just because I have.

The thing that makes me want to climb a tall tower with a high powered rifle is the people who are in such a hurry that they either roll their eyes when they try to get past me at the mall, who cut in front of me and cause me to freeze up, or—as happened on Christmas Eve, yet—actually BUMP INTO ME and then keep walking while Gail and I try to keep my fat ass from falling into a row of mannequins.

Most people, I've observed, are very nice and respectful of a person with obvious disabilities. Thank goodness we have the jerks out there to keep my cynical streak alive!

Like I Said...

January 11, 2009

As I write this, it's 31 degrees outside. That's about as warm as it's been this year so far. It's been cold and windy and not much fun for someone who hates the cold to be stuck outside.

Unfortunately, walking with me these days means getting stuck. Outside.

Gail and I just got back from the store where we bought some lunch. Because of our uneven sidewalk, I always tend to freeze up when walking to the car. (Thank goodness for Gail and my walker - - they keep me from falling.) When we got to the store, I found myself freezing up every few steps.

I try not to even think about the terrain. I try to make each step as automatic as possible. And it works, too! For about 5 or six strides. Then, I go to raise my foot for the next step and... nothing. Same for the other foot. I'm generally able to unstick myself by letting the walker roll forward just a little bit, and then I can follow it.

But on a windy, freezing late morning in a grocery store parking lot... freezing of gait also means freezing of mate! (I almost wrote Freezing of Gait means Freezing of Gail... but I think I like the previous version better. How about you?)

It's OK when I freeze up in the store. We're inside. It's warm. But to and from the car as the winter winds blow and howl (and sometimes, it's the wind itself that makes me freeze up...), it's frustrating on several levels. One, I know my wife hates the cold even more than I do. And she waits, patiently, for me to unstick myself. I would tell her to go on ahead and get into the car, but I know she wouldn't do that. She has this idea that she can stop me if I fall... which is true if she catches me just as I start to tilt (which I did, going into the store and we hit an upslope and I leaned backwards and my walker started to roll backwards—but I was able to grab a cement post to steady myself). Many is the time when I've frozen up, started to tilt one way or the other and Gail has braced herself against me to stop the fall. God, how I love her.

Anyhoo...

It's all part of the colorful tapestry that is Parkinson's disease. Along with tripping over dogs, having trouble getting out of bed in the morning (and I mean that PHYSICALLY, not cuz I'm tired), the hassle of trying to roll over in bed, missing the car seat with my butt when I try to sit down, bumping into the wall in a narrow passage, needing an alarm to remind me to take my pills throughout the day, needing help to get out of a chair, having to sit while taking a shower, not being able to close my eyes while standing cuz I'll fall, being careful not to tilt my head too far backwards when taking a drink cuz I'll lose my balance, having to take little steppy steps to turn around instead of just pivoting, not being able to back up without falling, inhaling little hunks of food into my windpipe, having a runny nose all damn day, zoning out at the computer when I'm supposed to be working, forgetting what the hell it was that I was just about to do, having the "stares" (one reason why I stopped driving—I will focus on something outside and STARE at it until I realize I'm doing it and stop myself) and my general stumblebummery.

But hey... it's nice and warm in the house! And lunch was good.

Every Day, a Surprise!

January 21, 2010

I must admit that, being new to this later stage of Parkinsonism, almost every day brings a new surprise. Like waking up in the morning with something hurting and having no idea what you did to hurt it. Taking your shower and seeing a scratch on your leg and not remembering when or how you got scratched. Looking in the mirror and seeing a scratch or a bruise on my head, having no idea who's beating me in my sleep. Having an ankle that's so sore it's hard to walk on it, but you don't recall having done anything to hurt it. There was one famous incident last Valentine's Day weekend when we were at a hotel and I left blood on the sheets and in a trail to and from the bathroom because I had somehow cut myself on the back of one of my heels.

This morning, it's my chest. Actually my ribs, right below the pectorals. More on the right than on the left. I feel like I've either been lifting weights or doing pushups in my sleep. Which, if I had, would be a good thing because medical experts agree that exercise is beneficial for those of us with Parkinson's disease. But I would think that if I were engaged in such strenuous exercise during my sleepy-time hours, I would have disturbed my wife and my dogs would have wanted to participate.

So, knowing that I did NOT do pushups or lift weights in my sleep, I'm left to wonder just what the hell I did that made the right side of my chest feel like I had been exercising past the point of all prudence.

Oh. And my ankle hurts, too, if anyone cares. :(

LATER THAT DAY

Gail and I just got back from our near-daily trip to the grocery store. I was standing there, leaning on my walker, deciding which frozen pizza I wanted to get. I made my selection and opened the freezer door, to hear a young voice behind me...

"Mommmmm! I can't GET a pizza! That MAN is in everyone's WAY!"

I turned and looked, and there was Little Timmy Asshole! So, I put my pizza on the seat of my walker and rolled away. That's when I heard Timmy's mom, Mrs. Asshole, speak.

"It's OK, honey. He's gone now."

I turned and glared at them, then just rolled away because I know that if I beat their skulls into a mushy pulp with a frozen ham and then hid their bodies in the freezer, it would be ME who went to prison.

Such is the state of fairness in America today.

Am I OK?

January 24, 2010

One question I hear a lot from my beloved... usually when I'm seated in my recliner and my 1000-yard stare is focused on the TV and I haven't moved or blinked in awhile...

"Are you OK?"

I snap to attention and smile. "Sure. Just having a bad face day. Feeling Parky!"

She knows what that means.

To the uninitiated, the blank, expressionless, sometimes pissed-off looking face of a Parkinson's patient is mistaken for something else... like "The Lights Being On, but Nobody's Home."

In truth, it's more like "The Lights are All Out, but EVERYBODY's Home."

When I sit, staring what the experts call a "reptilian stare," that doesn't mean my mind isn't going a mile a minute or that I'm not in a good mood. A masked expression is usually one of the earliest symptoms of Parkinson's. It gets worse as time goes on, as shown by recent pictures of Muhammad Ali and later pictures of Pope John Paul II.

Here's the official explanation:

One way that we express emotion is via facial expression. Facial expression of emotion is made possible by the working of complex muscle groups in the face. In some people with Parkinson's disease, these facial muscles no longer work properly, and so facial expression of emotion is more difficult. The person's face is not as expressive as it once was and sometimes resembles a mask.

So, when you see me, and I'm just sitting there with that 1000-yard stare and I'm not moving or blinking or smiling or showing any emotion whatsoever... worry not.

I'm just having a bad face day.

Self-Testing is Revealing

January 26, 2010

Hmm. I finagled a free download trial version of the CNS Vital Signs neurocognition test battery. Gave myself a patient name, tested myself, and here's what we came up with.

In the verbal memory test, the computer screen shows 15 words that you have to memorize. Then, it shows a longer string of words and you have to hit the space bar when you see a word that was on the original list. Then, later in the test, they show another long string of words and—once again—you have to hit the space bar if you see a word you recall from the original list.

In the visual memory test, they show 15 different abstract symbols. Like the verbal memory test, you have to memorize the original symbols. Then they show a longer list of symbols and you have to hit the space bar if you see a symbol that was on the original list of 15. Later in the test, you repeat the process.

In the finger-tapping test, you tap the keyboard with your right index finger, then your left index finger, as fast as you can for 20 seconds. (I scored 50 on the right [18th percentile] and 53 on the left [40th percentile].)

In "Symbol Digit-Coding" you see a line of symbols, each with a number under it. Then you get a row of symbols, and you have to match the symbol with the number.

In the Stroop Test, first you tap the keyboard when you see a color, spelled out as a black word—BLUE, GREEN, etc. Then, you have to tap the keyboard when the COLOR of the word MATCHES the word... a blue BLUE, a green GREEN, a red RED, etc. Then, you have to tap the keyboard when the color of the word does NOT match the word... a green YELLOW, a blue RED, a yellow BLUE, etc.

In the Shifting Attention test, you see red or blue circle or square at the top of the screen, and a circle and square—one red, the other blue—at the bottom of the screen. If the computer tells you "Match Shape" you tap either the right or left shift key, under the correct shape. If the computer tells you "Match Color," you tap either the right or left shift key under the shape with the correct color.

In the Continuous Performance Test, you're shown a single letter, one letter at a time, two seconds each for 5 minutes. You press the space bar whenever you see the letter "B".

Afterwards, you see the results.

The Neurocognition Index (NCI) - An average of the five neurocognitive domains and a general assessment of the overall neurocognitive status of the patient. I scored "100" which put me at the 50th percentile for my age group.

They combine the Verbal Memory (which I scored a woeful "41" which put me in the 1st percentile [very low] and the Visual Memory, (in which I scored a slightly less miserable "38" which put me in the 7th percentile [low]) to come up with a Composite Memory score of 79, which places me in the 1st percentile (very low). Yaaaaay for my BRAIN!!!

In Processing Speed, I wound up with a score of 40, which put me in the 13th percentile (low).

My Psychomotor Speed, indicating problems with slowed information processing (i.e., perceiving, attending/responding to incoming information, motor speed, fine motor coordination, and visual-perceptual ability—I scored a 146, which puts me in the 18th percentile (low average).

Everywhere else, I did pretty well.

Executive Function, which refers to the capacity for autonomous behavior beyond the structure of external guidance. In clinical terms, this refers to initiative, motivation, spontaneity, planning, judgment, insight, goal-directed behavior, the ability to operate in favor of a remote or an abstract reward, the capacity for self-monitoring, and the flexibility required for self-correction—I scored a 63, which put me in the 95th percentile (above average).

Reaction Time—scored a 576 which put me in the 84th percentile (above average).

Complex Attention, which refers to attending to multiple stimuli at the same time. Ability to maintain focus, track information over brief or lengthy periods of time, performs mental tasks quickly and accurately—I scored a 3, which put me in the 79th percentile (above average).

Cognitive Flexibility, which refers to shifting attention between two stimuli. Ability to adapt to rapidly changing directions and/or to manipulate the information, I scored a 63, which places me in the 96th percentile.

So, my Executive Functioning, Attention, Reaction Time and Cognitive Flexibility are doing great.

My Processing Speed and Psychomotor Speed are low average.

My Visual Memory is below average, my Verbal Memory is WAY below average, totaling in a Composite Memory Score of WAY below average.

So I can still figure things out, but it takes awhile to process the info, and then I'll forget about it.

What were we talking about again? Where are my keys? Did someone say "cake"?

And now, we notice the onset of a NEW symptom. In most folks with PD, their voice problems consist of having difficulties with volume, as well as slurring and word-finding deficits. I'm still nice and loud. Thirty-plus years in broadcasting have seen to that. I slur. And I stutter.

Homina Homina Homina

February 1, 2010

Parkinson's disease, thou art a WHIMSICAL affliction!

Having a particularly Parky morning... if I didn't push myself, I would be completely satisfied to sit here, staring at the computer screen, motionless, listening to blues on Music Choice on the cable. But that ain't what they pay me the big bucks for, so I manage to force myself to log into my work e-mail account and update the press log to reflect some activity over the weekend.

I force myself out of my chair and make my slow, halting way into the living room to get my slippers. Gail volunteered to get them for me, but I told her no because "I have to push myself."

Got the slippers, turned to walk back to the kitchen and get back to work. My left foot was more than happy to comply. My right foot stuck to the floor. I managed to keep from falling. This is nothing new .

I noticed Gail looking at me with concern. I said, "Here in the house, that's how I come close to falling. I'll start to walk, one foot will move and... and... and... and..."

I forced my mouth shut and closed my eyes so I would stop saying the word "and."

"And the other foot gets stuck?" Gail added helpfully.

I felt flush. I got STUCK on a WORD! I knew full well what I WANTED to say, but like an old fashioned record in an old fashioned record player, the needle in my brain got stuck in the groove of my language center.

I looked it up on my NIH-linked computer. It's called "palilalia." It's a subset of "bradykinesia"—or slowness of movement in Parkinson's disease.

Speech and swallowing may be affected. The speech may be slightly softer, muffled, and less distinct. In more severe disease, the speech is rapid, monotonous, and slurred. Palilalia, repeating the initial syllable of a word similar to stuttering, also can occur in patients with more advanced disease and can be a side effect of medications. Sialorrhea and dysphagia are common problems in patients with more advanced disease.

Swell. I am feeling slightly drooly this morning (dabbing at the corners of my mouth with a napkin to contain the overflow) – no trouble swallowing yet today, but I am clearing my throat a lot and my voice is thin, hoarse and scratchy.

Oh, Parkinson's! How I DESPISE thee!

UPDATE: Seems like "palilalia" might be too specific—what happened this morning seems to fall more neatly into the category of "repetitive speech phenomenon". According to an article in the National Library of Medicine:

In idiopathic Parkinson's disease repetitive speech phenomena seem to emerge predominantly in a subgroup of patients with advanced disease impairment; manifest dementia is not a necessary prerequisite. They seem to represent a deficit of motor speech control; however, linguistic factors may also contribute to their generation. It is suggested that repetitions of speech in Parkinson's disease represent a distinctive speech disorder, which is caused by changes related to the progression of Parkinson's disease.

So, there.

More Funky Speech Fun!

February 2, 2010

Ak! Ak! Ak! Ak! Ak!

My speech problems continue for another day. Last night as Gail left the bedroom to use the facilities, I meant to ask her if she wanted me to turn on the bedside lamp. What I said was...

"Would you like me to turn the... the... the... the..."

I pointed at the lamp and Gail said, "No." Thank goodness, or else I'd probably STILL be saying the word "the."

So far, I'm noticing that the problems fall into a couple different realms.

1. When I talk casually, I'll start to say a word—but begin it with the wrong syllable. For instance, instead of saying, "It's getting dark outside..." I'll say, "It's getting nark...." and then I freeze up, close my eyes, concentrate on what I want to say... and then say it.

2. Also when speaking casually, I'll run words together until it's all garbled. I sound like Popeye. When this happens, I have to

close my eyes, take a deep breath, and say the words I want to say with definite breaks between each word.

3. When under pressure to say something, I tend to just freeze up. It would be FINE if I just stayed silent, but I start making babbling noises with the "aaaaah" and the "errrrrr" and the "uuuuhhhhh" and I sound like a moron. When this happens now, I force myself to shut up, then say "I'm trying to think of the right word."

So, what to do? Well, other than being breathy and hoarse, I'm not really having trouble with volume (hypophonia). It just seems like I've picked up a stutter (neurogenic stutter) in my old age.

Gail says we can make a little extra money by taking me on tour to do Popeye impressions. She LOVES me!

It's Not a Temporary Thing, I Guess
February 3, 2010

I may as well stop complaining about it. Seems like my Parkinson's disease-related vocal difficulties are here to stay.

After Gail took the photos that you can see in a previous entry from today, she asked if I could print one out so she could frame it.

"I'll see if we have any pho... pho... pho... pho... (shut my eyes, take a breath, concentrate) photographic paper."

There's been other examples throughout yesterday and today. Just now, Shiloh—our neurotic German shepherd—was nosing my elbow as if she needed to "use the yard." I went back to the other office where Gail was browsing the web and asked how long it's been since the animals have been outside.

"I just brought them in," she said. "I guess I could just hang Shiloh out on her cable for awhile."

"Tha... tha... that... tha... (close eyes, concentrate) That. Would. Be. A. Good. Idea."

I guess this is just something I'm going to have to get used to. That's all, folks!

She's a FUNNY Lady!

February 7, 2010

The other night, my wife and I were conversing over one thing or another and I kicked into my newly found Parkinson's stutter.

Gail said, "I'm going to have to start calling you Elmer." "Elmer? Why?" "Isn't he the cartoon character who stutters?" "No," I said. "You're thinking of Porky Pig."

"Oh, that's right," she said.

"Yeah, Elmer has problems with his "L" and "R" sounds. I don't have that problem."

"Not yet," she said without even looking at me. My wife. She woves me vewy, vewy much!

I admit, I became a bit of a nut for the "self testing" earlier this year. Just trying to figure out where my progression ranks in the scheme of things. I'm at the point now as I approach disability retirement where I think more along the lines of "que sera, sera."

I Guess I'm Doing OK, Considering the Alternative

February 16, 2010

I've been doing a lot of griping about my Parkinson's disease symptoms on this site as of late. It's been a rough few months— from the death of my older sister (who would have been 58 years old today), to the recent horrible weather. I'll be seeing my neurologist day after tomorrow. New since my last visit in October? Trouble swallowing (dysphagia), voice difficulties (hoarseness and stuttering). I haven't fallen since then, so that's good. I don't feel like I'm any slower than I was, so that's good, too.

In fact, all things considered, I think I'm doing fairly well for a fella who has been diagnosed with Parkinson's for over 10 years now. I'm still working. Studies show that after 5 years, 25 percent of us can't hold down a job. That figure jumps to 80 percent after 9 years. I passed 10 years on Jan. 30. True, I'm not digging ditches, and I'm not doing all the duties I was hired to do (I can't do media escort anymore), I'm still able to do most of the stuff in my job description, and I can do it from home.

I have a wonderful caregiver, partner, friend and wife. All in the same person! She motivates me to do my best. I reward her by giving her a headache most evenings with my constant throat clearing. She is always there for me and I could not do this without her. My stepson, TJ, is great as well. During the recent snowpocalypse, he lent his hand and his back to keep us shoveled out. Gail helped, but TJ was the work horse.

THE PDQ-39

There's an excellent measuring device to show where you are in the progression of Parkinson's disease. It's called the Parkinson's Disease Questionnaire, or PDQ-39 for its 39 questions. I took it the other day (after researching how to score it), and it showed mixed results.

The 39 questions are broken into 8 different areas. Each item is scored from "0" (meaning "never" or "no problem") to "4" for "always" or "can't do at all.") You add up your responses to the questions, and the physician gets a good idea of where to place you on the progression scale.

The first 10 questions deal with "Mobility". I scored a "35" where "0" would be perfect and "40" would be worst-possible.

The next 6 questions center on "Activities of Daily Life." I scored myself at "6" where "0" would be perfect and "24" would be worst case. (I can still button me own buttons, tie me own shoes, cut me own food and wipe me own backside.)

The following 6 deal with the "Emotional" aspects of PD. I scored a 10 in the "0-to-24" range.

The next 4 are for "Stigma"—meaning, how embarrassed are you by your symptoms. I rated myself at "4" on the "0-to-16" scale.

There are 3 questions dedicated to the "Social" aspects of the disease. Am I getting the support I need from friends, co-workers and family. I scored a perfect "0" on this one!

In the 4 questions dealing with "Cognition", I gave myself a "7" in the "0-to-16" scale.

There are 3 questions about "Communication." Gave myself a "6" on the "0-to-12" scale.

Finally, in the area of "Discomfort", I graded my 3 questions at "8" on the "0-to-12" scale.

Then, to get an overall PDSI or "Parkinson's Disease Summary Index", you total up all the scores from all 39 questions (76), divide that number by 4 (the most possible points for each question) times 39 (the number of questions), then multiply that number by 100.

My PDSI is 48.72. That would put me just a tad over the limit for the Stage IV area in the Hoehn & Yahr PD rating scale. (The dividing line between III and IV is 48.59.)

I'm guessing that's about where I should be after a decade since diagnosis.

ALL IN ALL...

Bottom line... my hands still work pretty well, thanks to the medication and the deep brain stimulation I had in 2007. My legs? Not so much. I take little steps, I walk slowly, I freeze when I walk. I need a cane in the house and a walker outside. Mentally, I'm just starting to notice some slippage in the area of cognition. My speech is just now becoming affected (oft times, it's the FIRST symptom). My posture sucks, and you could push me over with a finger poke to the sternum. (Please don't.)

But when I go to bed at night, before I fall asleep with a dog at my feet and the sound of my wife breathing in her own bed, I thank God that I have it as good as I do.

Whoops! iPhone alarm just went off. Time for my 11am Sinemet.

Another Visit with the Doc

February 18, 2010

Had my four-month visit with Dr. Grill today. The guy is great.

We did all the little tests we always do, and it turns out my hands are actually faster than they were before he adjusted my deep brain stimulation devices in October. So that's good.

We did all the movement tests... the first time he did the pull test, I fell right back into his arms. He told me to really try to stop myself by taking a backwards step and we tried it again. This time, I took backwards steps until I hit the wall. They call this "retropulsion."

I did well on the open and close your hands, finger taps, turn your hands like flipping a burger thing. I had a HUGE problem with the heel tapping thing. With my left leg, I was tapping away like a pro! With my right leg, it was like "tap-tap- (pause) -tap- (pause) (pause)- tap-tap-(pause)". Dr. Grill said, can't you do that in a more regular rhythm? "I'll try," I said. And I tried again... my right heel would strike the floor, I'd raise my leg, I'd try to lower it and it wouldn't lower all the way... then it would finally tap the floor and bounce right back up, and down again, and up, then hang up again on the downward stroke.

"Hmmmm....." Dr. Grill said.

We discussed my gait and balance, my recent speech and swallowing issues. He prescribed a visit with a physical therapist who has been dealing with Parkinson's patients for 20 years. So, I guess she knows her stuff!

We discussed my medication, and decided to drop the Sinemet and replace it with Stalevo. The benefit of Stalevo is that it contains entacapone, which causes the levodopa to be delivered to the brain in a smoother, steadier, extended and more consistent manner. This will help the symptoms I have that are helped by levodopa. It won't help the gait, the balance, the speech, the swallowing. I also got a script for Ambien to help me get to and stay asleep at night.

Speaking of gait, I still have a slow, heel-to-toe walk, but my stride is short. Dr. Grill says physical therapy will help that as well as my posture. I'll also get a swallowing evaluation and a voice eval. The

Lee Silverman Voice Treatment is designed to help Parkinson's patients speak louder.

"Forget the louder," Gail said. "We don't need the louder."

Dr. Grill smiled at Gail's other suggestions, such as a prescription for Drano to help clear out my windpipes at night, and for a cattle prod to get me moving when I freeze. Well, he shot down the Drano idea, but he didn't SPECIFICALLY nix the cattle prod, so Gail still holds out a modicum of hope.

We had a nice chat. I explained that the last thing I want to be is a "full time patient." Someone who lives next to the medicine cabinet, who needs a Sinemet at 6, a Mirapex at 7, Entacapone at 7:30, another Sinemet at 10, another Mirapex at noon, something for the dystonia, something for the depression, something for the cramps, yada yada yada yada...

"I realize there will never be such a thing as 'normal' for me again," I said. "I know this is a progressive disease, it will get worse. I just want to be able to function as best as I can and to go into this thing as gracefully as possible." He said he thought I had a good attitude about it.

I guess I do. It helps to have a partner like Gail.

"He didn't specifically say no to the cattle prod," she reminded me as we walked to the car.

I love her so!

Again, when you get to where I am in the progression of a disease, it's all a matter of choices. Am I going to get better?

No. Will eating the ice cream make my Parkinson's worse? Probably not. Easy choice.

Who Do I Listen To? The Doctor? Or the Ice Cream?

February 24, 2010

One voice is stern and scolding. The other is soft and soothing.

When I visited with my neurologist last week, he gave me a gentle scolding for putting on some weight. "It's gonna catch up to you as the disease progresses," he said. He advised more exercise and less of what he called "the bad food."

And I know he's right. It makes all the sense in the world. If I were lighter and more muscular, I would still have Parkinson's disease, but it wouldn't be such a heavy bulk for me to lug around.

But the soft, soothing voice of ice cream tells me differently.

Yes. I can hear ice cream.

It happens when I'm waddling down the aisle at the grocery store, my walker in front of me. That's when I hear the voice. I turn to the freezer display, and at first I have to wonder how that tub of Ben & Jerry's "Cherry Garcia" knows my name.

It draws me closer. The pint of ice cream sparkles like a glittering diamond in a jeweler's display case.

"Hi there, Bill," the ice cream says. I say nothing, because I know the voice is meant just for me—and besides, if folks see me holding a one-way conversation with a pint of ice cream, I'll be in "the home" sooner than I really want to be.

I decide it will be OK if I communicate with the ice cream telepathically.

The ice cream seems concerned about me. "What are you afraid of, Bill?"

"You're BAD for me," I think at the pint. "My doctor says I shouldn't eat you anymore."

"Oh, piffle!" the ice cream says. "You have Parkinson's disease. You're ALWAYS going to have Parkinson's disease. And even if you DO lose weight, you're still gonna end up in the wheelchair sooner or later."

Now, I know I'm the only one who can see this, but the ice cream slides just a little bit closer to the edge of the display case, nudging aside the frozen yogurt and sorbet.

"Now, if you buy me and take me home and EAT me, you'll STILL have Parkinson's disease. You'll STILL have trouble walking and balance difficulties. But for a moment—just a BRIEF portion of your evening—you'll have a cool, tasty, creamy treat that will make you FORGET about the stiffness, the soreness, the slowness. Think of it as a brief vacation from reality, Bill."

I have to admit. The ice cream is making sense. I begin to back away from the display case.

"No, no, no," I think at the tempting pint of deliciousness. "You're telling me what I WANT to hear, not what I SHOULD hear! You're giving me bad advice," I think as I slowly retreat.

"Ah! Ah! Your doctor said 'No backing up!'" the ice cream scolds - - but ever so sweetly. "You don't listen to THAT advice, but you WILL listen to advice that would deny you my rich, sweet, cold and creamy goodness?"

I feel something snap in my mind. Call it the "breaking of resolve" if you will. I prefer to think of it as "making an executive decision."

"No!" I shout telepathically. "I will NOT be ruled by fear! I WILL buy you, ice cream! I will take you home and EAT you at a time that is convenient for ME!"

I open the display case, withdraw the pint of Ben & Jerry's. It's cold and heavy in my hand.

"Wise decision," the ice cream says, as I place it in the shopping cart my wife is pushing.

So, spare me your lectures. I know it's bad for me. So is Parkinson's disease. I can exercise more. I can eat less. But none of that is going to make a WHIT of difference at the end of all things. When the end comes, as it certainly will at some point no matter WHAT I do—whether it's from aspiration pneumonia (the leading cause of death for Parkies) or falling and breaking a hip (hey, if I'm padded well with adipose tissue, won't that make my hip HARDER to break?), I will NOT lie on my deathbed regretting that I enjoyed the cool, creamy, fruity goodness that lured me to the display case at a grocery store.

Death awaits us all. Some of us sooner than later. Will YOU lie on your deathbed wishing you had eaten one less cheeseburger, one less order of fries, one less pint of ice cream?

Not ME, Mister! Not ME!

Again, it becomes easier and easier to pick out the jerks from the nice folks when you're hobbling around a mall with a cane or a walker.

Hey! Don't Worry! Just STEP on Me!
February 27, 2010

One thing I like about Saturdays is that Gail and I usually do something fun together. Today, it was a trip to the Mall in Columbia, Maryland. For one thing, I really NEED the exercise. For another thing, I really NEED to get out of the house. For another thing, I really NEEDED some new jammies!

I also, it seems, need to expose myself to rude morons so I can truly appreciate nice people when I meet them. Last time we parked near Macy's and walked through the store, I was nearly knocked off my pins by a young chickie baby who actually bumped into me—bumped IN to an OLDER MAN with a

WALKER—and just kept going. I was able to keep from falling, but barely.

This time, heading into the mall, there was the typical assortment of the walking dead looking for skinny jeans and skinny t-shirts to cover their fleshless asses and breastless chests. I saw a young, tattooed fellow trundling my way with a push cart. He saw me and stopped. Then he politely motioned me past him. I thanked him for being a gentleman, and we made our way through the store.

So, first we toddled to the food court. Gail ate Chinese. I ate Japanese. Mine had more teriyaki, but that about spells the difference.

Afterwards, we strolled in my typical leisurely fashion down towards the Big and Tall store. I try to keep close to the wall when I walk, because people—being jerks—just love to cut me off, bump into me and score points by making the old man fall so they have something to "ROTFL" and "LMAO" about when they text message their idiot friends. Gail veered away to look at something towards the center of the aisle and I had to veer around an obstacle. This young 100-lb. teen chickie baby darts right between me and Gail because GOD FORBID she should have to WAIT a frickin' second for some OLD MAN to dodder his useless ass out of her way. She was in a HURRY! She caused me to freeze, and I almost fell as a result. Had to throw the brakes on the walker and steady myself.

I told Gail what happened when she was looking at the sparkly things, and she said, "Just keep close to the wall, Rat Boy." (See, rats and other vermin tend to scurry along the baseboard of a wall to avoid notice.) "I can only protect one side of you at a time," she said.

She made her point.

We got to the clothing store, I got some new PJ tops and bottoms. ("What does this say about my life," I asked Gail. "I no longer shop for clothes to wear to work. I just shop for stuff to sleep in.")

After that, out to through the Macy's where young waifs, looking like the starving cat mannequins they strive to emulate, cut in front of me, around me, beside me, not so much as an "excuse me." That is, until an elderly African American gent needed to make a left turn in front of me. He waited until our eyes met, and he made his turn. "Pardon me," he said. "No problem! Have a great day!" I replied. "You do the same," he said as he walked away.

See? You need to expose yourself to the jerks so that you will really appreciate the nice folks when you meet them.

(The next morning, Gail and I went grocery shopping. I toddled out to the car while she went through the checkout. As she came out of the store, this young chickie baby in an Acura rolled past the stop sign, honked twice at Gail as she was in the middle of the crosswalk, then – without waiting for Gail to get to the other side – she curved around her and zoomed down the parking lot. I don't understand why it's the young people who are always in such a freakin' hurry. They have all the time in the world. Us older folks – WE should be the ones in a hurry. Who KNOWS how much time WE have left...)

Parky "Masking"

February 28, 2010

Did our weekly grocery shopping today. One thing I'm grateful for is the fact that my walker has a seat on it so I can sit and relax while Gail peruses the kidney beans.

So, I'm seated on the walker and after a few minutes of examining the kidney beans Gail walks up with a big smile on her face. "Well, don't YOU look like the poor beleaguered husband waiting for his wife?"

"Not at all," I said. "Actually, at the moment I was thinking about how grateful I am to always have a place to sit."

Gail understands the philosophy of Parkinson's disease "masking."

"I know," she said, "but nobody else does."

So after we got a few more things, she gave me the car keys so I could toddle out to the car and wait while she went through the checkout. And I decided to take a picture of myself to see just how bad of a "face day" I was having.

"Yikes!"

This is one of the hallmarks of Parkinson's disease. No matter what kind of mood you're in—and I'm in a fairly decent one—this is how you look when your face is relaxed. I can make myself smile and show emotion if I want to, but it takes effort. This is why people get the mistaken expression about Parkies that "the lights are on, but nobody's home."

Actually, the truth of the matter is, "the lights are out and EVERYONE is home." Behind the sullen, angry-looking, granite face of a person with Parkinson's disease, the mind is still working at full speed... more or less, in my case.

At least I didn't drool on my shirt.

(ADDENDUM: I just read this to Gail. "I still think a cattle prod would help that," she said. She loves me.)

Now THAT's a Hallucination!
March 7, 2010

Rough day for Billy, and it's barely 10 am!

I've been congested and hacky all morning because I have trouble with my night time, shall we say, "secretions." We were at the grocery store and I had a throat spasm. I bent over and hacked like I had a lung coming up. And, to my horror, I watched in slow motion as a long string of drool cascaded from my lower lip to the

floor. I looked up and saw the horrified faces of customers around me.

Gail suggested I might want to start carrying paper towels with me.

You can tell she loves me.

Then, on the way home, we approached the off ramp to US 1 from Highway 100. I saw a guy standing on the shoulder, between the highway and off ramp, and it looked like he was waving down a car. He watched as the car went past him, then he turned and walked onto the off ramp.

"Watch out for the guy on the off ramp," I said to my wife. She looked and looked and saw nothing.

I looked again, and the guy turned into a shadow on a light post. I swear, I could almost see face detail, tell you what kind of clothes he had on, and his hair color. I saw him waving and walking. And then... he wasn't there.

"God, I'm afraid to tilt my head one way or the other because my brains will come pouring out my ear," I said.

"Just make sure to have those paper towels with you," Gail said. I can FEEL the love coming off her in WAVES! :)

Oh, Parkinson's disease. Truly thou art an ENTERTAINING affliction!

Rainy Days and Mondays Almost Knock Me Down
March 22, 2010

It's Spring in Maryland. We just had a few glorious days of sunshine and 70s. Then we pay for it with a week of cold, rainy days. Today is such a day.

It was barely sprinkling when Gail and I left for the store. If it had been raining harder, I would have just stayed home... not so much for my dryness sake, but for Gail who feels compelled to walk along side me getting just as soaked.

As we made our way through the store, my walker proved its worth once more. I've been having a bit of foot drop today— mostly on the left side. Toodling down the dairy aisle, my left toes dug into the tile. I managed to throw on the hand brake as Gail grabbed me around the waist. The walker kept me from falling. If I had just been using my cane, I would have been kissing the tile, with Gail likely laying beside me on the floor.

THEN who would take care of us? :(

On our way out of the grocery store (where we picked up the fixin's to make some tasty ham, egg and cheese sammiges for Billy—yum!), it began pouring. I told Gail to go on without me, but she said no because she had to put the walker in the back seat anyway.

So, we made it eventually to the car, getting soaked. Got home. Gail helped me peel out of my hoodie so she could throw it with hers into the dryer.

And so it goes, another day in the life of a Parky and his Caregiver.

A Bad Case of the "Yibble Bibbles"

March 24, 2010

Feels like this is gonna be a rough day.

Generally, the first words I speak on a given morning are potty instructions to my dogs. "Go potty, Raven. Go potty, Shiloh." Pretty simple stuff. Then, when they've done their deeds, I urge them back to the house with instructions such as, "That's a good girl, come on now, let's go in the house."

This morning, that instruction came out like, "That's a guh... that's... that's a guh... guh.. good girl. Get... Get... Get... in the house."

OK, maybe that's just a passing thing and I'm over it.

Nope.

Gail gets up, we hug and kiss, I tell her I had a good night's sleep, we talk about the stuff we usually talk about in the morning, except she's finishing sentences and questions for me because I'm talking like Porky the freakin' PIG this morning.

It started again last night when we were discussing something we were watching on TV... I couldn't get a word out, so I just pointed at Gail and she guessed the word I was trying to say. (There's something to be said for knowing someone for 22 years.)

I should try to get some of this on tape so you can hear what I'm talking (or not talking) about. But as soon as I turn on the camera, all of a sudden I'm like Walter Cronkite.

Parkinson's disease. How I loathe you!

Stumblebummery, Mufflemouthery and Seeing Stuff

March 24, 2010

This hasn't been one of my better days. The language difficulties I described this morning are continuing. When Gail and I went to the store for lunch, I was even freezier than usual. And I had three episodes of seeing things that weren't there.

Episode the First: We were still in the trailer park, and through the driver's window, out of the corner of my left eye, I saw someone walking down his driveway to the street. I turned to look. No one there.

Episode the Second: Moments later while waiting at a stoplight, out of the corner of my right eye I noticed something moving on the windshield. It was small, and I took a closer look to see if it was a spider or an ant. It was a nothing.

Episode the Third: Walking into the store, out of the corner of my left eye, I notice a reflection in the glass and it looks like some guy in a jacket and a baseball cap is trying to squeeze around Gail to get into the store ahead of her. I turn around, he's not there. Just me and Gail.

Since we've been home, there's been a lot of me talking, stopping, waving my hands as I urge Gail to guess what the fuck it was that I was going to say. She usually gets it right. We would have been GREAT charade partners.

Nope. Not a good day. So far.

"Don't Inhale That Wine!"

March 26, 2010

Sitting in my recliner last night, settling in for the evening, getting ready to watch Countdown. Had a nice little glass of port wine next to me that I was about 1/3 of the way into.

Picked up the glass, took a sip, and poured a mouthful of delicious, sweet wine right into my lung.

This wasn't a case of a little bit of liquid sneaking past the seal made by my epiglottis and pharynx. It poured STRAIGHT DOWN!

My epiglottis didn't even TRY to close.

This was the first example of my Parkinson's disease actually trying to kill me. They call it dysphagia. And aspiration pneumonia, along with injuries from falls, are the leading causes of PD-related death.

I immediately bent over and started hacking up the wine from my lung. (Oddly enough, it only went into my left lung. Didn't get any in the right one. Wonder why that is.) If you don't think wine burns when you get it in your trachea and lungs, think again.

For some reason, I was very upset about this. That feeling was furthered by the fact that my wife has to sit and wear wireless headphones to block out my constant coughing and throat clearing every night or else she gets a headache. Is this what it's coming down to? Is this how I'm going to spend the rest of my life?

I have a consult for a speech therapist. Had it for awhile, but I've kept putting it off. Nothing like getting a couple teaspoons of wine in your lung to motivate a fella! I don't think I need any work on my "loudness." I still have the "loud". But I better get to work on this swallowing thing before I inhale something I can't cough back up.

One of the truly positive things to come from my experiences with Parkinson's disease is my blog and the way it has allowed me to reach out to others in the community of

Parkies. Unfortunately, not all of my Parky brethren and sistheren see things politically or religiously the same way I do. I've done my research on Parky Blogs. A lot of them are smarmy, flowery, "O Lord, Thank You for Showing Your Love with the Gift of Parkinson's So That I May Testify to Your Great and Enduring Mercy by the Evidence of my Grace During the Struggle to Swallow my Oatmeal."

May I just politely remark, "Bull Hockey!" I don't believe in a God who "gives disease" to "test your mettle." For one thing, if God is omnipotent and knows HOW you will react to adversity before he gives it to you, WHY GIVE IT TO YOU IN THE FIRST PLACE??? But I understand that there are folks who need their version of God to provide them with a source of comfort – and someone to blame. MY version of "God" isn't involved in any of this but is more than happy to help you gain the strength to deal with whatever happens. Still...

I Did It Myyyyyy Waaaaaaaaaaaay!

April 1, 2010

I got a VERY nice note from a friend of mine on Facebook. I won't reveal her name, but the note moves me to comment. The occasion of the note seems to be my status update on Facebook about right wingers practically praying for the downfall of America so they can blame it on Obama.

Here's the note...

I suppose you could classify me as one of your new "right-wing" friends if that is what a follower of Jesus Christ is. I am Christian and have been since I was 4 ½ and I am now 54. My husband Larry is Christian as well. Speaking as one, I would like to tell you as all apples in a basket are not rotten; it is unfair to place all of us "right-wingers" in a basket. Speaking for myself alone, I do not pray for the fall of America....though many an empire in history has fallen due to turning from God and turning to moral decay as we witness in America. I pray the LORD God will change all our hearts back to Him. As far as electing a Republican, I am a registered Republican, however I do not vote now or ever for the party...I vote for the man running - His integrity, his political experience, his heart for God. If he follows the laws of God as in our New Testament Bible - this nation will become strong again and be one we can be proud to be a part of. I am a firm believer that if the morals of a country are corrupt...then so shall the decline and decay of the government evidence itself. Every man has the power and the right to choose what he thinks is true and right....as only that one man will be eternally responsible for the result of that thinking. In true love, we must give every person the right to choose for himself what he believes and thinks is right.

Deep set anger with name calling ("Bill Schmalfeldt never ceases to be amazed at how his right wing friends hope and pray that America fails, just so they can elect Republicans"), will not solve the issues at hand. I will pray you can be set free of all your anger expressed whether in blogging or day to day life. As life and death can be given from our tongues...what we say is what we become. Our words written and spoken have much power as I am sure you know and realize. Many read what we say, many are influenced by what we say, and ultimately we are responsible for that influence. I sense in the midst of your humor - fear, cynicism, and hopelessness. I care about you, Bill, though we have just barely met. I will have hope for you....and I will pray your fear will cease, your hope will grow, and you will come to know the love and peace of God. There is so much more waiting for us after this life. My husband, Larry, whom also has Parkinson's, shares in my feelings and views. He does not enjoy computers in his daily endeavors, however, but wishes to express his support and friendship through this letter as well. We have enjoyed 29 wonderful years together on April 4th, and it is a gift to share a life with someone whom your heart is bonded with forever. I so appreciated reading of your family. You are blessed.

It was a truly lovely note and beautiful sentiment and is greatly appreciated. But she's wrong in a couple of areas. She's also RIGHT in a couple regards.

Blessed? You BETCHA!

Am I a cynic? Oh, YES I am! Ever since I was a kid, I've always been one of those "question authority" types. I used to get kicked out of Sunday school classes for asking questions—not smartassy ones, either—that the priest couldn't or wouldn't answer. I spent more than my fair share of time with the principal (who turned out to be a very good friend of mine) when I challenged my teachers on the things they taught us from their books.

So, "cynic?" Guilty as charged.

But "hopeless"? "Fearful"? You got da wrong man, lady!

I admit to some anger. Anger over this disease that has taken over my life. Anger over the eight years wasted in research because President Bush chose superstition over science in the Embryonic Stem Cell Debate.

I admit to frustration when I try to say something and end up sounding like Porky Pig. When I swallow a sip of something and it ends up in my windpipe. When I try to record a podcast and have to edit the hell out of it because of the phlegm that gets caught in my vocal cords. When I try to walk and my feet freeze to the floor. When a slight, playful tap from my wife makes me have to grab on to her arm to keep from falling.

But dear friend, and gentle readers... I don't have TIME for "fear" OR "hopelessness." If you were to read my book about DBS surgery (and if you haven't bought your copy yet, why not?) you would know that I charge headlong into the breach in the fight AGAINST fear, AGAINST ignorance, AGAINST prejudice, AGAINST hopelessness. If there is any story that I would hope my life would tell, it is that I LIVED.

I was thinking about this very subject last night as I was drifting off to sleep. Look at this list of things I have done in my life -- (not all of them are what one would call "family friendly" but are included here).

I have traveled nearly ¾ of the way around the world.

I've dangled by my crotch from a helicopter, and have jumped out of said helicopter into the ocean wearing full 782-gear.

I was once almost killed by a mistakenly-thrown white phosphorous grenade.

I lived in Japan for 18 months. I've been inside the Great Buddha in Kamakura.

I once took a train ride from Pusan to Seoul, South Korea, because I didn't want to hang around with my friends and chase hookers.

I once had sex on a revolving stage in Japan. In front of paying customers.

On New Year's Eve, 1983/84, I had drinks in a Tokyo disco with a guy from Libya. We clinked glasses and toasted each other. "Ronald Reagan is an asshole," he said. "Yer right," I said. "So's Khadafi!" "You're right," he said. Later that night, I was so wasted I asked a girl to dance with me and it turned out to be a guy.

I've had a kneecap removed. I've been in all 50 states.

I've been married three times. This last time for 20 years and counting. (She's a keeper.)

I've had a novel published and have self-published four other books I've written.

I had a national radio audience when I worked at XM Satellite Radio.

I have six children—some of which love me, others of whom are ambivalent at best, others who hate my guts. I have two grandchildren, one I haven't seen since he was a baby, one I've never seen.

At the stroke of midnight on New Year's Eve 1974/75, I kissed a stripper in a Jacksonville Beach strip club who was old enough to be my mom and had half her nose missing from skin cancer.

I had a national radio audience when I did the "NIH Health Matters" segments heard on XM and on radio stations around the country.

I've stood in Dealey Plaza and on the grassy knoll where President Kennedy was killed.

I've been a newspaper editor, columnist and reporter.

I've been on top of the Empire State Building.

I've been a radio station program director, news director, talk show host and disc jockey.

I've participated in the search for a cure for PD by having volunteer brain surgery as part of a Phase I clinical trial.

I've been to Disneyland.

I've flown in a plane that landed on an aircraft carrier, grabbing the cable with a tailhook.

I sat in a grass-roofed bar with no walls in the Philippines, sipping 10-cent rum and cokes during a torrential rain storm.

I've done stand-up comedy in New York City. Manhattan, yet! I've been to Tokyo Disneyland.

I've set foot in Spain, Italy, the Vatican, France, Lebanon, Mexico, Canada, the Philippines, South Korea and Japan.

I've been to the NFL Hall of Fame in Canton, Ohio

I once ran for elected office, coming in second out of four candidates.

My ex-wife and I were on the pilot for a game show shortly before we broke up.

I've been to the Green Bay Packers Hall of Fame. I've stood in the majesty of the Sistine Chapel.

I've walked in the Roman catacombs, seeing the bones of early Christians.

I had late night sandwiches with a German couple a friend of mine and I met during a performance of Beethoven's 9th Symphony in an ancient ampitheater in Taormina, Sicily.

I've been propositioned in the apartment of a beautiful German girl in Naples, Italy—and said no.

I took part in the evacuation of Americans and Lebanese nationals from Beirut in July 1976.

I once saw a guy get his head lopped off by a helicopter blade.

I once took my wife for a drive all the way around Lake Michigan. I went to Wrestlemania XIII with my late twin brother and his son. I was once a contestant on "The Price is Right".

I mourned the death of my father, a twin brother, an older brother, an older sister, and the abandonment of her family by my youngest sister.

I've had Parkinson's disease for 10 years.

And I'm only 55 years old.

When my time comes, which I hope is no time soon, I will leave with no regrets. I've already donated my mortal remains—all of 'em—for the furtherance of medical science. (Actually, I hope I get "plasticized" and posed in some bizarre fashion to be placed on display in some art gallery where someone I knew while alive, checking out the exhibit, will tell his companion, "doesn't that one kinda look like Bill?")

To quote "Old Blue Eyes..."

"I Did it All. And I Stood Tall. And Did it My Way!"

So, dear Facebook friend, thanks for your offer of "hope". I'll take it and add it to the pile I already have. And best wishes to you and your lucky husband.

And now, your gentle author steps down from the pulpit to talk about other stuff.

I Loves Me Some Speech Therapy

April 7, 2010

Had my first appointment with the speech therapist today. Olivia is a sweetie! She is a Marquette grad, so she knows her way around Milwaukee... another point in her favor. And she pretty much confirmed everything I suspected is going on—voice and swallow- wise.

First, my voice is still strong. Three decade as a broadcaster have seen to that. I already know how to project from the diaphragm, so I'm not prey (yet) to the thin, whispery voice of the Parkinson's disease sufferer. I do, however, seem to be a "silent aspirator." She had me take sips of water (without tucking my chin) and spoonfuls of yogurt and sure as heck, my voice got all gargly and bubbly. I'm still clearing my throat from all that.

She gave me some good tips on what to do when I get hung up on a word or find myself trying to say too much, too fast.

She wrote a note to Dr. Grill, my neurologist, suggesting a video flouroscopy to see how much is getting past my epiglottis. And she gave me a bunch of exercises to work on daily.

I always feel good after appointments like this one. It makes me feel like I'm fighting back, not just sitting there and letting it happen to me.

I have my first physical therapy appointment on Tuesday. That should be fun, too!

Take THAT, Parkinson's!

No Way for a Man to Die!!!

April 12, 2010

When I die, as I know I must someday, I want a nice respectable death. I want to steal away, quietly, with my family by my side, with a minimum of pain and a maximum of "let's make him comfortable" drugs. I want soft music playing in the background. I would like my last words to be directed to my wife. I would like to hold her hand and say, "See ya on the other side, beautiful. I love you." I'd give her a little Bogie-esque chuck on the chin and then, quietly, peacefully, close my eyes and—as they say—join the invisible choir.

Now that you know how I WANT to die... here's how I do NOT want to die.

I do not want to drown in ice tea like I almost did last night.

"ELKRIDGE, MD—Bill Schmalfeldt, 55, died in his home Sunday night, April 11, 2010. He was drinking a glass of iced tea, choked on it, and died. His wife identified the brand as 'Lipton's Brisk Sweet Tea.' 'I tried to get him to drink Snapple, but he was stubborn that way,' the Widow Schmalfeldt said."

Honest to God! Sitting there, watching TV, sipping a tasty glass of iced tea, and my epiglottis doesn't even TRY to close. I can feel the cool, cool tea pouring right into my lung—just the left one, again, like when I inhaled a sip of wine a couple weeks ago. At least iced tea doesn't burn like wine does. Good thing it was the tea, because a few hours earlier I was sipping some tasty 12-year old single highland malt scotch, and that would have burned like the Great Chicago Fire!

(I can hear my nephew, Tommy, right now. "You gotta tuck your CHIN when you sip and swallow! Liquids move FAST." Yeah, yeah, yeah, I know. My speech therapist told me the same thing.)

It could be worse, I guess, when I think of other things I ate yesterday and what kind of obituary THAT would make...

"ELKRIDGE, MD—Bill Schmalfeldt, 55, died at his home Sunday, April 11, 2010 when he inhaled an entire bratwurst into his left lung. 'I've always been after him to chew more carefully,' his grieving widow said. 'I kept telling him, it's not a contest! You're not fighting off six brothers and sisters for the last scrap of food anymore.' Doctors said Schmalfeldt's death was hastened by the catsup and shredded cheddar cheese that accompanied the bratwurst. 'It was that 'triple cheddar' kind of shredded cheese,' the Howard County Medical Examiner said. 'That gets right into the blood stream. It was already too late by the time the paramedics arrived.'"

When I go, I want it to be a natural death at a very old age. I do not want to be referred to as "another senseless food-related death."

Comical Ways to Kill Myself

April 13, 2010

I can picture it in my mind. Someone driving down the street in front of my house. They hear a crash, and see my fat ass come a-tumbling out the front room window, onto the BBQ grill, flopping over backwards on my head.

That almost happened yesterday. In fact, I almost fell quite a few times yesterday. But the closest I got was when I was schlepping through the living room, my right leg gave out and I lurched right toward the window... with only the screen between me and a BBQ- grill related neck-breaking.

Well, there was a kitchen chair parked in front of the window. And it saved me. I was able to grab it, steady myself, get my feet under me, and contemplate my near doom.

Yesterday was that kind of day. I almost tipped over backwards like a falling redwood yesterday morning when giving my wife a kiss. At the store, my feet froze but my walker kept rolling. I had to slam on the brakes, pull the walker back towards me, get my feet under me, and proceed.

I seem to be far more steady on my feet today than I was yesterday. But I know this is a fleeting thing. This house is full of danger—active dogs swarming about my feet, a German shepherd who seems determined to kill me by dropping toys and balls in my path as I walk (she's easily amused) -- and that's just the start. Getting out of a chair, I am likely to flop back down onto it. Sometimes, two or three attempts are needed. Sometimes, I just give out.

But, like I said, today is pretty good. Maybe that is because I've kept my fat ass planted in this chair for most of the day. But 7 pm approaches. That means "The Daily Show" re-run from last night, and a glass of wine.

I just hope I survive.

Now, we add **ANOTHER** difficulty one experiences in the mid-to-later stages of Parkinson's.

Do not read this while eating.

The Benefits of Working @ Home

April 16, 2010

Working from my home has really turned out to be a benefit for me. For one thing, since I don't drive anymore, I don't have to get jammed onto crowded trains and fight perfectly capable people for the few handicapped-only seats... for another, I'm only steps away from the office and easily accessible. If the fatigue sets in, I can take my cell phone with me into the bedroom and get a bit of a restorative snooze.

Then, there are other benefits.

For instance...

It was 11 am this morning. Both of my dogs were hinting that they wanted to go outside. Gail was doing laundry, so the LEAST a fella can do is take his girlies out into the yard. So, I got Raven onto her leash, opened the door, and...

How do I put this delicately?

...immediately noticed I was "filling up my diaper."

There was no urge. There was no "need to go." I just stood up, walked to the door, bent over to put a chain around a dog's neck, opened the door, and...

Pooped 'em... just a bit before my Parkinson's addled brain realized the horror that was being perpetrated in my underwear and snapped everything shut.

Now THERE'S a benefit of working at home. If something like that happened at WORK, I would have to sit there in my filth, await the next shuttle to the Metro, take the Metro to Union Station, wait for the next MARC train, sit for the 40-minute trip home, have Gail pick me up for the 10 minute ride home... all the while "marinating" in my own "gravy."

Yes. For the boy with Parkinson's disease, the federal government's "work at home" plan is a good deal, indeed.

Now, to explain the reason why I write about stuff like that.

Something My Mom Asked Me Today...

April 17, 2010

We're in Milwaukee and having a wonderful time... even though I had an embarrassing moment. Tell you about that in a few.

The flight was uneventful. We got the rental car, a 2010 Ford Fusion. Had a great brekky with Becki, then over to Mom's. Where I—uh—had a repeat of a previous gastrointestinal incident that I wrote about yesterday. This time, it soaked through the pants and into the chair I was sitting on... something every adult child dreams of. Poopin' on one of Mom's chairs.

Of course, every boy can remember the first time he purchased adult diapers for himself. Today would be that day for me.

Muz asked why I write about stuff like that. I said it's because I know I'm not the only person with Parkinson's disease who has this trouble, but I am one of the few with a blog. And if I can make one reader who is suffering the same problem feel less alone, a little less "weird" about it, then I'm serving a higher purpose.

You get used to 'em after a while.

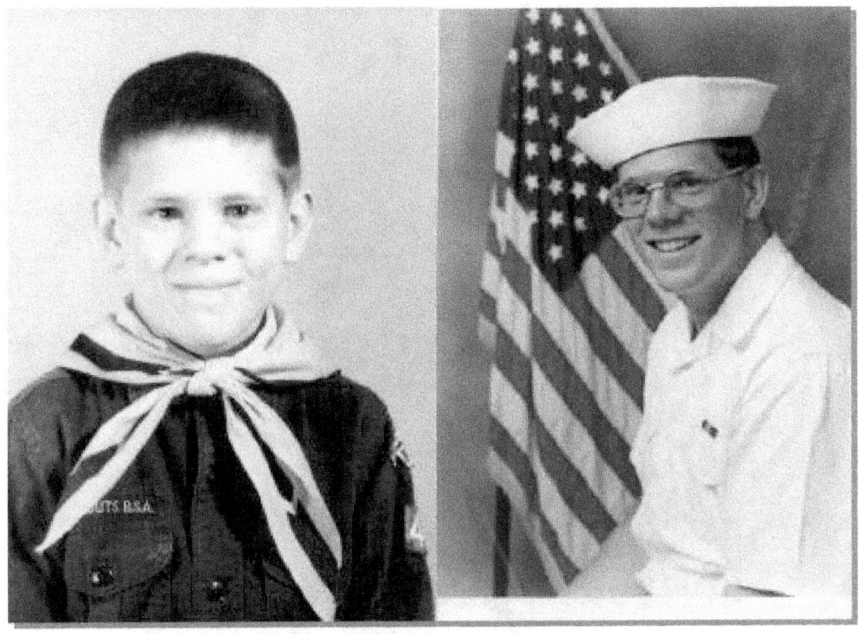

Girls LOVE a Man in Uniform!

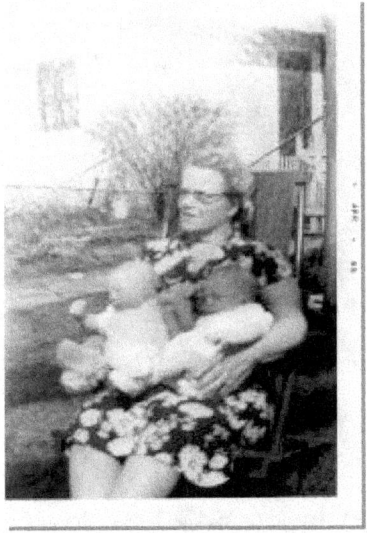

I'm Not Sure Which is Me and Which is My Twin
Brother Bob in This Shot, Taken with my Mom's
Mother in 1955

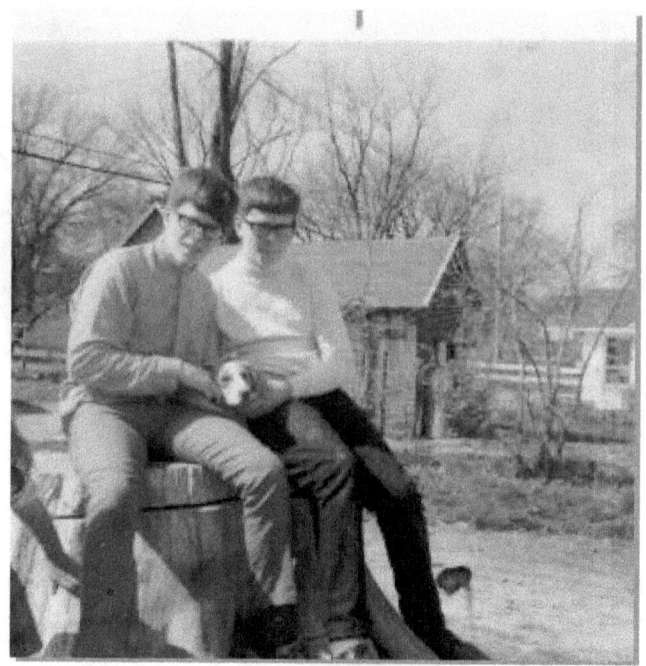

My Twin Brother (in white) and Me in 1969.
Groovy!

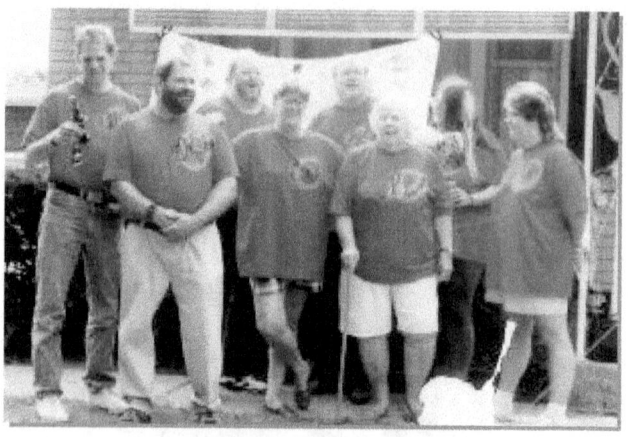

Schmalfest 1994 – the Last Time We Were All
Together. (L to R) Jack (died 2008), Joe, Me,
Cindi (died 2009), My Twin Brother Bob (died
2004), My Mom, Becki, and Micki (who changed
her name and abandoned the family in 2010.)

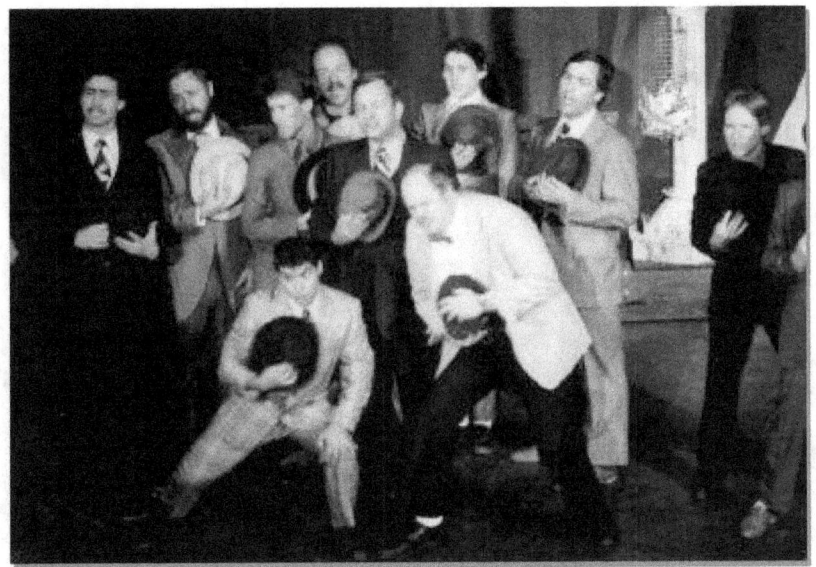

Me (front right) as "Nicely Nicely Johnson" in a
California production of "Guys and Dolls, 1996

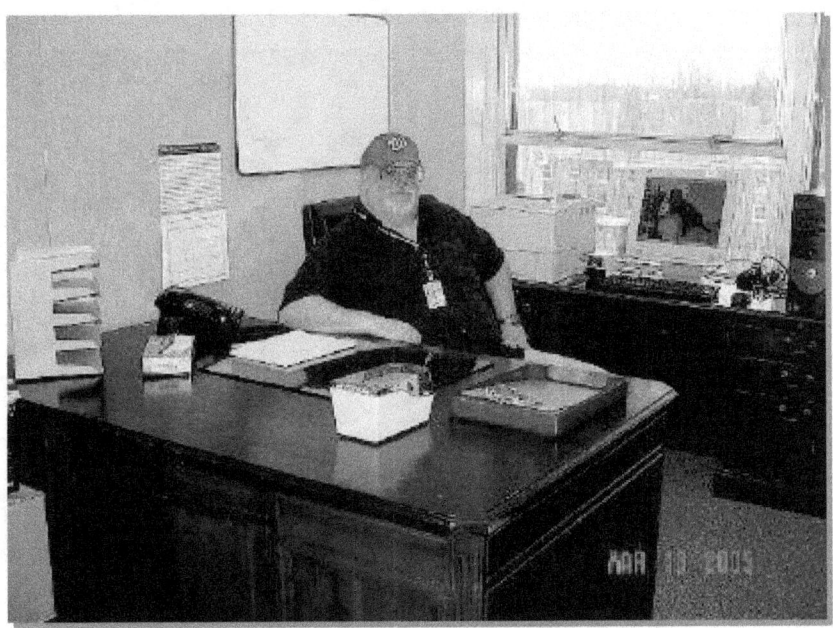

New Guy On the Job at the National Institutes
of Health, 2005

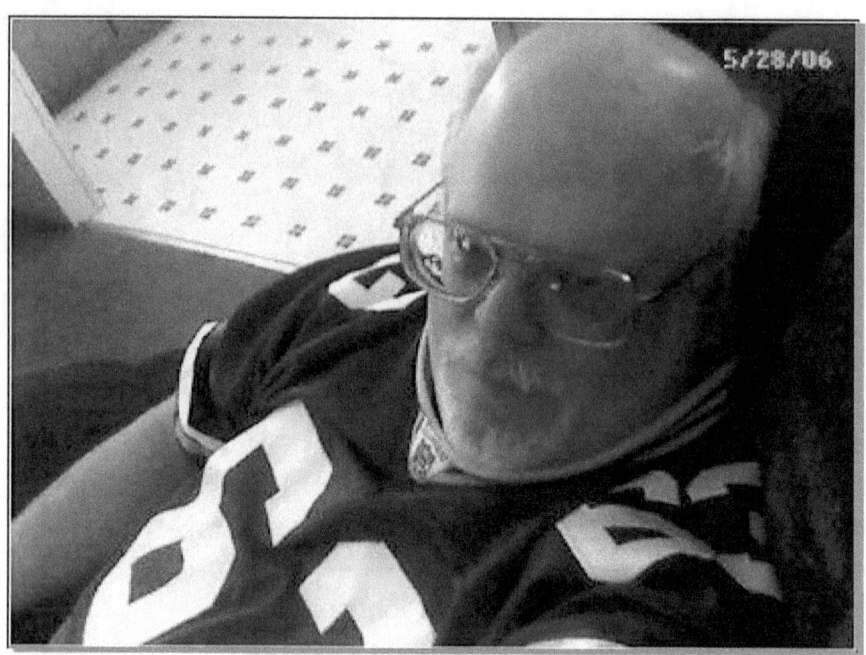

Such A Beautiful Head of Bone I Had...

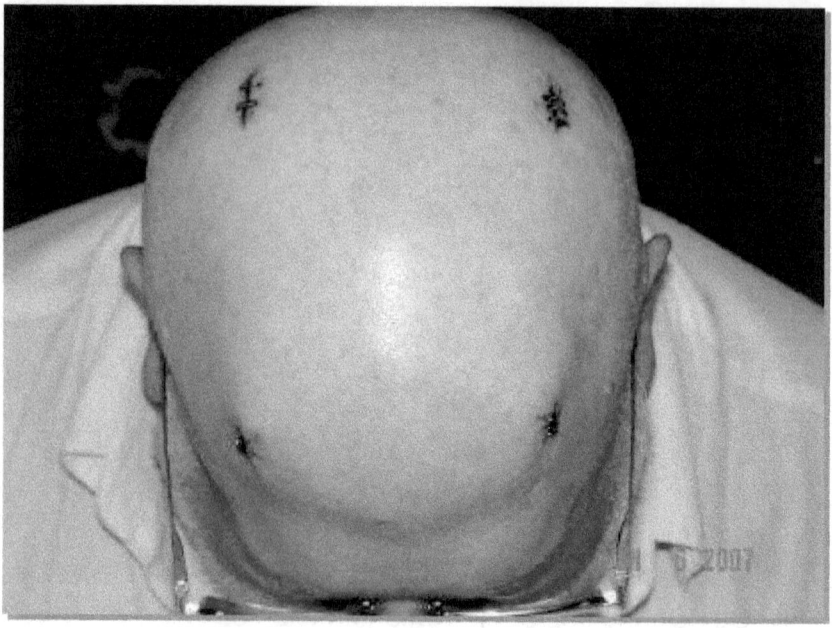

Until They Did This to It... Insertion of the Bone
Markers for Stereotactic Brain Surgery

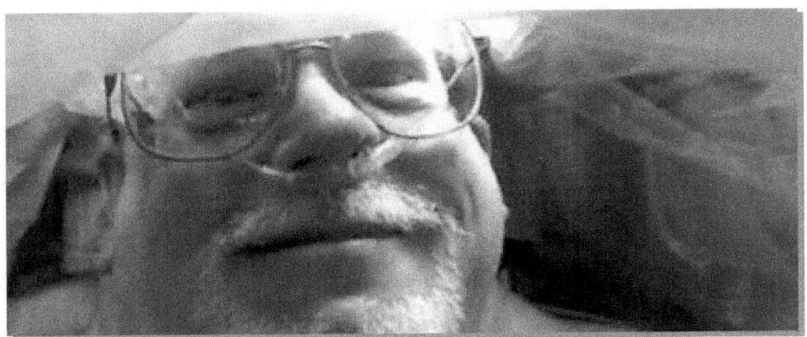

Happy, Smiling, with Two Holes in My Head

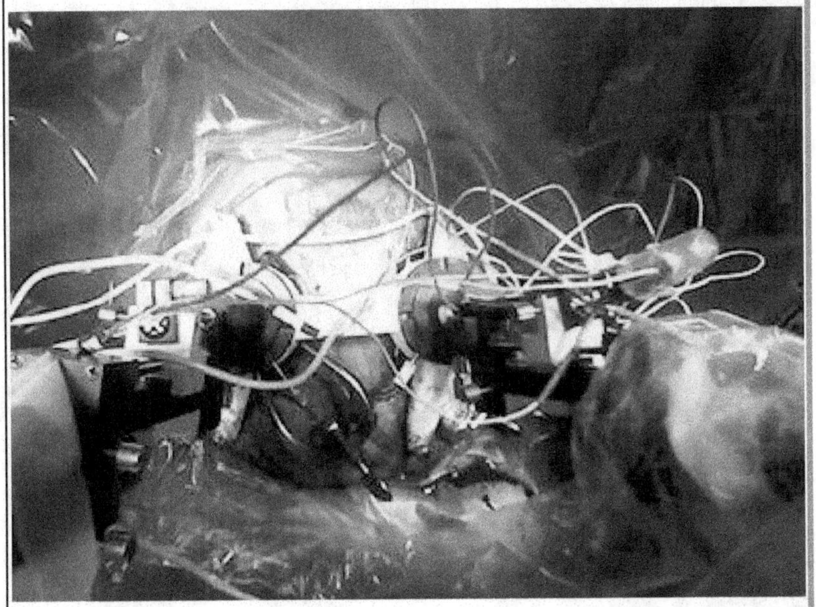

Here's How Things Looked on the OTHER Side
of the Plastic Sheeting

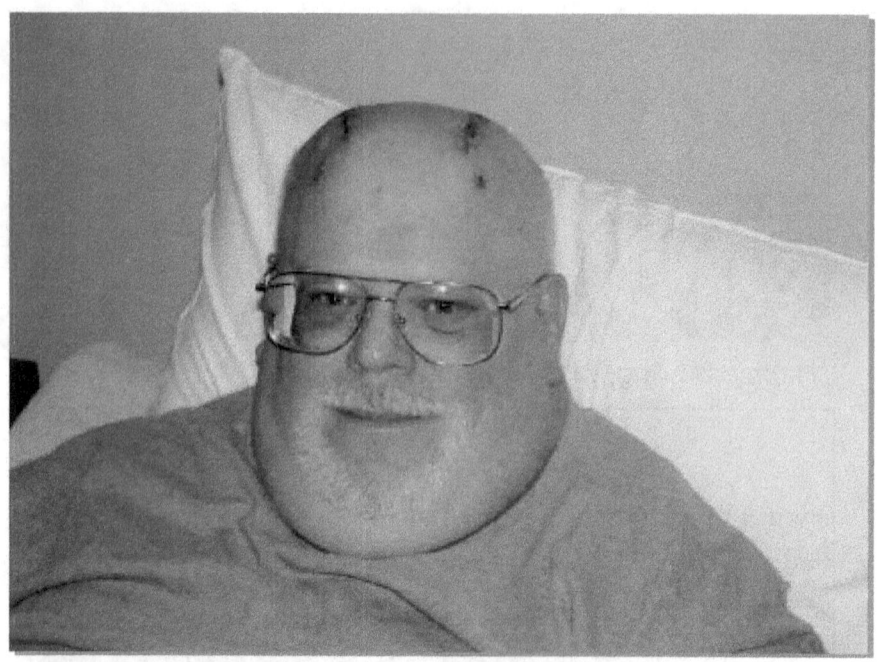

Incredibly Jovial, on the Night After Surgery

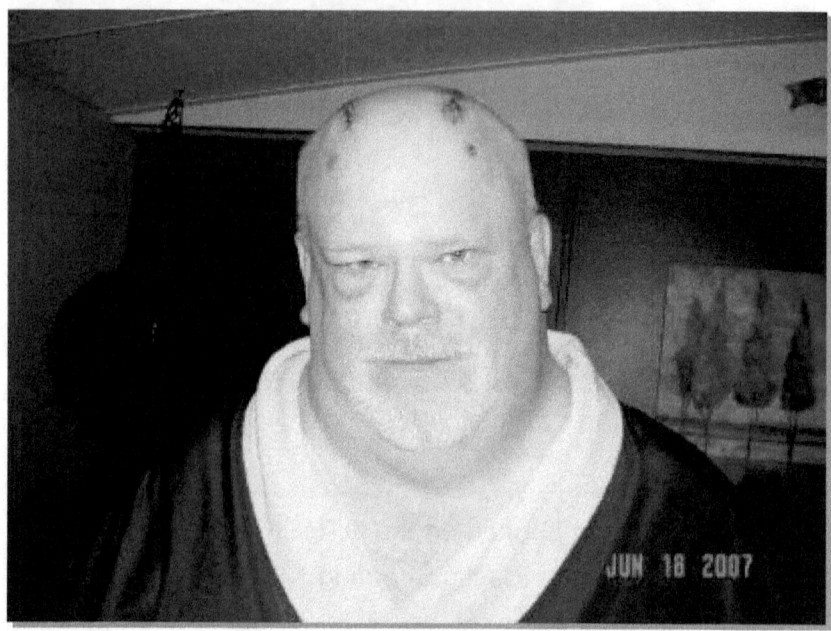

Several Days Later, the Fluid that Gathered
Under My Scalp Migrated to My Face!

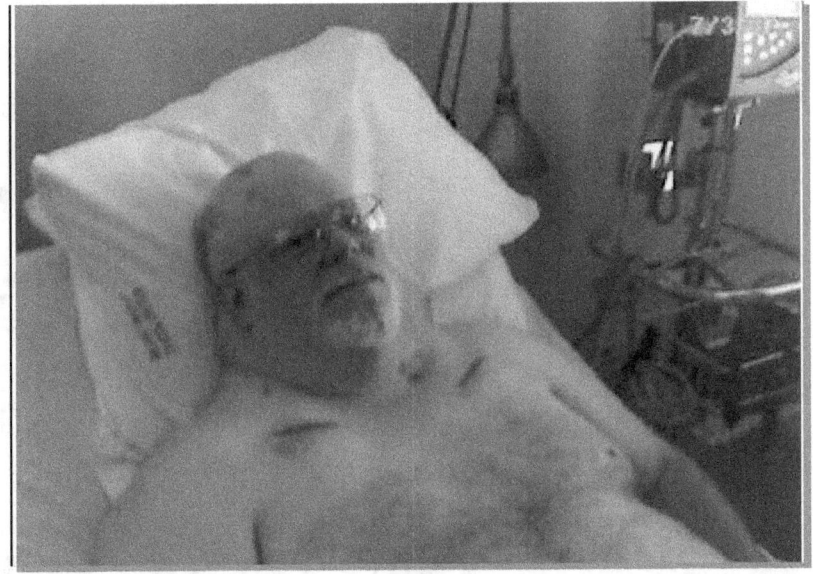

A Couple Weeks Later, They Inserted and
Connected the Neurostimulators

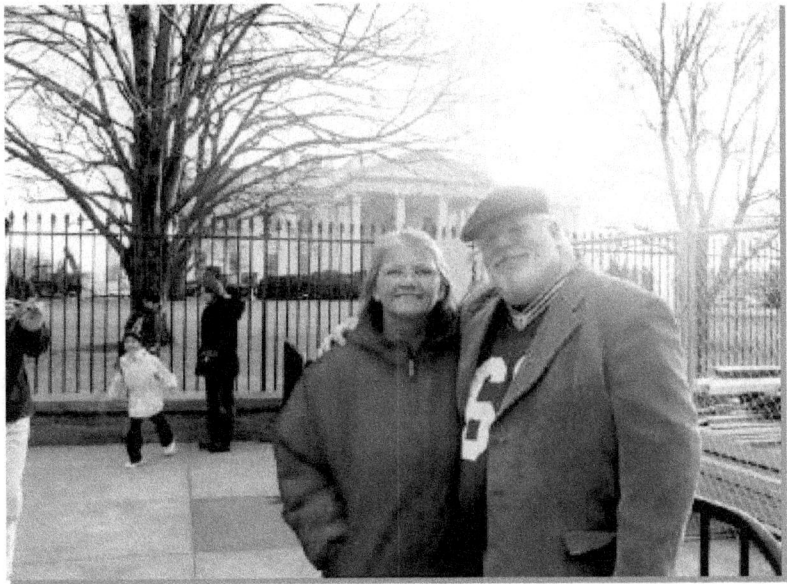

Here's Gail and Me in Front of the White House,
Valentine's Day 2009.

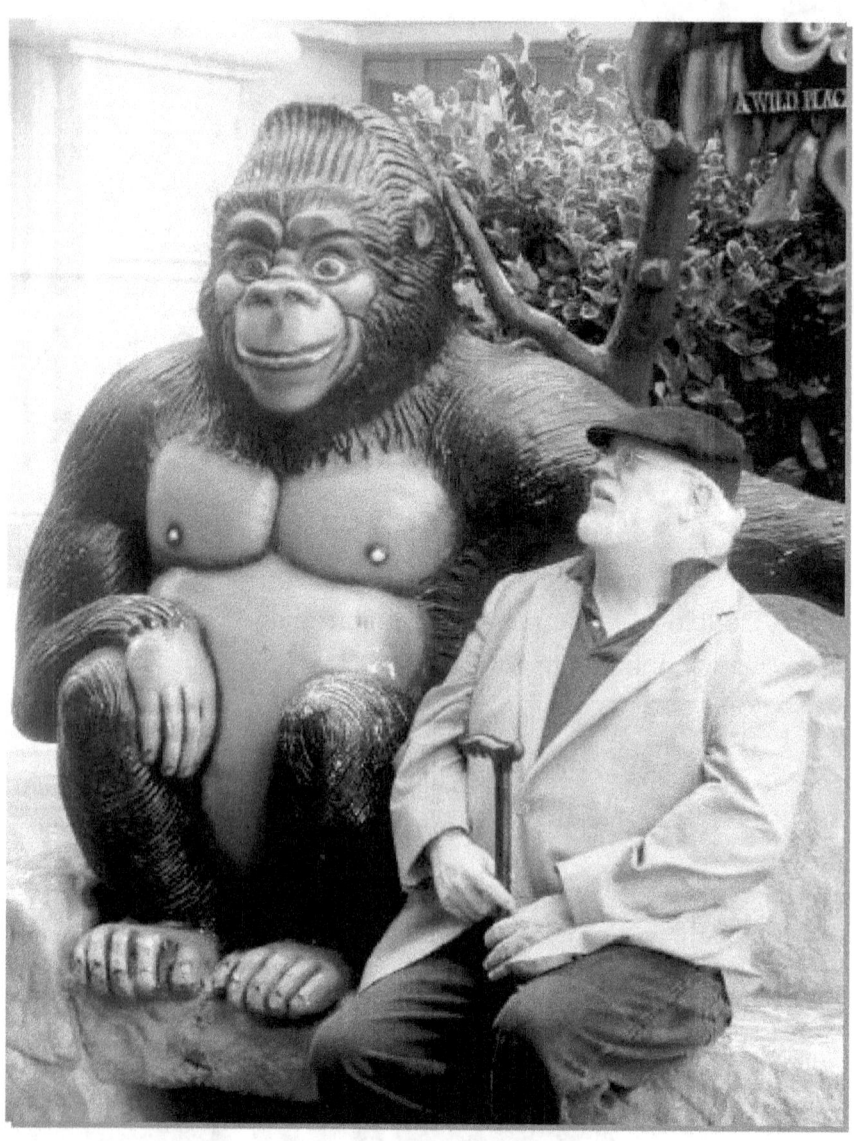

Over the Years, the Things DBS Could Help, it
Helped. The Things it Couldn't, it Didn't.

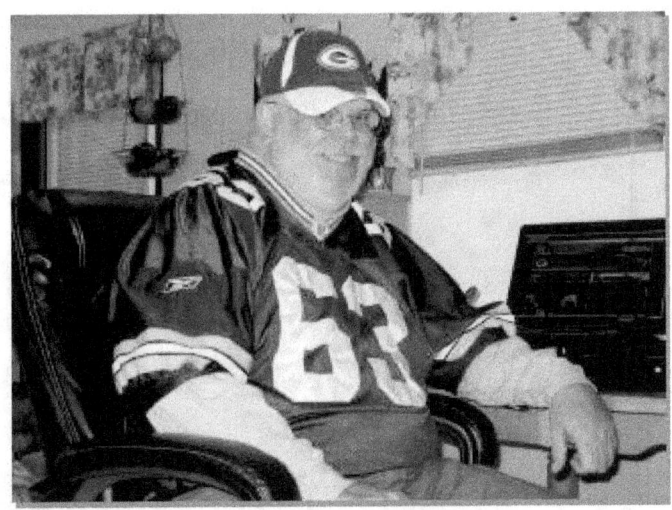

When the Hassle of Commuting Got to Be Too Much, NIH Allowed Me to Work From Home – from June 2009 Until I Retired in March 2011.

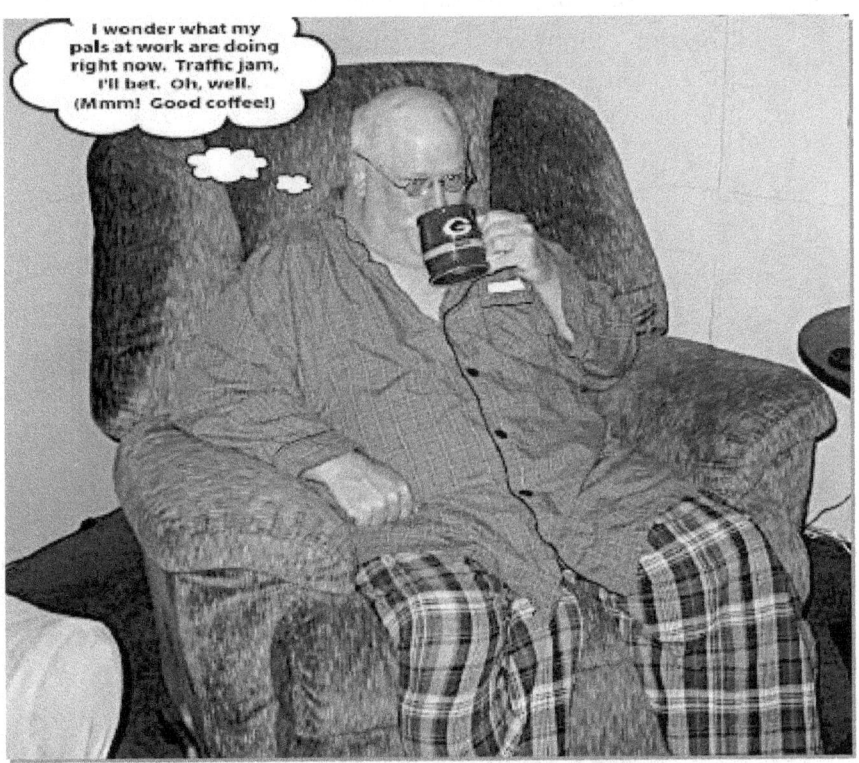

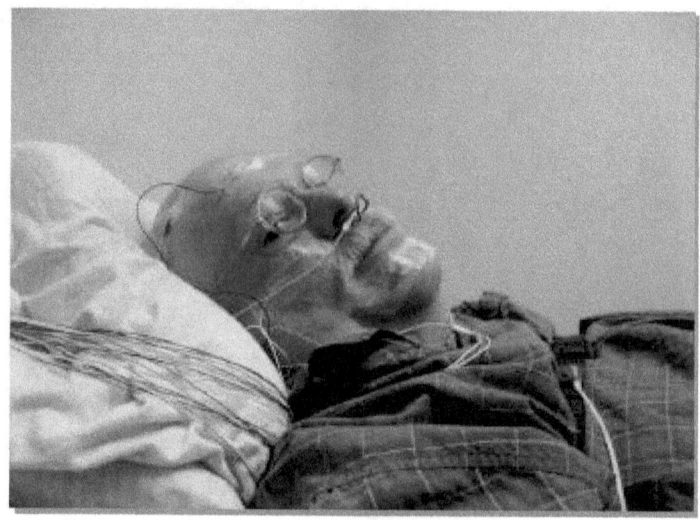

Parkinson's Disease is a Multi-Faceted Thing. I Had a Sleep Study Done for Sleep Apnea in early 2011. No Apnea, just REM Sleep Behavior Disorder, Controlled by Clonazepam.

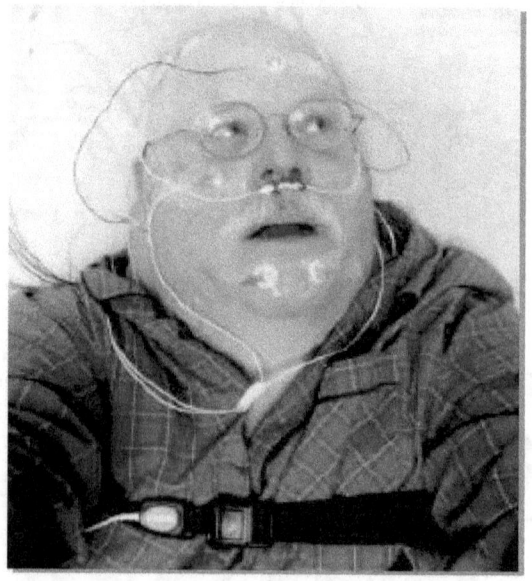

Although I Was Acting for the Camera, My Sister Asked Me to Take This Photo Down from My Facebook Profile Because I "Looked Dead."

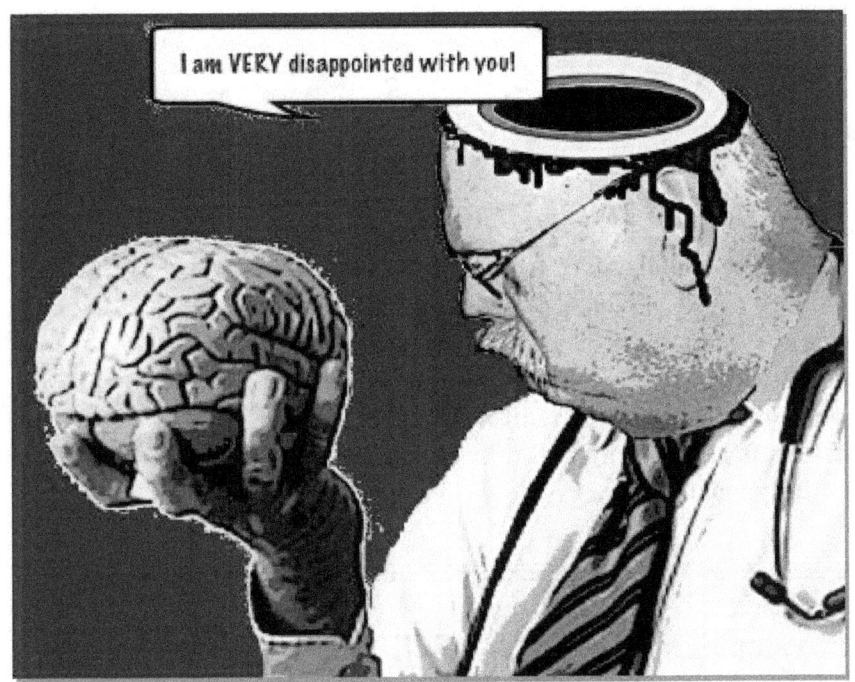

Executive Dysfunction is Starting to Set In. It's a LOT of Fun!

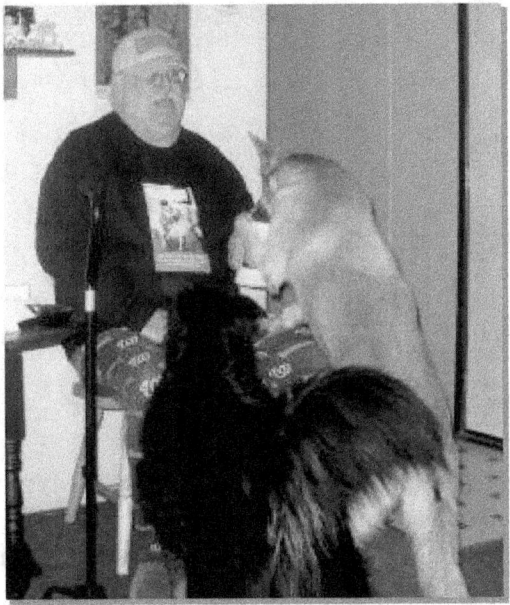

But I Still Look Good!

CHAPTER 5

Fighting Back – to a Degree

After years of letting things happen, it was a real boost to the old fighting spirit when Dr. Grill prescribed some physical therapy. I finally felt like I was fighting back. I know PD is and always be a progressive thing and all the PT in the world won't make it "better." But it did give me some tools to walk better, to stand up straight, to take larger strides. So, it was entirely worthwhile.

Physical Therapy—IT BEGINS!

April 26, 2010

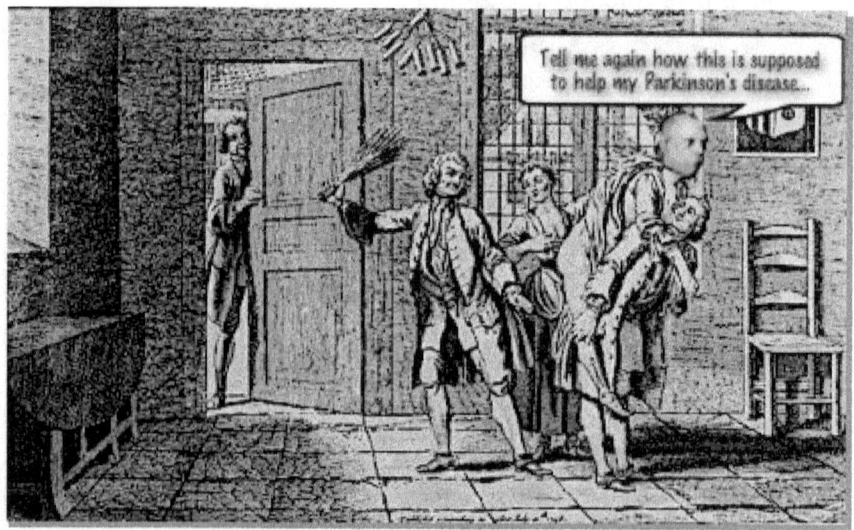

OK, the time for lollygagging is OVER! Time to start physical therapy to see if we can improve any of my Parkinson's disease-related balance and gait problems. Gonna get as much out of this old Parky body as I can before it gives out on me all together.

Had my first appointment today. Guess what. I'm wobbly. And slow .

After filling out paperwork and handing over my $30 co-pay, I met with the therapist. We discussed my condition, she asked a bunch of questions, and she did some strength assessments. Then, it was out into the gym so she could conduct the Berg Balance Scale.

We went through 15 different tests, and I scored a 42. Here's what that means, according to the BBS, that I would have a 91 percent chance of falling at any given time.

She gave me homework. Twice a day, I must do this...

Practice rolling in bed (Count to three, throw your hand in the direction you want to roll, follow it. Five times, each side).

Put my back against the wall, with my shoulder blades and butt plastered against the wall, reach up 10 times as big as I can, getting bigger with each try.

Walk in the hallway (I call this my BIG BOY walk) with big steps reaching with my heel with each step, 5 times up and down the hallway.

We're also going to work on the pain and tightness in my left shoulder.

It feels good to be fighting this thing instead of just sitting around waiting for it to get worse. I mean, I know it WILL get worse, but I'm gonna work this body while I'm still able to do so!

I go back on Wednesday, then three times a week.

I Faw Down. Go Boom. Again.

April 28, 2010

I've foiled yet another attempt by Parkinson's disease to KILL me this morning.

I fell down today. First time in quite some time. Since last September or October, I believe. I've had numerous close calls, but always managed to catch myself while still more-or-less vertical.

Not this morning.

Oh, I'm fine. Didn't hurt a thing. Not even my pride. I was practicing my "big boy walk" when I froze. When one foot freezes, it's a simple matter to get the unfrozen foot under you and center yourself, then start over. When both feet freeze and you're legs are in full stride (not the shuffling side-by-side little footie steps I've been doing), then your base of balance is skewed. I tried freeing at least one of my feet and toppled over to my right, catching myself on the chair we have in front of our front room window.

Then I got up, assured Gail that I was fine, and finished my exercises.

I suppose I'll have to tell my physical therapist about this when we see her this afternoon. When I first started doing this "big boy walk" stuff, it was clear that I was overextending my stride in an exaggerated "John Cleese in the Ministry of Funny Walks" sketch sort of way. With Gail's advice, I shortened the stride to a more normal sort of walking step length. But still... the feet freeze, I get stuck, and today I fell while trying to unstick myself.

Maybe I should wear a football helmet when I do this stuff...

American Academy of Neurology Says.... YAAAAH! BUGS ON MY KEYBOARD!!!

April 28, 2010

Got an interesting e-mail from the "We Move" folks today. Seems that we folks with Parkinson's disease pretty much ALL have hallucinations of some sort at 10 years into the disease.

Few PD patients do not have hallucinations after 10 years of disease progression, according to this study.

Eighty-nine PD patients were followed for 10 years. At baseline, 20 had normal sleep without hallucinations, 20 had sleep fragmentation only, 20 had vivid dreams or nightmares, 20 had hallucinations with insight, and 9 had hallucinations without insight. Follow-up evaluations were conducted at 6 months, 18 months, and 4, 6, and 10 years.

After 10 years, 62 patients were deceased or too ill to interview, while 27 were available for interview. Four patients remained without hallucinations after 10 years. Hallucination prevalence increased over time, with severity correlated with baseline hallucination status and cognition. Hallucinators had more exposure to dopamine agonists than non-hallucinators.

"The prevalence and severity of hallucinations in PD progresses over time, and few surviving patients at ten-years' follow-up escape this disease complication," the authors conclude.

I'm getting used to them. The other day, a chip in the enamel on my stove grew legs and crawled away. It's kinda like being on acid, but not as much fun (from what I've heard).

Awakened by a Cartoon Dog?

April 30, 2010

So it's just about 6:30 this morning and I'm lying there in that zone between awake and asleep. My eyes are closed, and I hear a voice. Not loud or obnoxious. I wasn't dreaming because there was no visual component. The voice of a cartoon dog, almost like Disney's "Goofy."

"Hello!"

Loud and clear as if it were right next to my bed. Just the one word.

"Hello."

I snapped my eyes open and looked around. Gail and Raven were already up. I was in the room by myself.

I figured I'd better get up before the voice started ordering me to set the house on fire.

I looked it up, and people with Parkinson's disease who have visual hallucinations may also have the occasional auditory hallucination. Like their visual counterparts, these hallucinations are rarely threatening or paranoid or "evil" in anyway. And what could be less evil that a cartoon dog voice saying, "Hello"?

Ah, Parkinson's disease. You never fail to entertain.

My Lazy, Lazy Epiglottis!

May 5, 2010

Well, we figured out what the problem is. It's not that I aspirate food and drink on every swallow. But, according to the delightful speech pathologist who fed me barium in various forms and explained the video she shot, there seems to be some weakness around my hyoid bone (the only bone in your body, by the way, that is NOT connected to another bone. Save that for your next Trivial Pursuit game) and my epiglottis—that flap that's supposed to close off your windpipe when you swallow—closes enough (most of the time) to keep stuff out of my larynx... but it doesn't close all the way! So, from time to time, when I'm not careful, some stuff is gonna leak through.

See, the muscles around the hyoid bone control the motion of the epiglottis. My hyoid is supposed to move up and forward further than it does. As a result, the way I understand it, the epiglottis inverts... but not completely.

And that, jolly readers, is that!

I will continue with my speech pathology and physical therapy in my ongoing effort to improve this thing that is me!

Consulting the Family Speech Pathologist

May 5, 2010

My genius nephew, Tommy, of whom we all love and his sainted mother would be so proud, had a thing or two to say about the video I posted here earlier today. He's a grad student, a future speech pathologist.

I just had 4 different speech paths look at your MBS. We all agree your epiglottis is indeed very naughty!

MBS means "modified barium swallow." I asked him to elaborate.

I saw penetration with the thin and thick liquid, but no aspiration. (Although the movie is very fast.... most of the time we watch it slowed down) But that makes sense. It sounds like you have more trouble with liquids. Liquids move very fast, so if you have weak muscles the epiglottis will not close off in time for the liquids to pass. I would be interested to see the report. Did the speech path recommend a chin tuck when you drink liquids? That will make it so your epiglottis doesn't have to travel as far.

I had to look it up to see what he was talking about.

The delineation between 'laryngeal penetration' and 'aspiration' has been better agreed upon recently, with the term 'laryngeal penetration' reserved for entry of materials into the laryngeal vestibule but not below the true vocal folds and 'aspiration' for when material passes below the vocal folds...

So, it's like the epiglottis doesn't keep the slop from getting into the TOP of the airway, but during the act of swallowing, that slop gets stripped out of the vestibule and down the hatch... as it were.

Tommy further elaborated that "swallowing" is "gross" and that he prefers to work with communication. But without "swallowing," Thomas, how will one have the nutrition with which to communicate? Hmm?

Anyhoo... I did some MORE looking up. This from my friends at Viartis.

Silent Laryngeal Penetration is when material enters the top of the airway and is subsequently removed during the swallowing. People with Parkinson's Disease who produced excessive saliva during the day were evaluated. Of those in which Silent laryngeal penetration or silent aspiration (SLP/SA) was observed, most developed respiratory infection. Some of them died of it. The authors claim that the results suggest that patients with Parkinson's disease with diurnal sialorrhea (excessive saliva during the day) and SLP/SA have an increased risk of respiratory infections, which is the main cause of death in Parkinson's Disease patients.

Oh, well. Gotta die of sumthin'.

P.T. Reveals the Current Extent of PD Spazzery

May 6, 2010

So far, through my physical therapy, I've learned little things about myself, little tricks I can use to make my life with Parkinson's disease easier. She's showed me ways to unfreeze myself when I get stuck. She's gotten me to try to keep my arms and torso loose when I walk. She's even loosened up my painful left shoulder.

Today, PT revealed the extent of what a frickin' spaz I am.

Every time, they add a little something new. Today, in addition to walking my "big boy" walk, taking large steps, leading with my heels, she had me look to the left and to the right with each step.

It was a nightmare.

I noticed this more than a year ago, that I was having trouble walking with someone, then turning to say something to him. Today as I walked in that hallway, turning my head back and forth with each step, I froze, I had to grab stuff to keep from falling. The therapist had to hold on to the back of my belt. I was a total spaz.

Then she had me do it again, this time looking first up and then down as I walked. Same thing. Freeze. Grab something to keep from falling. Stumble. Spaz.

She also had me stand with one foot directly in front of the other, first the right foot, then the left, between some balance bars. I wove back and forth like a drunk. I had to grab the bars to keep from falling.

Every now and then, it just slaps you in the face. All the stuff you used to do without even thinking about, now you can't do it without falling or freezing or looking brain-damaged.

Not a good day. Not at all.

NAUGHTY, LAZY EPIGLOTTIS!

May 6, 2010

Looking again at the video from yesterday's modified barium swallow, something finally caught my eye. Something my wife noticed yesterday when I first played it. ("You never listen to me," is what I THINK she said, but I don't think I caught all of it because there was a reflection of sunlight on my computer screen that distracted me.)

The epiglottis doesn't even TRY to close until most of the barium- laced applesauce is past it.

Yes, the epiglottis is controlled by muscles attached to the hyoid bone which is attached to other muscles and ALL muscles are affected by Parkinson's disease. That's why so many of us develop swallowing problems. This isn't actual "aspiration." You can only call it that when the stuff gets into and past your vocal cords. This stuff is just penetrating my larynx (hence the term, "laryngeal penetration") and gets swept out before it can do any real harm.

But it's NOT even supposed to GET in there!!! Do you HEAR ME, epiglottis?

BAD epiglottis! NAUGHTY epiglottis! You'll be the DEATH of me YET!

(Probably...)

Adventures in Physical Therapy: Or, "Hey! I Learned Something NEW!"

May 7, 2010

Had my third physical therapy session of the week earlier today. I learned that my sore left shoulder isn't just a sore left shoulder. It's called "frozen shoulder syndrome" or "adhesive capsulitis."

Frozen shoulder, also known as periarthritis or adhesive capsulitis, is a syndrome consisting of spontaneous onset of pain and progressive restriction of movement in a shoulder, in the absence of any demonstrable intrinsic joint abnormality. The onset is followed by a chronic phase in which the pain recedes but the shoulder immobility remains marked, and finally by gradual spontaneous resolution.

I also learned that it can be caused by Parkinson's disease.

We have found that frozen shoulder is indeed a common complication of Parkinson's disease, occurring in 12-7% of our patients. The incidence may actually be higher, but we were unable to be certain of the diagnosis in other patients with suggestive histories. Men were affected out of proportion to their numerical majority in our population, contrary to the predominance of women found in other studies of frozen shoulder.

So. I learned something new. And that explains why they're beating the hell out of my shoulder. Deep tendon massage, stretching, bending, twisting, turning. I feel like a Stretch Armstrong toy.

Oddly, "frozen shoulder" is commonly the first presenting symptom in PD. But I didn't get mine until about six months ago. But then, I've never been the kind to do things in the typical way.

My usual therapist was gone today, so I worked with Karen, who proudly refers to herself as "The Queen of Pain." After the shoulder workout, we did the balance and walking things.

It's still alarming to me to see how uncoordinated I have become. I'm so used to doing my little shuffle with my arms hanging limp by my side that when I'm told to swing my arms when taking big steps—I have to give it careful thought to accomplish this thing that most folks do all the time without even thinking about it. In fact, Karen had to stop me and start over a few times because I was swinging the left arm and left leg, then right arm and right leg instead of the way YOU walk, which is right arm, left leg, vice versa.

We had me take the "big steps" while turning my head side to side. I froze with every second step... usually when turning my head to the left. I was walking like a cheaply made toy robot. Nodding my head while walking is easier, but still challenging and requiring a great deal of thought to accomplish.

We did the "stand with one foot in front of the other and turn your head from side to side" thing, too. I was wobbly with my left foot in front of my right leg. I could barely stand with my right foot in front of my left leg.

This physical therapy has been a real eye opener. I have at least two more weeks of it. I don't know if it's helping anything (other than my shoulder, which does feel looser...)

But I'm sure learning stuff.

I take a lot of pills for my Parkinson's disease and other related and non-related stuff. I take four Stalevo 100s each day. I take two clonezepam and one Ambien at bedtime, the latter to help me GET to sleep, the former to help me STAY asleep without kicking and slapping and screaming and the other stuff that comes with REM Sleep Behavior Disorder.

Funny thing about pills... If you forget to take them... they don't work!

A Night I'd Rather Forget Caused by Forgetfulness
May 9, 2010

It was 1 a.m. I woke up as Gail came back into the room from going potty and taking the beasts out to the yard. I settled back and waited for sleep to come over me again.

And waited. And waited. And waited.

And lay there with stupid songs running through my head. (For some reason, last night's selections were from Gilbert and Sullivan's wonderful creation, "The Mikado.")

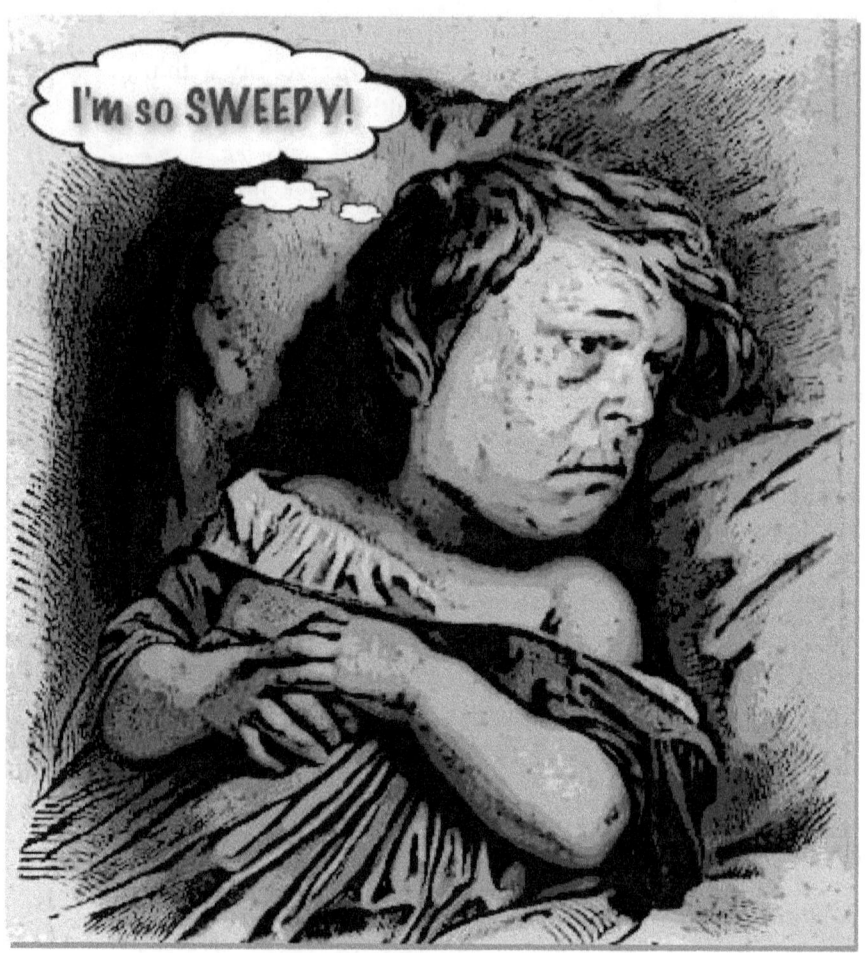

And waited. And sleep just wouldn't come.

I was comfortable. Well, my left shoulder aches a bit, but not enough to keep me awake.

3 a.m. went by. Then 4 a.m. Around 5, Raven began walking from bed to bed doing that ear flapping thing she does when she wants to wake you up without being TOO obnoxious about it. Gail told her to lay down.

I drifted and dozed a bit. I wondered why I was having such trouble getting back to sleep.

At around 6:10, Raven came by my bed and flapped her ears again. I figured enough was enough, so I struggled out of the sack, took her out, took Shiloh out, then went to take my morning pills.

Mystery solved.

The reason I had such a crappy night was right before my eyes. Despite the alarm on my iPhone set to go off at 8:30 p.m. to remind me to take my nitey-nite pills, I had forgotten to take them. We were having so much fun watching TJ play with the dogs last night, and were enjoying a nature show, and I just turned off the alarm when it went off and forgot to take my Ambien and Klonopin.

Duh. Me so stoopit sometimes.

So Far, it's Been an Interesting Monday

May 10, 2010

Slept pretty good, but only after getting up at 10 to down another Ambien. Sometime around 1:30 or so, I was sound asleep, I don't recall dreaming anything. And I kicked off my covers and yelled at the top of my lungs. I sat up in bed, wondering why in the hell I had just done that. The Klonopin has all but eliminated that sort of nutty behavior. Gail got up, went potty, took the dogs out, came back in and got into her bed.

"By the way, sorry about that," I said. I didn't have to explain what I was apologizing for.

"No problem," she said as she settled back to sleep.

For the rest of the night I had fitful dreams and woke up for good around 6:10 when Raven clambered up onto my bed with an "I gotta go potty" look in her eyes. I grabbed my walker and stood, almost falling back onto the bed, then struggled to the door and let Raven into the hallway.

Both girls did their business, I checked the previous evening's e-mails...

And there was a note from work that an entry had been made into my electronic personnel file. So, I checked that out. And it was good news.

I think it was back in January that my boss told me that I had received an "excellent" performance rating for 2009 and I was given a choice between time off or a cash award. I took the cash award. I think the last time I got a cash award, it was something like $900. This time it was more than that. SIGNIFICANTLY more than that. And it will be in my paycheck this Friday.

Gail and I are going to use the money to get something we've both always wanted! Tempurpedic Beds! Mine will be adjustable so I can raise my head and legs as needed. Gail's will be flat. We will both be very, very happy!

Shot an e-mail to my neurologist asking if I should double my Klonopin dosage from 1mg to 2mg. That's the stuff that's SUPPOSED to keep me from yelling, hitting and kicking at night.

Did my 20 minutes on the exercise bike. Took a shower. I don't have physical therapy until 6:30 tonight. So, time to get some work done.

Nighttime Ain't the Right Time for Physical Therapy
May 11, 2010

I'm no big fan of physical therapy at night. Had the first of my three PT appointments this week, all at 6:30 p.m. I'm already tired from just moving around all day by then, so add that to the fact that I'm expected to exercise when I get there and you can understand my lack of enthusiasm.

But a man's gotta do what a man's gotta do even when he doesn't feel like doing it.

And it's still good. The "Queen of Pain" worked out my shoulder again... it is getting looser. We did all the "big walk" and "reach for the stars" and "ride the bike" and "stretch the calves" and "put one foot in front of the other" stuff and I didn't fall and crack my skull or anything.

Came home, and for the first time took 1.5 mg of Klonopin for nitey-nite time. I don't know if the late night exercise (and I just noticed I referred to 7pm as "late night." Jesus, I'm so old.) or the

Klonopin, but I slept like a lord! Best night's sleep I've had in weeks.

Just did an interview for a podcast, got dressed and did my PT exercises. Almost fell several times but managed to keep myself more-or-less upright and unhurt. This time.

Gotta go back tonight. But no PT tomorrow. Just a speech pathologist visit.

I live quite the life!

Oh, You Lazy, SLUGGISH Epiglottis!

May 12, 2010

Had my follow-up appointment with the speech therapist this morning. She hadn't received a copy of the radiologist report from last week's Modified Barium Swallow. So, we discussed generalities and agreed that—so far—I'm doing all the right things, and she said she would try to get a copy of the report faxed to her.

Gail and I decided that as long as we were in the area, we'd head out to Howard County General Hospital to get a copy of the report. But they wouldn't give it to me, because it's still in "draft" form.

So as we were driving home, Olivia (my speech therapist) called and shared the high points of the report she had faxed to her.

1. For one thing, the radiologist disagrees with my nephew and the other speech paths who looked at my videos because the report says there was NO laryngeal penetration.

2. The report indicates that there seems to be some weakness in the muscles near my hyoid bone since it doesn't move up and forward as much as it should. But it DOES move BRISKLY!

3. The report indicated that there was one instance of my epiglottis acting "sluggishly" when swallowing, but that my airway remained uncompromised regardless.

4. They suggested that I should just quit with the throat clearing, something Olivia disagrees with.

5. They suggested a regimen of exercise to strengthen the muscles around my hyoid. Olivia said she would have to do some research because she's not aware of any such exercises.

So... my hyoid doesn't move far enough when I swallow, but it does move BRISKLY! My epiglottis was sluggish on at least one occasion (the applesauce swallowing episode where my epiglottis didn't even TRY to close until most of the applesauce had passed it). But the report said there was no sign of Parkinson's disease-related dysphagia.

So that part's good, anyway.

On Wii, I'm an Athlete! Here in the Real World? Not So Much.

May 17, 2010

Last night before watching the Simpsons, I fired up the Wii and bowled a few frames. My first game was a 195, my second was a 192, and finally a 224! That's a 204 average!

In the Wii World, I am a CHAMPION!

In the real world, however, I remain a staggering, halting, slurring, stumblebum because of my Parkinson's disease. If I were to attempt a REAL game of bowling, I would lose my balance and paint the lane with my face every time I tried to hurl the boulder.

This afternoon, for instance.

We're done with physical therapy and we're making our way to the car. I've just spent over an hour working on my balance and walking and having my sore left shoulder worked on. I'm standing up straight and taking big steps and cruising along fairly well—slowly, but relentlessly. Then my cane hits something. I look down. I'm not SUPPOSED to look down while I'm walking. But it was because I WASN'T looking down, my cane got stuck into something. It's a crack in the sidewalk. My feet see this crack and squeal like little girls.

"WE can't step over THAT!!!!"

And they freeze solid. I start to rock myself in an attempt to urge my cowardly, frozen feet onward.

And I feel myself starting to tip backwards. I try to use my leg muscles to move my body mass forward, but all I'm doing is poking my butt out backwards and taking my center of gravity in the wrong way. I reach the tipping point—the point of no return—and I take five or six tiny little backwards step as I start to fall and the only thing that kept me from cracking my freshly shaved and beautiful head on the sidewalk like an egg is the fact that Gail rushed up to grab me and use her body to stop my retropulsion.

If I had fallen on that sidewalk, I would have been seriously injured. Gail saved me. And not for the first time.

This is why I can't go anywhere by myself. One second, I'm cruising along nicely, the next second I freeze and in the effort to unfreeze myself, I fall and crush my skull or break my hip.

But in the WII world... I am KING! Ya takes what ya can gets!

No Doorway Wide Enough

May 18, 2010

In 1981, I was a young Hospital Corpsman just beginning my second hitch in the Navy. I was assigned to what was then the U.S. Naval Home in Gulfport, Miss. It was sort of a retirement home for Navy and Marine veterans who had no other place to live.

As was true for most of my first hitch, as soon as someone in charge learned I could type, I was assigned to office duties. But every 4th night or so, I had the duty section which meant I was on the job for sickbay. Mostly minor stuff, little injuries like bumping your head on the bed stand, that sort of thing. If someone was in real trouble, it was the duty corpsman's job to call the ambulance and keep the patient as stable as possible until the paramedics got there.

It was during this time in Gulfport that I noticed something about older folks. It seemed that some of them just could not walk through a doorway without sizing it up first. They'd shuffle to a door, stop, look it over, and then shuffle their way through.

I thought that was a riot. I shared this observation with some friends of mine and really floored them with my spot-on demonstration of how these older folks looked when they came to a doorway.

Yet, I wondered. What in the world is there about getting older that makes a person question his or her ability to fit through a door?

Now, 10 years and nearly 4 months into my diagnosis of Parkinson's disease, I understand fully. It's not that you're wondering if you can fit through the door. Your brain perceives the doorway as a narrow passage and causes your feet to freeze in place. It's the same thing YOU would do if you were walking toward a crack in the wall and had to stop before hitting the wall. I know the doorway is wide enough. But my midbrain has trouble conveying this information to my legs and feet. Eventually, somehow, they get the message and moving through the doorway becomes possible.

I experience something like this every day, especially during physical therapy. When my mind only has to concentrate on one thing—taking big steps, for instance—I'm able to navigate a narrow hallway with minimal difficulty. But when I add something to the mix, like turning my head side to side or up and down as I walk and I have to concentrate on taking big steps, swinging my arms and coordinating the movement of my head...

I freeze with practically every step. It's like my brain allows me to move, assesses my position, checks my balance, makes sure my head is facing in the proper direction, observes the area surrounding me, then allows me to take that next step after which it assesses my position, checks my balance, makes sure my head is facing in the proper direction, observes the area surrounding me, and allows me to take that next step where it all happens again and again and again.

During these "big walks with head turns," if it feels like I'm losing my balance... I freeze completely. One arm in front of me, one arm behind me. One foot in front of me, the other behind. My head looking either to the left or the right. Frozen. Like a statue. Then, once I have my balance, I concentrate. I make the mental decision which of my limbs I'm going to move.   And each step is a challenge and I'm exhausted by the time we're done with PT.

But that's not all! We also do this thing where I stand between padded bars, put my feet together, my arms at my side, and close my eyes. I can generally maintain that position for 30 sec. or so. Then I have to put one foot halfway in front of the other and close my eyes. I can't go for more than a few seconds without feeling myself tipping one way or the other. One foot completely in front of the other is difficult, even with my eyes open. Almost impossible with my eyes closed.

So now, almost 30 years later, I understand why those older folks had to size up the doorway before passing through. The thinking mind knows what it has to do. But the things you do automatically are anything BUT automatic to the Parkinson's patient. We have to THINK our way through the doorway. And it's tiring work, my friend.

Tiring work, indeed.

Wrapping Up the First Round of Physical Therapy
May 26, 2010

Yesterday at physical therapy I was treated by the center's clinical director. She told me that when they get a patient with Parkinson's disease, she likes to do at least one session with that person to see how he or she is progressing.

Looks like my therapy has definitely done some good. For one thing, my left shoulder is much looser. Still sore, still stiff, but I can put both arms behind my head now where I could not when I started PT. My "big walking" is much better. I told her how freaking "unnatural" it felt for me to stand up straight, swing my arms when I walk and take big steps, and she said she has never had a PD patient who didn't tell her the same thing.

We worked on some balance exercises, including some I did for the first time. I didn't fall, and I got kudos for my efforts to right myself when I was tipping from side to side.

She had me walk up and down the aisle. When I froze, she said I did the absolutely correct thing by just stopping. Too many Parkies try to jostle themselves free and end up falling or taking a bunch of tiny little forward steps (festinating) until they DO fall forward. She said my strategy of just stopping and waiting for the freezing episode to subside should save me some falls. And, she said, that is the be all to end all in doing PT with Parkies — to give them coping skills to keep them from falling since broken hips lead to immobility, which leads to pneumonia, which leads to death for most of us.

Tomorrow will be my last visit for the time being. They'll do a repeat of the assessment they did on my first day back in April and give me a comparative score. They'll send a report to Dr. Grill. Then, in about three months or so, we'll do another round of PT.

As she explained, PD is a progressive disease. All they can really do is work in the issues that are present at the time. Then it's up to me to go home and keep doing the exercises. As new issues arise (which they will), further sessions of PT will deal with THOSE issues, and further sessions will deal with the issues that arise months from now, years from now...

For the rest of my life.

Frozen Custard + No More PT = Happy Billy!

May 27, 2010

I can't believe my Mom and little sister, Becki. I've whined so much about not being able to get frozen custard here in Maryland that they sent 10 pints of Kopps Frozen Custard, along with hot fudge and pecans.

2 Swiss Chocolate.

3 Vanilla

1 Mint Chip

1 Red Raspberry

1 Chocolate Almond

2 Milky Way.

Deliciousness all around! The dry ice was fun, too!

The box was sitting in my office chair when I got home from physical therapy. No more PT for at least three months. My balance has shown some marginal improvement in some areas and my "big stepping" has caused me to shave 10 seconds off my "Timed Up and Go." So, they'll check me again every 3 months or so, tuning up what needs tuning up when it needs tuning up.

Gotta go. Gonna order some pizza and then eat frozen custard. Mmmm! Frozen custard!

New Cappuccino and a Realization

May 29, 2010

Purchased a new Cuisinart EM-200 Programmable Espresso Maker. Turns out I may have been packing the grounds in our old espresso maker too tightly, and that ruined the pump. When I first tried making coffee in this one, the water wouldn't pump through the grounds. So I watched the DVD that came with it, and it said to pack the grounds firmly—but not TOO tightly. Made a nice cup of coffee. Problem solved.

Then, the realization. I had planned to go down to Bethesda for our staff meeting by myself, sparing Gail the task of having to drive me down and back. But walking through the mall proved that I'm a subway tragedy waiting to happen. I freeze up when people suddenly come up alongside me. I freeze when they walk in front of me. And the subway is a pushing, shoving, get-out-of-my-way sort of environment. Even before things progressed to where they are now, I was a moving obstacle to the other rush hour rushers. Once, this little cutie even yelled, "Get out of the way!" at me. How charming.

So, we finally decided that I am unable to travel on the trains by myself. Gail will take me to Bethesda for this meeting. And maybe we'll even get home alive.

Going IN to Work Today

June 2, 2010

For the first time since August 2009, I'm going to Bethesda for a meeting at the NIH Clinical Center today. This is an important meeting about bringing in a new service that will affect all our lives, so it's imperative that I be there rather than just hear it on a conference call.

As I had mentioned earlier, I planned to make this trip by myself. But Saturday's adventure at the mall showed that to be impossible... well, not IMPOSSIBLE, actually, but very difficult without getting myself hurt or killed by freezing up in the middle of a rush-hour crowd.

Gail will drive me down there and wait in the comfortable lobby while we meet, yell and throw things at each other in an upstairs conference room.

It will be good to see these wonderful, supportive people again! Seriously.

If I ever needed a reminder of why I'm glad to be allowed to work from home because of my Parkinson's disease, I got it today!

Gail and I headed out of the house a little after 8. After making our way through the rush hour traffic on I-95 and the Beltway around DC, we finally slid into the NIH Campus around 9:45. We had to wait awhile until we could get the car through security and a temp ID badge for Gail. Then we drove to the Clinical Center, used the valet parking, and I was about 10 minutes late for a 10 am meeting.

I haven't been down there since August. It was great seeing everyone again, but the meeting seemed aimed at breaking down the resistance of employees who are not thrilled about the addition of the call center to our office responsibilities. It makes sense to me, so sitting through all these charts about "Why Change is Hard" and the like struck me as a little bit much.

Maybe it's just the military or Midwest work ethic. If you're getting paid, and the person paying you says, "You have to do THIS now," you frickin' DO it. And if you don't like it, you find another job.

Personally, I think that our patient recruitment efforts will be well served by this move. I think it will take some "come to Jesus" sort of talk to get those who are resisting to come around. But it will be done.

I was my usual, comical and serious self during the meeting. When giving a response of more than a sentence, my voice was halting and slurred. I'm sure folks noticed.

Afterwards, I took Sara (my boss) down to meet Gail—who was happily involved in "people watching" in the lobby. They seemed to hit it off, which makes sense since Sara is my boss at work and Gail is my boss at home, so they have ME in common...

Then we met with a co-worker of mine, slogged over to Bldg. 61 where I fixed the microphone she uses for podcasting. After which, we gathered up my stuff leftover from last August and drove home to let the dogs out and eat some Chinese food.

I'm exhausted. Traffic wasn't bad going in and was better coming home, even though the outer loop of the Beltway was jam-packed all the way from I-95 past Bethesda (opposite direction from our trip home), and it made me remember all-too-easily why I am so happy that I am allowed to work from home.

Croaky Voice, Porous Brain

June 4, 2010

Waking up with a croaky voice and a bunch of podcasts that need doing. Proof that God has a sense of humor.

Had a few more instances of that "in and out of alertness" phenomenon yesterday, making me wonder if Parkinson's disease is beginning to affect the mind as well as the body. When we went to the grocery store to get lunch, I needed to get some creamer for our coffee. I saw some "white chocolate mocha" creamer and thought, "Mmmm! That would be good with the espresso!" So I got a bottle. Then Gail caught up to me. Then I got a bottle of "Sweet Italian Creme" creamer and saw a bottle of the "white chocolate mocha," and thought, "Mmmmm! That would be good with the espresso." So I got another bottle.

Imagine my surprise this morning when I saw that I had two bottles of "white chocolate mocha" creamer!

Then after 4pm yesterday, around the time Gail takes our next door neighbor to work, I was sitting in my recliner—looking at the TV and none of it was registering. I watched the beginning of a Law and Order episode where a woman was in a confessional, confessing to a priest. During the commercial break, I turned to Gail and said, "I watched that whole thing, listened to every word, and I'll be damned if I can remember what the woman was confessing about."

I settled back into my chair, and when Gail left to take our neighbor to work she had to startle me out of my fugue to let me know she was leaving.

A couple hours later? I was fine! I wrote that witty piece about Obama's "failure to show the appropriate amount of anger," then went to bed and slept like a lord.

This morning, my voice is almost gone. I feel slightly fuzzy-headed, but functional. And I'd better be, cuz I have work to do.

UPDATE: Screw it. I wrote and recorded the Rec Therapy podcast and sounded like a drunk with bronchitis. I am neither. I will write whatever needs writing today, but no more recording. Not until my voice gets better. My voice box actually hurts when I try to talk. To hell with this.

Things to Discuss with the Neurologist

June 7, 2010

My next visit with my neurologist is a week from tomorrow. I gotta put together a list of things that I want to discuss with him, things that have changed for the better, for the worse, and things that I have questions about.

My top concern is this fluctuating attention thing. Even now, I feel less focused than I did when I got up this morning a couple hours ago. I go from being sharp as a tack and able to write witty, compelling copy, to sitting here staring at an empty screen and the useless keyboard without a thought in my head.

Then there's the question of apathy. Late last week, I was like a man on fire. I wanted to get as many podcasts done as I could — even though I had a slurry, raspy voice. I felt energetic and rarin' to go. When I'm at the other end of that scale, it takes an imminent deadline to move me into action. If I don't have to do it now, then to hell with it. At the moment, I'm sorta swinging from the high end to the low end of that scale. So I'd better get as much done this morning as I can.

Then there's this "losing my train of thought" thing. I'll be working on the blog or on a podcast or on some other writing project and something will occur to me that I need to fix, or check, or take another look at, and just as quick as I think about it... I forget. I'll see something in a widget or a misspelling or an improper punctuation and go to the page in the edit mode to fix it, and when I get there, I've forgotten what I've come there to fix. I have to retrace my steps and hopefully remember what it was that needs fixing. For instance, there's a "/" in the middle footer of my landing page now that I've been wanting to remove since yesterday afternoon — and I keep forgetting to do it.

My motor symptoms are about the same as they were at my last visit, I suppose. My hands still work pretty well, although I find myself hitting the wrong keys a lot more these days. I've learned new ways to walk during physical therapy — remembering to do it is another thing. I know I'm supposed to stand up straight, yet I slump unless I either remind myself or am reminded. I can take bigger steps, but unless I remind myself, I still shuffle. It feels unnatural and it's hard to remember to do it.

So, we'll see what else I can think of in the 8 days until the appointment. In the meantime, I'd better get to some of this work that's piling up and get it done while I still feel a little bit of steam in my engines.

Frustration—Plain and Simple

June 9, 2010

Here's how my day has been — so far.

Is "frustration" a symptom of Parkinson's disease?

I don't know if it's fair to call it "constipation" since I "make bigs" nearly every morning, regular as clockwork. And when I say "bigs," I mean "BIGS". And therein lies the problem. One is reminded of the Daniel Day Lewis movie....

"There Will Be Blood."

Then there was the two-hour telephone call — another meeting about bringing the "call center" functions in-house. When I spoke in sentences of three or fewer words, I did OK. But when I tried conceptualizing that we're not being asked to do anything that will be impossible to do, I stammered, I stuttered, I strung out words, I struggled to FIND words, I sounded like a spaz.

Then Gail and I went to the grocery store. On our way out to the car, I caught a flash of white out of the corner of my right eye that looked just like a little bunny running away. I turned to look, and it was a small piece of paper on the road. But even now, I can remember seeing its grey fur and it hopping away.

When we got to the store, I tried to do everything my physical therapists said to do. Stand up straight. Take "big boy" steps. Swing my arms. Not only did it wear me out, but I kept digging my toes into the floor because of foot drop. I almost tripped a couple times, and once I froze and festinated. (Took several tiny steps to regain my center of gravity.)

Now I'm home. Gail is asleep on the couch. And I'm frustrated as hell.

So what else is new? Meh...

My PDQ is FUBAR

June 9, 2010

Back in February, thanks to the kindness of Dr. David Churchman, a project manager for Health Outcomes — part of Isis Innovation Limited, I got a copy of the two premier Parkinson's disease self-assessment rating tools. The PDQ-39 (Parkinson's Disease Questionnaire with 39 questions) and the PDQ-8 (same thing, but with 8 questions.

I wrote about my self-assessment in a previous version of this blog, which can now be seen at Wellsphere (where I am one of the Health Bloggers in the PD Community).

When I took the tests in February, I scored a PDSI (Parkinson's Disease Summary Index) of 48.72. This correlated very well with the PDQ-8-SI which came in at 46.875. According to a rating scale that can be found here, the first score placed me just over the line between Hoehn & Yahr stages III and IV, while the second score put me on the III side of the line.

Well, I retook the tests again today. Keep in mind, this is a total self-assessment in the areas of mobility, activities of daily life, emotional well-being, social support, cognition, communication and discomfort. This time, I landed squarely on the Hoehn & Yahr Stage IV side... my PDQ-39 PDSI came in at 53.205. My PDQ-8- SI was 53.125. The line between III and IV is 48.59. That dividing line for the PDQ-8 is 47.86.

This squares with what I've been noticing over the months, as chronicled here in the blog. It's not good news, but it's certainly not unexpected for a person more than 10 years past diagnosis.

The thing to keep in mind is that both of these PDQ's are self assessments. You check the proper box that most closely matches your symptoms over the past month. So ya gotta be truthful with yourself to get an accurate score.

Another Fun Day

June 10, 2010

Oh Boy! It's another fun day with Parkinson's disease! Day #3,783 since diagnosis.

I was the first one up this morning. At around 5:45, Raven began her regime of "head flapping," which is a technique she uses when she wants to make noise and be noticed without going as far as "barking." She did this for awhile. Then she sat on the floor and scratched herself, making sure her leg pounded the floor like she was Thumper. Then she started with the flappity-flappity-flappity again. Then I felt something press down on my mattress. I looked. It was a very sad dog face. She noticed that I had looked at her, and suddenly the JOY returned to her face. She started making whiny, happy, "I gotta go potty" noises. She went over and bottle-nosed Mom's bed, as if to say, "It's OK, Mom. DAD's got me!"

I grabbed the handle of my walker and pulled myself into a standing position. Then I had to grab it again to keep from falling back- wards back onto my bed. I shuffled to the door, let Raven out, went and released Shi-loh from her prison. (There was a "blue bag of shame" on the porch this morning, meaning Shiloh went poopie in the kitchen during the night. We give up.)

I'm feeling down and discouraged this morning. I feel like the only people who really care are my family and close friends.

And besides, I'm having a bad Parky day. Right now, my shoulders and upper arms are tight and sore, just from typing this.

So, I guess I'll stop.

CHAPTER 6

Random Thoughts from a Parky Brain

LET'S BEGIN WITH "THINGS THAT ANNOY ME"

Now, more things that annoy me, culled from the popular media's reporting on Parkinson's disease!

"Eeeeew! Grampa is OLD and SHAKY and DROOLY!!!"

Saw this note in the online Washington Post on June 14 from a whiner, whining about bringing an   elderly parent into her home.

My father lived with my family for nine months, following the onset of Parkinson's disease. His depression settled over the whole house. Dad clearly didn't want to be there, and the kids, 16 and 8 at the time, avoided the living room, where dad hung out and slept in the chair constantly, refusing to take any interest in life. Both of the kids essentially quit inviting guests over. They were not immune to the depression and, not to be melodramatic, the feeling of death that surrounded us.

I was driving home from work three or four times a day to check on him, feed him and monitor his medications. My husband was a saint about it, but eventually even he said, "We can't keep this up. We are raising our children in a nursing home."

Once his illness was diagnosed and he began medication, Dad was actually able to move for a year into an independent living facility, and I truly think he was happier there. He eventually had to go to a nursing home, and has since died.

You THINK he was happier there? Did you ASK him? Did you even frickin' VISIT him?

Sweetie? I guarantee ya! Nobody was happier about getting out of your house of whiners than your dad was. You poor, sweet little slackers and your snot-nosed kids could learn a thing about family by learning how to care for an elderly member who needed your help.

And here's how she winds up her note.

I guess what I am trying to say is that in spite of our best intentions, we can't stop the natural course of life, and that also we as parents have to be acutely aware of the effect on our children when a household changes so dramatically. And, too, it is not always the desire of an elderly parent to be in their child's home. My father had been extremely independent all his life and it was almost more than he could take to have the balance of the relationship change so drastically.

Nobody was ASKING you to "stop the natural course of life." Your friends calling your husband "a saint" didn't make you GOD! And I am more than sure there were nights when your crappy little diaper needed changing or your little cough kept your parents awake all night or you had a fever and your dad ran to the drug store to get something for you. And yet you talk about your father like he was some sort of malignant presence in your home. Shame on you. Shame on your husband. Shame on your children. And congratulations to your dad for dying and finally being rid of you.

Now, would you trust a news report that misspells a simple word like dementia? (http://www.kusi.com/health/96488854.html)

Each Wednesday during Good Morning San Diego, KUSI provides the latest research, advice, and health information.

New research shows that Parkinson's disease doesn't only affect the motor system, it can also cause dimentia in about a third of patients. This coming Friday, UC San Diego will be hosting a free memory screening clinic. Dr. Joanne Hamilton, from UC San Diego Medical Center, was here to tell us how this screening can benefit Parkinson's patients.

TV News. Meh.

Oh, Goodie! Another PD Preventative!

CoQ10, Glutathione, a handful of Pomeranian fur—seems like everyone has something that will make your PD better or keep you from getting it. Coffee (which I've been drinking since I was 14), nicotine (I've been smoking cigars since I was 17) -- they're all supposed to be neuroprotective.

Now this.

(http://www.allvoices.com/contributed-news/6078534- small-amount-of-vitamin-b6-may-help-prevent-risk-of- parkinsons-disease)

The latest research reported in the July 2010 issue of Life Extension magazine, page 74 (print edition is published in June) notes that vitamin B6 may help prevent Parkinson's. See the article, "Latest Research: Vitamin B6 May Help Prevent Parkinson's." The recent study revealed that "inadequate dietary intake of vitamin B6 may increase the risk of developing Parkinson's disease by 50%."

Scientists examined the relationship between dietary intake of folate, vitamin B6, vitamin B12, and vitamin B2 as it relates to the risk of developing Parkinson's disease. After adjusting for other factors, scientist found that low intake of vitamin B6 was associated with an approximately 50% higher risk of Parkinson's disease.

Meh. I suppose it's like chicken soup for a cold. It couldn't hurt... And now, something ELSE I coulda told the researchers...

PD affects the tummy.

New data from a retrospective cohort study showed that up to three quarters of patients with Parkinson's disease (PD) developed gastrointestinal disorders (GID) that can have a substantial adverse effect on major PD-related clinical and health economic outcomes. These data were presented at the 14th International Congress of Parkinson's Disease and Movement Disorders in Buenos Aires, Argentina (June 13-17, 2010).

"The new retrospective cohort study suggested that the prevalence of gastrointestinal disorders among patients with Parkinson's disease was high, increased over time and had a significant impact on clinical and societal outcomes," said Dr. Florent Richy, Head of Epidemiology, UCB & Adjunct Professor of Epidemiology, University of Liege, Belgium. "Gastrointestinal disorders can impair the onset of symptom relief by Parkinson's disease drugs and these data help us to better understand the prevalence and consequences of such disorders amongst patients diagnosed with Parkinson's disease."

The study found that gastrointestinal disorders in PD patients were associated with significantly higher rates of neuropsychiatric and motor disorders, as well as increased emergency room admissions, number of concurrent drugs and non-PD healthcare costs.

So THAT'S why I'm having cognitive problems. It was the ICE CREAM!!!

FELL ON THE BED, BROKE MY HEAD

Well, not really. My head isn't broken. But it is sore.

I was doing my PT balance exercises in the kitchen, and I noticed that I was particularly wobbly, even doing the easy stuff like two feet together, side-by-side. Felt like I was gonna fall. Knocked the plastic flowers and their vase off the counter.

So I decided to go into the bedroom, so if I fell it would be onto something soft. Like a bed. Or a dog.

I did the one-foot-half-in-front-of-the-other thingie. Closed my eyes, crossed my arms over my chest, and immediately began to wobble. I over-corrected from a lean to the right and fell to my left. Right onto the bed. Right onto a dog on the bed. And the back of my head crashed into the bedroom wall with a loud "WHUMP!"

I said the only thing I could think of. "OWWWW!" From the bathroom, Gail hollered, "Are you all right?"

I said, "Yeah," and flopped back on the bed, closing my eyes so the room would stop spinning.

I didn't lose consciousness. But for a little while it was more difficult than usual to speak.

I'm still wobbly, still moving slower than I usually do, but I think I will be OK.

So will the wall.

(The Next Morning...)

I don't seem to be suffering any ill effects from bashing my skull on the bedroom wall yesterday. I don't feel any particular increase in wobbliness or dizziness. I'm still slow, still talking KINDA slow, but at least I'm making sense.

Banana border tickle mafia. Weasel preen glue, whiffle hamburger purchase in the glade.

Besides that, I will have to overcome the fear of falling when I do my exercises again. When ya fall off the whore, ya gotta get right back on.

Staple umbrellas for the hyoid principalities. And that just about says it all.

WANDERING WILLIE

I suppose I should point this out... for the record, at least... as we track my slow, insidious slide into dementia...

When Gail and I went to Best Buy last night to get the second of the two computer modems we ended up having to buy (we had to return the first one), she parked the car in a handi-crippable space, I hung up the placard, opened the car door, and started walking away. In the wrong direction. Towards the back of the car. Then I heard a voice.

"Bill? Where are you going?"

I turned around. It was Gail. She was on the sidewalk. The sidewalk that leads to the Best Buy front door.

Fact of the matter is, I had NO IDEA where I was heading! I was just walking. Seemed like the thing to do.

I smiled sheepishly and hobbled over to where she was. She shook her head. "IT BEGINS!" she said, laughing. "It began a long time ago," I replied, also laughing. "Yeah, but it's beginning BAD now," she replied.

Oh, Parkinson's disease. Where will you lead me next?

Now... let this be a lesson to all you young, strapping studs or beautiful chickie babies who are thinking about settling down with someone for the rest of your life. Look at that person and ask yourself...

"Will she (he) be there for me when my mind starts to slip? Will she (he) take care of me?"

It's an important consideration, young'uns. And, in my case, in the final analysis, after two mistakes, it seems I lucked out!

A BAD CASE OF THE EMPTIES

I got a bad case of the empties. The blanks.

Gail is at the store. I have a black border collie at my feet, using my right foot as her pillow. In the absence of any outside stimulus, I would be perfectly content to sit here and stare at a blank screen. All day.

I'm not sad. I'm not happy. I'm nothing. Flatlined. My brain seems to be just kinda occupying space in my skull. Last night, I had particular difficulty speaking... getting stuck on syllables, words coming out in a rush. That's not so much of a problem today.

Parkinson's disease. My lifetime companion.

Gail is my soulmate. She's my OTHER lifetime companion. She's gonna come home with chicken. Did I mention that?

Really enjoyed my interview with Warren Krech at KWOS Radio in Jefferson City, Mo. yesterday. Total books sold since then? Zilch. Zip. Zero. Maybe I'm just a shitty writer with nothing interesting to say.

If I hear a TV commentator say "Larry King is hanging up his suspenders" ONE MORE TIME, I shall run amok.

Not that I'm hung up on selling books. I'd love to make a less-than-embarrassing donation to my PD charities. But if folks ain't interested, then they just ain't interested.

If Parkinson's disease happened only to attractive redheads with knockout gazongas and the disease caused uncontrollable nymphomania, betcha THEN it would get some notice. But most of us are old, a lot of us can't hit the ball out of the park anymore (wink-wink), we're twitchy, we drool, we talk funny, we walk funny, we remind people of their own impending death.

Try writing a funny book about THAT!

Where's Gail with that chicken?

Did my 20 minutes on the bike this morning. Still have to do my PT walking/balancing exercises. And the Wii Fit is a naggy little bitch if you miss a couple days, so I suppose I'll have to do some of THAT, too!

My Day.

Up at about 6:30.

Take pills. Losinipril and Metoprolol for blood pressure. Stalevo for PD. Zoloft to keep from jumping (very slowly) in front of a bus. Prilosec, because it works.

Check work e-mails. Open the Patient Recruitment/Public Liaison mail folder.

Toss out the spam, divide the "good" e-mails to whoever is supposed to get them for that day.

Check out blog to see how many dropped by during the night. (Take a few minutes to get over the disappointment.)

See if I sold any books overnight. (A couple more minutes to get over the disappointment.)

Make cappuccino for Gail. Make cappuccino for me. Drink said cappuccino.

Twenty minutes on the exercise bike.

Shower. Shave.

Plant myself here at the computer and put out fires as they flare up.

If things are slow, do my PT walking and balance exercises.

Take 11am Stalevo.

Eat Lunch.

Plant myself here, record podcasts, put out fires as they flare up.

If things are slow, do my Wii Fit workout.

Take 4pm Stalevo.

Watch Law and Order reruns.

Have a glass of wine.

Watch the Daily Show replay. Then Colbert rerun.

Have a glass of wine.

Take nighttime pills. 2mg of Klonopin to stop the nighttime screaming and slapping and kicking. Ambien to get me to sleep in the first place. Dulcolax to make the following morning less of a blood festival.

Go to bed.

No WONDER I'm usually so friggin' tired allatime!!!

BUT IT FEELS GOOD WHEN I STOP!

I think it's time I say "Enough with the Balance exercises." I'll keep doing the walking, I'll keep doing the bike riding, I'll keep doing the Wii, but the balance exercises are gonna kill me. Literally.

Monday, I fell and hit my head while doing the exercises.

Tuesday, I fell onto my mattress, no harm done. Same thing Wednesday.

Today, I fell onto my mattress and gave the back of my head a glancing blow against the wall. Then I fell against the OTHER wall and bruised my arm against the corner of a print Gail has hanging in the bedroom. I use the walker, of course... but the walker falls WITH me.

Face it. I'm not gonna get my balance back. It's gone. Practicing with something you don't have just doesn't seem to make any sense to me. And I don't want to keep hurting myself.

Now, when Gail gets back with my ham & cheese sammich, I'll feel better. :)

EVER BEEN IMPALED BY A DOG'S TOY BOX?

I almost killed myself—or so I thought, at first. After Wednesday's power outage (100 minutes, no power, 97 degrees, THANK you, BGE... that's how they do it each summer... "OH NO! THE GOVERNOR NEEDS ICE CUBES! SHUT DOWN THE TRAILER PARKS!")

Excuse me. I was ranting and rambling.

Anyway, the power outage killed my son's cable box. So Gail took it down to the Comcast place and swapped it out for a new one. And since TJ has a HDTV now, we decided to cough up the extra $7 to get him HD service. I gave him our old cable box and was trying to put in the new one on our TV. I tried to get down on the floor, but as I was doing so, I fell and stabbed myself on my left side, just below the ribs, on the corner of the doggy toy box. It's a canvas box with a metal frame, and I was certain I had impaled myself liver-deep on the damn thing because I COULD NOT MOVE to get off of it. When I finally COULD roll to the floor, I just laid there in extreme pain while Gail stood over me asking, "What did you do? What did you do?" (Note: She did not ask "what happened?" She asked "What did you do," indicating that I had done something stupid and was suffering the just consequences of my action. It was a fair assumption, so I'm not complaining.)

It was a few moments before I could speak. I asked Gail to lift up my shirt and tell me how much of my intestines were protruding. Gladly, the answer was "none." I have a dinky little "owie" on my left side, under my ribs, and it hurts. Might bruise a little.

So upset was I about this that I launched into a delirious state where I believed that LeBron James had gone to the Miami Heat and I actually cared about it.

Ah. Parkinson's disease. You are the tricky one!

THIS IS NOT A FATAL DISEASE!

Let's get one thing clear. Parkinson's disease is not a fatal illness. You die WITH, not OF Parkinson's disease. It's one of my pet peeves, newspaper or other media stories that say someone "died of Parkinson's disease." It spreads a false believe that this is a fatal condition.

Fact of the matter is, more people with Parkinson's die of cardiovascular disease than any other single cause.

People who die from COMPLICATIONS of Parkinson's disease are folks who fall and break a hip and develop pneumonia and die. Or folks whose swallowing difficulties cause them to inhale a turkey leg and they get pneumonia and die.

But the cause of death is something ELSE! Parkinson's didn't kill the guy. Falling, breaking his hip, becoming bedbound and getting pneumonia did the trick.

Let's look at how several different news organizations wrote about the same death of the same guy—Jim Bohlen, one of the founders of Greenpeace.

The Province, a Canadian publication leads with:

Greenpeace Founder Jim Bohlen died from Parkinson's disease last Monday. He was 84.

Well, actually, no he didn't. Seven paragraphs into the story:

He was diagnosed with Parkinson's disease four years ago, his wife Marie said.

Five weeks ago, he had fallen off a chair while exercising and broken a hip.

"He just went downhill from there," Marie said. He died Monday at St. Joseph's Hospital in Comox.

That'll happen! And my first question is, what in the bloody hell is a 84 year old with PD doing exercising ON A CHAIR??? My neurologist is CONSTANTLY telling me to avoid things that could even POSSIBLY lead to a hip-breaking fall. EXERCISING ON A CHAIR?

This guy didn't die of Parkinson's. He died of complications of a broken hip, caused by a fall that was caused by PD.

The Vancouver Sun does a better job of it.

Jim Bohlen died Monday at the age of 84 after a long battle with Parkinson's disease.

Absolutely true... but still leaves the impression that it was the PD that killed him.

The Old Grey Lady, the New York Times, is more accurate.

The cause was complications of Parkinson's disease, his daughter, Margot Bradley, said.

But the story says nothing about the fall, the broken hip and the pneumonia that killed him.

If a man walking down Park Avenue is killed by a falling piano that fell because the rope hauling it up to an open window 10 stories up was cut by a shard of metal caused by an exploding transformer that blew up when a bus hit the telephone pole, you don't say the man was killed by a bus! The bus set off the chain of reactions that led to the man's death. The man would not have been crushed by the piano without the bus accident, but it wasn't the bus that killed him.

Same thing with Parkinson's. If you can keep living without falling (from a chair while exercising) and breaking your hip and getting pneumonia or choking to death on a piece of stew meat because your dysphagia made it go down the wrong hole, or your dementia caused you to forget it's not a good idea to stick a fork into a plugged in toaster, then you will live a long, parky life.

Parkinson's is a life sentence, not a death sentence.

Just don't put yourself into situations that could lead to your hurting yourself... like I did... yesterday... because I'm a moron.

(Friggin' thing STILL hurts...)

PILLS DON'T WORK IF YOU DON'T TAKE THEM

I've been forgetting to take pills. I have my iPhone set to go off when it's time for my 11 am Stalevo, my 4pm Stalevo and my 8:30 pm Klonopin and Ambien. I rarely forget to take my pills in the morning, because it's all part of the morning routine. It's the first thing I do every day. But if I happen to be involved in something at work, or writing a blog post, or examining my navel for lint that I don't think came from MY clothes, if I don't get up IMMEDIATELY and take that 11am or 4pm Stalevo, I WILL FORGET! Usually, I will remember an hour or so later. But about twice a week, I forget it completely and just recycle the unused pill back to the first open slot in the pill box.

I had a horrible night's sleep last night. (Trust me, there's a point to this sudden shift in narrative.) I went to sleep just fine, then woke up at 11-something and just laid there. Nothing bothering me. Very comfortable. Just not sleeping. I eventually drifted off long enough to have a little dream, then I woke up again. Around 3 this time. Laid there until about 5. Not anxious. Not worried about anything. Just wondering why I was having such a rough night.

After Gail got up with Raven at around 5:30, I drifted off again. Had a dream about being a new kid in high school. There was only one desk available and I took it. But it turns out that it was John Goodman's desk, and he wanted it back. So I had to sit on a heating vent in the back of the classroom. The teacher said not to worry about it, they'd try to get a desk delivered as soon as possible. At lunch time, I was angered to learn there was no cafeteria. "What kind of high school doesn't have a cafeteria," I complained to anyone who would listen. When I got back to the classroom and sat on my heating vent in the back of the room, the teacher gave me two wiggling little puppies... they may have been Yorkies, not sure. It was going to be my job to take care of them.

Then I woke up again, saw that it was a bit past 6 and decided, "That's enough of THIS crap." Got up, made my way out to the kitchen. My two girlies circled around me trying to get THEIR kisses before I could give Mom HER kiss. Everyone got kissed, I went into the kitchen and took my morning pills.

And there they were. My last night's "Nitey-Nite" pills. My Ambien, to help me get to and stay asleep! My clonazepam to make sure that I have NORMAL REM sleep, the RESTFUL kind of sleep you need to feel refreshed in the morning. When my 8:30

alarm went off, I took my iPhone into the kitchen, plugged it in for the night, turned off the computer, and went back to the living room to watch the last half-hour of "Cops." The thought of taking pills never even entered my mind.

This is it, kids! This is the onset of Parkinson's Disease Dementia! This forgetfulness, this inability to focus, this—wackiness!

Better communicate with me while I can still understand you.

THE MOST FRUSTRATING PART IS...

It is the single most frustrating thing about my current state in Parkinson's disease progression.

It's not the hallucinations. I can deal with the occasional hallucination (or, "illlluuuuuuusion" as my neuro doc calls them). I had another auditory hallucination yesterday. This would be the second such. The first is documented here. Yesterday afternoon, while seated at this very computer, I heard a rather loud "MEOW!" coming from the living room. The TV was on, but it was Andrea Mitchell talking to somebody about something, and she RARELY meows on her show. I looked at my two dogs. Certainly THEY would have been alerted by such a loud meow. They both laid there, sleeping. But I HEARD a LOUD MEOW! So, we chalk it up to auditory hallucinations.

It's not the walking, the freezing or the balance problems. I'm used to that now. I know how to get myself free when I freeze. I know to try to keep my center of gravity balanced at all times. I refrain from doing things that will cause me to tip over.

It's not the slowness. I'm in no hurry to get anywhere... although it is a hassle when a sudden "potty emergency" comes on and I have to make my slow way down the hallway to the bathroom while the urgency grows. But that's what the "Depends" are for.

It's not even the onset of dementia. It's frustrating not being able to figure things out sometimes and lacking focus and not being as quick on the uptake. But I figure when it fully sets in, it'll be everyone ELSE's problem... not mine. :)

No, the single most frustrating thing about where I am in my Parkinson's progression is the WAY IT'S MESSING WITH MY TALKING! It's not the typical whispery, throaty, hoarse PD kind of speech. It's just that I've got a case of the "yibble bibbles!"

Just now, for instance.

Gail said she was going to try to tackle cleaning TJ's office today.

What I wanted to say was, "Feeling energetic today?"

What came out was, "Feel.. feel... feel...um... feeling..."

Gail finished my sentence for me. "Energetic? Not really. But it has to get done."

I started saying something else, I don't even remember what it was, but it was all garbled and nonsensical so I put my face in my hands and moaned. "JEEEEEEESUS, I hate this!" (That part came out quite clearly.)

For someone who has made a living with his voice, with his ability to be witty and humorous and snarky off the cuff, this inability at times to express myself is particularly frustrating. I don't even like talking on the phone any more because of it.

Maybe if I start walking around with a blue jacket, red bow tie and no pants, I can just tell people I'm doing a Porky Pig impression. Then we'll blame it in the dementia.

I'M NEVER, EVER, EVER GONNA WRITE ANOTHER BOOK AGAIN, NEVER, EVER, EVER, NEVER – Except for This One

Oh, don't blame yourselves. A few of you actually DID purchase a hardcover or paperback or Kindle or ebook cover of either "Deep Brain Diary" or "No Doorway Wide Enough." And as soon as I get my meager royalty checks for those purchases, I'll cut a fancy check for $45 each to the National Parkinson Foundation and the Charles DBS Research Fund at Vanderbilt University Medical Center.

My mistake was misunderstanding the market. And this would also explain why I had to take the self-publishing route. Agents KNEW folks wouldn't be interested in a patient's first-person story about Parkinson's disease. Publishers KNOW your name has to be Michael J. Fox before they'd publish such a book because otherwise they'd be wasting their money printing a book written by some unknown mook where the ultimate outcome for the writer would likely be worsening disease, dementia and then death.

I mean, Jesus! Who wants to read a downer book like THAT when there are Vampire/ Werewolf movies and Harry Potter and self- help books about how you can stop dating the wrong kind of man out there?

I've written about this before. You don't see telethons for Parkinson's disease because there aren't any cute, chubby little children with Parkinson's for Jerry Lewis to roll out on a wheelchair to make you feel sorry for. You don't see a coordinated "Susan B. Kolman Race for the Cure" effort to raise money for Parkinson's research, because there aren't a whole lot of vigorous folks at this stage of PD who look bright, clear-eyed, and seem otherwise healthy and vibrant except for that killer cancer that your donations will help cure. You don't see a national campaign for Parkinson's like you do for Autism because, for God's sake, Autism happens to KIDS! And who wouldn't want to do something for the KIDS? You don't even see the kind of campaign that the ASPCA has on TV now with the sad puppies and kitties in cages because who WOULDN'T feel sad about the sad puppies and kitties, and the little kids in Africa who have to get their daily drinking water from a stream full of water buffalo excrement, or little Maria Guadalupe who can't go to school because she has no shoes?

Best WE could do would be to show what Parkinson's does to people. And since consumer testing shows that, by and large, people don't LIKE even LOOKING at old folks... even HEALTHY ones... that idea is a loser.

Look at your TV, for God's sake. Even the commercials that cater to the elderly show older folks who look like they could run a 5K without even bothering to stretch first. Long, lean women with a few wrinkles and nicely greyed hair. Handsome, rugged men with rippling muscles and a thick crop of silver on their heads. THAT'S what the public WANTS to see in its old folks! THAT's the image that SELLS!

Maybe if we concentrated on Young Onset Parkinson's Disease. Show folks how 10 years of Parkinson's can turn a happy, carefree- looking young roustabout into a guy with just as much going on upstairs as before, as bright, as intelligent, as witty as he ever was, but due to Parkinson's masking, he can't show the emotions he's feeling, He has trouble sitting up straight, he's fully aware of how his body is betraying him and he tries to be cheerful about it—hell, he even wrote a BOOK about it—but to the public at large he's just another old man who shuffles when he walks with his cane or his walker, who stops and freezes when he comes to a doorway or a narrow passage or a change in the pattern on the floor, or a change from a level to a sloping surface. Just another old guy. Why bother. Old people are gonna die anyway.

Except, I'm not old. I'm 56 years old. I've had this bastard of a disease since I was 45. And if this year is like any other, 50,000 Americans... many of them in their early 40s... will ALSO get this diagnosis. And in 3 years, 5 years, 10 years, YOU could look like this... OK, maybe not quite so chubby and with a bit more hair on your head. But you get the picture.

And THAT is why you SHOULD CARE! If not for altruistic reasons, for SELFISH reasons. Don't wait for your dad or mom, your uncle or aunt, your brother or sister, your cousin, your SON or DAUGHTER for God's sake, to tell you, "The doctor says I have Parkinson's." CARE ABOUT IT NOW!

Here's where you can get more info.

The National Parkinson Foundation

The Michael J. Fox Foundation

The American Parkinson's Disease Association

The National Institute of Neurological Diseases and Stroke

OH, POOH! NOT AGAIN!

This is one of those things that's hard to write about, but since the purpose of this blog is to share my experiences with Parkinson's disease, if I only wrote about the nice stuff the blog wouldn't be worth much, now would it?

So brace yourself. I'll be as euphemistic as possible.

Gail and I were settling down to watch an "On Demand" movie. We were about 10 minutes into the movie when, without warning, I noticed I was...

"Making Bigs."

Now, this is not the sort of thing that you can really do without noticing it. So I said just about the only thing a person CAN say in a situation like that.

"Uh-oh!"

I made my way to the bathroom to assess the damage. Let's just say it was moderate. My brain eventually realized what my bottom was doing and managed to close the barn door after only SOME of the horses had gotten out.

Unfortunately, some of those horses had made their way up the back of my Depends where they soiled my underpants and the shorts I was wearing. My shirt was spared.

I got everything all cleaned up, the unfortunate adult diaper was bagged and tossed into the trash, the soiled clothing was dropped into the wash, I put on a new Depends, new shorts, and some long pajama pants.

I was a MESSY little baby.

And just the other day, I was wondering if I really needed to keep spending money on these things as it has been quite some time since my last...

Well... I guess they stay on the shopping list. I mean, if I would at LEAST get some kind of WARNING... Oh well. Them's the breaks.

WE GET LETTERS

Seems like I'm getting comments from all over the place... mostly on my Facebook account, but some here on the blog.

About my entry from yesterday, "Oh, Pooh! Not Again!" we hear from my Facebook pal and former XM Satellite Radio colleague, Dave.

I wish I could unread that. But if it is any consolation, three times in my adult life I have made dirties in my pants. And I have no excuse. I was not drunk, not suffering from a fit if lactose intolerance, or anything of the sorts. I simply went to break a little wind and apparently pushed a bit too hard.

Oh, can you send me the link to buy your books? I accidentally cleaned out my messages and your link went away like a soiled adult diaper.

My most excellent pal Ben was just as sympathetic to my plight.

"Making Bigs." Bill...I'm not gonna lie to you. Maybe I'm just a jerk but my first reaction to this story was complete full-body laughter. We go way back and I'm sorry to betray you as a friend by laughing at such a sensitive matter. Please accept my apologies...

Everyone's a comedian.

About my first review of the new Podiobook version of "No Doorway Wide Enough," we hear from Shantie—from across the pond!

Totally enjoyed this audio book "No Doorway Wide Enough" It is not just interesting and informative, it is also very entertaining with Bill's sense of humour. I bought the book too. It is nice to listen to the audio as Bill makes it so alive.

I would recommend this audio and the book also especially that it is helping raise money for research.

Well done Bill and thank you.

You can tell she's from the UK because of her funny spelling! :)

My pal and former XM Satellite Radio colleague, Matt, shared the following after reading my piece, "You Never Miss the Dopamine Until the Brain Runs Dry."

"I mean, Jesus! Who wants to read a downer book like THAT when there are Vampire/Werewolf movies and Harry Potter and self-help books about how you can stop dating the wrong kind of man out there?"

I'm afraid despite the subject matter of rejection I'm still laughing at this line. You are a gifted writer, Bill. Keep doing it til the well runs dry (or the dopamine does)

I saw a book yesterday at Borders on "Gay Astrology".....

You are right. No one wants to hear about what they themselves might just experience in the future. I had 2 near death experiences in the 90s, and it changed my life forever. I now know that our "personalities" survive death. I know this for certain, yet, I alienated my blood family and had a whole bunch of friends go "koo-koo" "Koo-koo..." and keep their distance after I told my story.

So I know fully well that people just flat out don't give a crap about important stuff like life and death.

That being said, there is a passage concerning "enlightenment" in the Bhagavad Gita....basically stating that karma yoga is doing the work with full intent, interest, and enthusiasm, but not being attached to the outcome.

Please consider this in your work. What you are doing is very valuable, though at this time through other peoples indifference it seems not to be. No matter. Keep slogging through, Bill. Keep slogging through.

Unfortunately, fools like me are out of work, so I had to go the cheap route and download your book. I still have to get your audiobook, though intend to....so even I'm a schmuck....

I hope life becomes a bit more gentle with you as the process unfolds, or at least gives you the wisdom of experience. . . and you write about it and leave it for selfish indifferent humanity.

much love, matt

It's good to have friends!

STUDIES THAT MAKE YOU SAY "DUH?"

Sometimes I'll stumble across one of these Parkinson's disease studies, and my first reaction will be, "Duh? You didn't, like, KNOW that? From LOOKING?"

Like this one.

A study on the impact and factors associated with drooling and Parkinson's disease.

Guess what they came up with as a conclusion?

PD droolers had worse quality of life and had more difficulty speaking, eating and socially interacting compared to PD non-droolers.

DUH!

Do you know a drooler who ENJOYS drooling? Did they think it was EASIER to talk when you've got a mouthful of saliva? Did they think EATING might just be a LITTLE easier with a yap full of drool? And social interactions? Margaret, PLEASE!

"Oh, hello Mabel. (Slurp!) That's a lovely dress you're wearing. (Sluuuuurp!) Oh, the bib? (Drool.) Whoops! Some got away that time. (Slurrrrrp!) Well, I guess that answered the question for you, didn't it? (Slurrrrrp.) So, what's the plan? (Awwwwk.... hawwwwwwk..... gag.... guh!) Sorry, A little went down the wrong way. (Slup.) What do you say we go get some corn on the cob? (Slurrrrrrrrrrp!)"

I'm sure there must be something I'm missing here, some deep scientific THING they needed to determine in this study, but the results just kinda floored me. I drooled in public one time, I mean REALLY drooled, bent over and had a string of saliva slip from my lips to the mall floor. I was humiliated.

Seems by using common sense we could save quite a bit of research money. But that's just me, I guess.

IS SOMEONE BEATING ME WHILE I SLEEP?

"What's gonna hurt NEXT," is a question I suppose I could start asking myself each night when I go to bed. I remember being told that Parkinson's disease was not a painful disease, and by and large it is not. But then you get something like the "frozen shoulder" I had before physical therapy (which still hurts to move, but at least it ain't frozen no more...). And then, Friday I'm hobbling around on a right hip that felt like someone kicked me and gave me a hip pointer.

This morning, the hip is fine! It's my RIBS that hurt. I must have been sleeping in some sort of scrunched up position last night

because the ligaments connecting my ribs to my sternum are aching with each movement, and my right neurostimulator implanted under my collar bone is painful to touch. AND, there's a spot on the ulnar side of my right forearm that feels like I whacked an iron bar with my arm.

Ibuprofen is taking some of the edge off. The Parkinson's drugs? They do nothing for the pain.

Not that I'm complaining, mind you... Oh, wait. Yes I am!

I'M A BIG BOY NOW!

Gail and I just got back from our midday runabout. It's been so freakin' hot lately that neither one of us really wanted to go out or do anything, but it's only 86 now, so what the hell. Went to the mailbox first. Then, I wanted a bottle of brandy. (On the Simpsons last night, Mr. Burns was clutching a glass of brandy. It made me want a glass of brandy. I am an easily-influenced person.)

Then we went to the grocery store. I got some chicken, Gail got some healthy stuff.

And as we were walking out to the car, Gail noticed I was taking little teeny steps.

"Are you taking BIG BOY steps?" she asked.

Right there, I froze. Thinking about what's involved in "Big Boy steps" totally confused my midbrain and we ground to a halt. Gail took my right arm, and I started extending my stride.

Then she noticed I was looking at my feet when I was walking. "Nuh-uh! No looking at your feet. Look up!" she demanded. "So much to think about," I whined.

See, the things you HUMANS do without even thinking about it, WE of the PARKINSONIAN race have to actually consider each action involved in a movement.

We got back into the car, and Gail said, "If you wanna have Big Boy Juice (meaning the brandy), ya gotta take Big Boy Steps!"

And she's right. Hopefully the day may come when I can start wearing Big Boy underpants again, too!

THIS, THAT AND THE OTHER

Just a few minor thoughts, observations and comments today.

1. There's something in the RSS Feed about Parkinson's disease in the middle column of my home page, about halfway down, about "MCI" or "minor cognitive impairment"—which seems to be a precursor to Parkinson's Disease Dementia. Earlier today, leaving the bedroom and heading for the shower, I saw a big, black bug for a fleeting second on the door jamb in the bedroom. It quickly vanished as I looked at it directly. Yesterday, something furry poked out between the couch and chair... both dogs were asleep at Gail's feet, so it weren't them. Today, I gets an e-mail from a colleague asking me to call an 800-number to record something on a draft she sent, but she asked me to review the draft first. I did and made comments and responded to her e-mail. She wrote back that she hadn't received the file yet. I thought she was talking about the file I would create by calling the 800 number. I FORGOT ABOUT THE DOCUMENT I HAD EDITED. I apologized and sent it to her just now.

2. My Mom went for about five days thinking I was mad at her. She sent a card with a very nice note telling me not to give up and to hang in there and not be like my brother Bob who just

gave up and let his condition take him over. I took the note for what it was... but the more Muz thought about it (she thinks about stuff a lot), the more she thought I was mad at her. So she called me yesterday and asked if I was done being mad at her yet. I assured her the last time I was mad at her was when I was 12 and she wouldn't let me buy a Suzy-Q at the store. Mommies can be silly!

3. As disappointed as I am that only 25 people have bothered to subscribe to my Podiobooks version of "No Doorway Wide Enough," I'm getting close to being finished with it. And I'm having fun recording my Podiobooks version of "Undercover Trucker" which I'll submit as soon as I'm done with "Doorway." If you're haven't read "Doorway" or are scared to because you think it's all gross and icky and sad, then you have no idea what you're missing. It's a fun book, and who knows.... ya might learn sumthin'.

4. Gotta stop drinking. Altogether. Immediately. Didn't realize I was rolling the dice. But I have been. I don't drink a lot. Two glasses of wine a night. On a weekend, perhaps three. After "seeing" the bug this morning, I did a search about Klonopin and Alcohol. Here's what I found about my nightly 2mg of clonazepam.

Drinking alcohol while on Klonopin can increase the risk of some side effects caused by Klonopin. These side effects include drowsiness, dizziness, unusual behavior, memory problems, and co-ordination problems. The heart rate and breathing rate can slow down due to the combination of Klonopin and alcohol. This situation can cause you to pass out and have difficulty breathing. It may even lead to death. Your body and mind can be more sensitive to alcoholic effects when you take it along with Klonopin. When you take Klonopin with alcohol, you may not be able to drink your usual amounts of alcohol, as it is not safe for you. Therefore, if your temptation to drink more overcomes your fear of danger, it can lead you to a disastrous situation.

Uh huh. And what about my nightly 5mg of Ambien?

Do not drink alcohol while you are taking this medication. It can increase some of the side effects of Ambien, including drowsiness.

Oh kaaaayyyyyyy... about my Zoloft and alcohol?

As per Pfizer, Zoloft did not increase cognitive or psychomotor effects with alcohol. However, it is strongly advised that alcohol is not recommended with the use of Zoloft.

Mmmm hmm. Any problems with my Metoprolol (blood pressure)?

Metoprolol may impair your thinking or reactions. Be careful if you drive or do anything that requires you to be alert. Drinking alcohol can increase certain side effects of metoprolol.

I see. How about my Lisinopril (also for blood pressure)?

Avoid drinking alcohol. It can further lower your blood pressure and may increase some of the side effects of lisinopril.

All righty. Any worries about my Stalevo and booze?

Do not drink alcohol or use medicines that may cause drowsiness (eg, sleep aids, muscle relaxers) while you are using Stalevo; it may add to their effects.

Well, that just about covers it. All my meds advise laying off the "big boy juice." Most say it could make side effects worse. One says it could kill me. And since I don't want to surprise my wife by waking up dead one of these mornings, I see what my choice has to be.

One glass of V-8 Fusion, please! And put it in a dirty glass!

DYSTONIA, THOU ART A CRUEL AFFLICTION!

OK, so I'm in bed last night. Gail is sitting up with Shiloh because there's supposed to be a line of thunderstorms coming through. (There wasn't a SINGLE clap of thunder, bolt of lightning and only a little rain, but my brave German shepherd freaks out during storms. She's so VERY brave.)

Raven is in the bed with me. She is generally made of sterner stuff. (Although she will hide behind my chair if a storm comes during the day.) But she's at the foot of my bed, panting heavily—and I have an attack of dystonia—the cruel twisting of muscles that sometimes accompanies Parkinson's disease.

My neck and back had been cramping since earlier in the evening. My left foot wanted to make like a parrot claw and grab a perch. My right calf wanted to ball up and clench. And I had a 70 lb. dog at the foot of my bed, making it difficult to get down there and rub the cramps out.

Raven eventually wearied of my fidgeting about and got up to lay on the floor. I was able to rub some of the cramping out, and if I lay perfectly still, everything was fine. But as soon as I would move one leg or the other, the cramping would start again. The last three toes on my left foot, my whole right calf.

I finally got to sleep. When I tried to sit up to get out of bed at 6:30 this morning, the right calf remembered it's supposed to be cramping and balled up. But only until I was on my feet.

Everything's fine now.

We'll see how I hold up when I get out of this chair to go do my "big boy walk" and balance exercises.

THE EXTRA STALEVO HELPS, BUT OY! THE DREAMS!

That extra Stalevo 100 at bedtime really helps with the cramps. But MAN, did I have a weird dream!

My first wife had died. She was working in a lumber yard and she had a forklift drop a load of 2x4's on her. Thing is, she had already been buried when I arrived in whatever town this was to attend her memorial service.

My dead twin brother Bob was there, too. We went to the lumber yard, and HE had a bunch of 2x4's dropped on HIM by a forklift. He survived, but had quite a headache.

Then I looked behind me and saw a forklift with a huge number of 2x4's on it just over my head. They started to drop them and I began running for the edge of the building, thinking "these are the last moments of my life." They just grazed me and tore my clothes a bit.

We went to, I think it was, some kind of fancy restaurant for the memorial service. Everyone's hugging me, telling me how brave I was being and how sorry they were for my loss. There was one chubby, older lady with gray, curly hair who hugged me and I noticed she had a little heart with the word "Avon" on it on her neck. It looked like it would be a necklace, but it was implanted directly in the middle of her chubby little throat.

Then it was time to go to the cemetery. We had to wade through knee deep water to get to it. "I'm sure she won't mind that we had to get our pants legs wet to come see her," I said. I could see the freshly turned dirt where her grave was...

And then I woke up.

Levodopa does encourage the vivid dreams that, in and of themselves, are a part of Parkinson's disease. Now that I'm taking one at bedtime, I image there will be a lot more of this.

According to the medical source information about Stalevo 100:

Psychiatric side effects have included reports of psychotic episodes (including delusions, hallucinations, and paranoid ideation), agitation, anxiety, confusion, dream abnormalities including nightmares, depression (with or without development of suicidal tendencies), somnolence, and dementia.

Fine. Just as long as the damned cramps stop!

WHAT A PAIN IN THE ASS!

...and I mean that literally. Right now, I feel like the Belle of the Ball at the Gomorrah State Prison Debutante Cotillion and Coming-Out Dance Social. (I was the most popular girl at the party!)

There's a reason for this. Parkinson's disease causes constipation. Some of the medications used to treat Parkinson's disease cause constipation.

I always thought the official definition of constipation was "fewer than 3 movements per week."

'Taint so, McGee!
(http://wichita.kumc.edu/hastings/constipation.pdf)

The Modified Rome Criteria defines constipation as = 2 of the following criteria present for =12 weeks during the last 12 months:

Fewer than 3 stools per week

Straining in 25% or more of defecations

Lumpy or hard stools at least 25% of the time.

Sense of anorectal obstruction or blockage at least 25% of the time.

Use of digital extraction or transvaginal pressure to assist evacuation.

If it's in bold italic, I GOTS DAT! (That 5th one... there was ONE time I hadda go in there and... well, never mind.)

Here's why. There are three muscles that have to relax in order for there to be a smooth transit of what those of us in the scientific community refer to as "the poopy" from the body to the potty. In Parkinson's, ONE of those muscles relaxes. The other two do not - - in fact, they tighten! This forces "the poopy" to FIGHT its way out of its confinement like a drunk sailor in a bar surrounded by Shore Patrol. Like the unfortunate drunken sailor, there is generally some bleeding when the whole affair is over with.

In Parkinson's Disease, involuntary rigidity afflicts striated muscle throughout the body including the muscles of defecation. Constipation occurs in 2/3 of patients. The internal anal sphincter relaxes normally during rectal wall distention, but this normal response is masked by an intense, prolonged, delayed spasm of the external anal sphincter and the puborectalis muscle. Treatment is complicated by the constipating effects of the anticholinergic drugs used to treat the disease, as well as the frequent development of autonomic insufficiency.

The key here, it would seem, would be to consume bulk laxatives like Metamucil, therefore rendering the aforementioned "poopy" into a softer, fluffier mass that WON'T rip its way out of my body like the Incredible Hulk through a police station wall.

We'll give that a try and see what happens.

DO I STILL *LOOK* LIKE ME?

With Alzheimer's disease, the patient often stops recognizing family. "With Parkinson's, it's like the family doesn't recognize [the patient] anymore," says Thomas Montine, a neuro-pathologist who heads the Parkinson's disease research center at the University of Washington in Seattle.

That puts is about as well as I've ever seen it put!

This comes from VERY interesting article in the Wall St. Journal Online. The subject: "How Parkinson's Disease Alters the Brain."

> *Unlike with Alzheimer's and other dementias, patients with Parkinson's don't lose their memory. Instead, they may develop trouble with planning, making decisions and controlling their emotions, and often exhibit changes in personality as a result. About one-third to one-half of Parkinson's sufferers exhibit some signs of cognitive impairment at the time they are diagnosed, but over time virtually all patients will experience substantial cognitive decline.*

All I really have to go by is Gail... and she says she hasn't noticed much change in me, personality-wise. She has noticed I am more emotional, moodier, and have trouble with planning and decision- making. If she had been in charge of the finances, I would not have spent as much money I did just to print a book that very few of you are interested in buying—even though the proceeds go to help fund the search for a cure. (Just in case, it's still available... and 100% of proceeds go to PD research... but if you wanted one you would have likely gotten one by now.)

So, I've had deep brain stimulation, I've increased the amount of levodopa I take every day. Why isn't THAT helping?

The motor symptoms of Parkinson's appear to be caused by decreased amounts of dopamine. Medicines like the generic drug l-dopa that boost dopamine can improve motor symptoms. Dopamine is also decreased in areas of the brain responsible for cognition, but dopamine-boosting drugs don't seem to work on cognition.

So, what is to be done about all this?

Biochemistry professor Richard Palmiter showed in published work that mice that lack the ability to produce any dopamine can't do even simple cognitive tasks, such as getting through a complicated maze.

Next, he will examine the cognitive effects of turning off the production of dopaminergic neurons in certain brain regions in mice that have the neurons intact. In order to turn dopamine production off and on, he will borrow a virus from a dog to transport a gene in the brain cells that will interrupt the ability to make the chemical.

With this experiment, Dr. Palmiter hopes to determine whether it's the amount of dopamine in the brain or the lack of dopaminergic neurons that affects cognition in Parkinson's patients.

While there are limits to what can be gleaned from such animal studies, the findings should provide insight into how critical it is in treating the disease to keep the neurons from dying, rather than just boosting dopamine in the brain, according to Dr. Palmiter.

It is so unusual to see such a well-written article about such a misunderstood disease. Kudos to Journal writer Shirley S. Wang.

Now... if we could only get people to CARE about it.

THE UP SIDE OF PARKINSON'S DISEASE?

Wanna know what's really NEAT about having Parkinson's disease?

It's the MYSTERY!

It's the getting up and walking into the living room to change the channel, but picking up the remote for the TV and not the cable, and changing the channel from "Input 3" (where the cable comes in) to "Channel 249" where NOTHING comes in, realizing your mistake, and then having to go one channel at a time back to "Input 3" so you can see an episode of "Law and Order" that you've seen a million times!

It's the working on a project for work and being distracted by an e- mail, then going back to your project and not remembering what in the hell it was you were doing before being distracted by the e- mail... the having to retrace your steps in the project until you get to the part where it was that you left off. That's COOL!

Know what ELSE is neat about having Parkinson's disease?

The sense of WONDER!

Wondering if what you're feeling in your lower gut is just gonna be gas, or reason to change your diaper. (But, by God, you're PREPARED!)

Wondering what you're going to feel like tomorrow. Next week. Next month. Next year. 10 years from now, God willing.

Wondering if one of your idiot dogs is going to see a rabbit next time you take them out and pull you off the porch, down the steps, and skipping behind them into the woods.

It's like living in a CIRCUS!

Trying to walk down a hallway without bumping into a wall. Trying to walk into an open room without freezing in place. Trying to walk down the aisle in a store without digging a foot into the tile and falling. The very act of WALKING with Parkinson's disease requires the concentration of an acrobat!

There's the way it can uncomplicate even the most COMPLEX relationships!

My wife and I have always been best friends, partners and soulmates since we met in 1988. I love her with all my heart. Only NOW we don't have those pesky "sex" complications that can cause disagreements and discordance in even the most STABLE marriages. If she's not in the mood, that's fine—cuz neither am I! We're no less affectionate—we hug, we kiss, we hold hands (especially outside when it looks like I'm going to fall) and we must tell each other "I love you" at least 10 times a day. So we're cool.

And it's as ENTERTAINING as HELL!

When I open my mouth, I never know WHAT the hell kinda babble is gonna roll out. Or whether or not I'm gonna get stuck on a syllable. Or freeze up and not be able to say anything. Fun, Fun, Fun! Especially for someone who was a professional broadcaster for 30+ years.

It's the "keeping people guessing" about what you're thinking.

Your face stays the same—a blank, almost grumpy Parkinson's mask. You could be thinking about Christmas and ice cream and soft, fuzzy puppies and carnivals, but your face looks like you don't have a thought in your formerly pretty little head. Neat!

But the really, most wonderful, most magnificently NEAT thing about having Parkinson's disease...

...is the support I get from my family, friends and co-workers. From my mom to my wife, to my brother, to one of my sisters. Everyone is on the lookout for my well-being. Even a goodly number of my Facebook friends. I have cheerleaders! My neurologist is fantastic. I don't feel like just a customer to him. My wife would throw herself beneath me to give me something soft to land on if I started to fall. My Mom writes letters to urge me to keep my spirits up. My sister Becki finds ways to tease and goad me into a good mood. My little brother Joe... same thing.

And I like the way it's freed up my creativity—to write, to dream, to think.

I really don't like the stuttering, the slurring, the shuffling, the forgetfulness, the difficulty making plans and staying focused, the fact that it takes me longer to type things because I keep mashing the wrong keys with my huge Parkinsonian fingers. The stuff with my balance sucks, the falling sucks, the occasionally lazy epiglottis that allows fluid into my lungs, I could live without all of that.

But who has a choice?

I have to life with it. The alternative is unthinkable. And as long as I enjoy my life as much as I do, I have no real problem with that.

Besides... my doggies would miss me. (For a minute.)

BILLY McHEAD BONK

Oh, Parkinson's disease! Your lack of body control has provided me with much amusement! Bashing my forehead on the kitchen counter this morning, pure hilarity!

Story of morning (so far).

Get up. Go to make coffee. See stove covered with ants. Me no like ants. Get ant kill spray. Spray ants. Ants die. Get paper towel, wipe off ants and remaining spray.

Then get another paper towel, and open cabinet door under sink. Reach under sink to get Windex.

Bend over too far and bounce forehead off of corner of counter. Bammo! See stars. It hurt.

Screw it. Think of pain later. Wife need coffee! Finish job. Wipe off stove. Make stove clean.

Finish making coffee. Pour coffee for wife. Add creamer. Take to her. Kiss wife. Wife NICE!

Then, fill own coffee cup. Grab creamer. Set next to cup. Pick up coffee pot again. Look confused.

"Why, coffee cup already full! No NEED more coffee! Why I pick up coffee pot?"

Pick up creamer. Put creamer in coffee. Go to desk and sit down. Wonder why brain acting like such numbskull this morning.

D'oh!

(As a side note, my wife said it's a sign of my devotion that I put my head into everything I do. God, how I love her.)

A FEW WORDS ABOUT SPEECH DIFFICULTIES

If you would have asked me a year ago, I would have said that it was my understanding that the only speech difficulty associated with Parkinson's disease is the way many Parkies speak softly with whispery, reedy voices. I never thought I would have a problem with that. Still don't. All my years in broadcasting have given me the habit of speaking from the diaphragm, not from the throat muscles.

Here's the part about PD speaking difficulties I did NOT know about:

It has been estimated that between 65-90% of Parkinson's disease sufferers will ultimately have troubles with their speech, and these problems can become apparent in explicit ways which include speaking in either a monotone or unintelligible gibberish. At times, patients hesitate before actually speaking which can give the impression that there is some memory impairment or dementia with the patient. At other times, the speech is faster than normal, and very often the same words are repeated over and over. Again, this can give the impression that the patient is suffering from dementia or memory impairment problems.

1. Unintelligible gibberish. There are times when I want to say something and all the words come out at once in an unintelligible jumble. For instance, if I want to ask Gail, "When were the dogs outside last," it might come out "whennerdogoudsidelas?" Then I stop, close my eyes, focus on the words and say them one. At. A. Time.

2. Hesitation before speaking. Last night, I was trying to tell TJ about something I saw on TV. Actually, I had two thoughts I wanted to convey: a) I may have told you this already; and b) I saw this thing on TV. I opened my mouth and nothing came out. So I forced myself to start, and I began with b), switching over to a) in mid-sentence. Stopping. Starting again. Same thing happens. So I closed my eyes, focused on what I wanted to say, and was then able to say it.

3. Speech is faster than normal. I think this is connected to #1.

4. Words are repeated over and over. I call this the "scratched record" syndrome. You can hear this for yourself on last Sunday's interview on "Boomer Nation Radio" when, early in the interview, I got hung up on a word and said it four or five times before stopping myself. I wrote about this the other day when I wanted to tell Gail, "Don't forget to check the mail," and it came out, "Don't forget chaa... chaa... chaa... chaa..." to which Gail (God love her) said, "I'll check the mail. I remembered." (She's getting very good at finishing my sentences.)

So far, I don't seem to have any trouble with conveying my thoughts in writing. In fact, I think I'm getting better at it, even though my fat, Parkinsonian fingers tend to mash all the keys at once requiring many corrections. And when I AM speaking clearly (and not slurring like I just drank a gallon of cheap wine), I am able to record a nice podcast (thanks to a great digital, audio editing program where I can clip out all the crap that I just wrote about). Love that editing software!

Now, I'm seeing evidence that the Deep Brain Stimulation may be the cause of some of these speech difficulties... or, at least, it can make a pre-existing problem worse.

DBS and its impact on speech:

- **There has also been a growing interest in understanding "speech" in individuals with PD who have undergone DBS-STN. Although some studies have noted that DBS can help speech by improving motor systems" involved in speech** production,9,13 such as helping individuals increase the motor force needed to produce speech and increase acoustic components of speech, the majority of studies comparing speech before and after DBS-STN have generally shown either no improvement or a decline in speech functioning following surgery.

- Some research has found that speech intelligibility (clarity in expressive speech) worsened following DBS, and speech sounded more slurred.

- DBS has also been found to have an adverse impact on intonation or rhythm, articulation, and intelligibility; the stimulation itself can cause changes in speech.

- Speech function is also very susceptible to micro lesions (damage to cellular structures in the brain) due to the surgical procedure itself.

- Krack et al. (2003) examined the long-term outcome of bilateral DBS-STN in 49 PD patients and found that speech functioning declined in these patients after five years.21 This result was interpreted as a reflection of the expected decline in speech that one would see in DBS-STN treated patients. According to this study, DBS-STN does not appear to offer any protection against declines in speech functioning in the long-term.

Yeah, well...

All things considered, with the dyskinesia I do NOT have because of the reduction in the amount of levodopa I need to take because of the DBS... I'm still glad I had it done.

THE MUTINOUS MID-BRAIN

With Parkinson's disease moving is a constant struggle between my mutinous mid brain and the frontal lobes—which are still (nominally) in charge.

Just got back from a delightful lunch at the Arundel Mills Mall with my beloved. We dined at the food court—Chinese for her, grilled meat with cheese on buns for me.

Then, it was exercise time... a walk to the tobacco store and back.

I generally start out OK. Doing the big-boy walk, stretching out my stride, standing up straight... but as we continue it becomes harder and harder to maintain this posture.

For one thing, the floor pattern keeps changing. My mid brain doesn't care for that. Not at all. And it sends a message to my feet, "HALT! We must assess this difference in the pattern on the floor so that we may decide what stride is best suited for you, the feet, to navigate this new condition."

I can almost imagine the rest of my brain, tapping its feet impatiently, looking at its watch, as my mid brain sorts out the various parameters. The floor is level... it just looks different. We may continue.

So, off we go. Then I notice I'm starting to lean forward. So I stop, force myself into an upright and locked position, and continue. I stick close to the wall in what Gail has coined my "Rat boy" position. See, with the wall to protect my right side and Gail to protect my left side, like the rat scurrying along a wall using my whiskers to judge the distance, I do just fine.

Then, I find myself coming up to an abutment coming out of the wall. This confuses my beleaguered mid brain and it pulls the brake switch yet again. The mid brain shoots an order to the eyes. "How much room between us and that thing coming out of the wall?" The eyes take a look and shoot their assessment back to the frontal lobes which signal the mid brain that we can make it past the obstruction with inches to spare. The mid brain checks its manuals, schematics and charts, then gives the feet the go ahead to continue.

Only I'm leaning forward again. See, what my mid brain REALLY wants to do is have me walk in a hunched over position and take tiny steps. Then and ONLY then will we truly be able to safely ambulate wherever we want to go. Until, of course, my center of gravity gets out ahead over my feet and I have to step even faster and faster and faster and I fall forward onto my face.

Fortunately the frontal lobes, the "Thinking Brain", still run the show. (How much longer that's allowed to be the case, we shall see in the years to come.) It shoots an urgent message to the mid brain, "STAND UP STRAIGHT! TAKE BIG BOY STEPS!"

The mid brain, responsible for the things you do WITHOUT thinking, flips a middle finger at the monitor screen but does what it's told. Until the next time the thinking brain sees something shiny and forgets about trying to keep an even keel and the mid brain can try—yet again—in its mutinous efforts to take over complete control of my ambulation.

I'm not sure which part of my brain is responsible for my speech... but that guy seems to be in on the mutiny.

None of these are issues that can be handled by DBS. These are so-called "dopamine resistant" symptoms, and DBS can only help in the areas where dopamine can help.

So we're on our own here, kids.

STEM CELL ROULETTE

I'm still in something of a state of shock over the recent ruling by a DC Circuit Court Judge putting a halt to federal funding of embryonic stem cell research at the request of a conservative group that argued ESCR "diminished the supply of available adoption babies."

I truly thought when we elected a progressive president and a progressive legislature that we were PAST the day when religious superstition could overrule science. Wrong again.

I think of the promise ESCR holds, not only for my exquisite little inconvenience, but for diabetes, spinal cord injuries, heart disease and other afflictions. I shake my head in wonder as I imagine what GOOD could have been done ALREADY if ESCR had been allowed federal funding between 2001 and 2009, back when religious conservatives held sway over the purse strings.

Now we're back at Square "0". We are once again second class citizens. Our rights are OFFICIALLY secondary to the rights of frozen blastocysts that will, inevitably, be thawed, scraped and burned as medical waste when Mommy and Daddy get the baby they want from in vitro fertilization. (And since IVF is the REASON these blastocysts are created and then destroyed, where is the right wing outrage over IVF? Why is it reserved only for the victims of Parkinson's and paralysis and diabetes and heart disease who could BENEFIT from these cells BEFORE they are destroyed—AS THEY WILL BE ANYWAY!)

Adoption agencies are actively seeking parents for children who need them. There is no shortage of adoptable kids. That was just an emotional ploy this conservative group used to get their case in front of this Reagan-appointed conservative judge.

The opponents to ESCR say, "Hey! We don't need it! Look at all the good things being done with ADULT stem cells."

I reply thusly:

1. Adult stem cells have to be put through a long and expensive process in order to be rendered pluripotent—able to become any kind of human cell.

2. Embryonic stem cells already ARE pluripotent. No added expense required.

3. And how do you KNOW adult stem cells are better than ESC's? There hasn't BEEN any serious RESEARCH with ESCs because of the LACK OF FEDERAL FUNDING!!! It's like you're opposing spending money to develop the automobile because "the horse works just fine." Only your reasoning isn't quite that advanced—or intelligent.

We had to wait 8 years for a progressive administration that believed in science over superstition. Now, we will have to wait again until some REASONABLE judge rules on the issue and federal funding for ESCR is resumed.

Given the 8-year delay, compounded by this new delay, it's probably wishful thinking to believe it could still happen in my lifetime. (The day I was diagnosed in 2000, I was told a cure was 10-years away... tops!) But I can still hope, if not for myself, then for the next generation. And the one after that, and the one after that, and how many other generations there are to come that will have to face disease, dementia and death because of the superstition of right wing Christian conservatives.

TIME TO PLAY: "MYSTERY BRUISE!"

Another mystery bruise.

No idea where it comes from. Was just changing my clothes and I noticed it there on my right ankle. It only hurts slightly. But I don't recall banging my ankle into anything.

Ah, Parkinson's disease! Always the riddles with you!

This, of course, is not the first time I've found bruises on myself with no idea how I got them. I used to get them a lot more back before I was taking clonezepam at night. Back then, I used to lash out, punch, kick and yell in my sleep. So, I'm guessing, at some point last night I must have smacked myself on my right ankle with my left heel and it didn't hurt enough to wake me up.

Whee!

IT'S ONE THING AFTER ANOTHER!

First, I'm nobody's sweetheart today. I have no patience for anything. I have a low grade headache and I'm grouchy. I bumped my knee into one of the handles on my exercise bike. I lost my balance and fell against our dresser, the corner stabbing me right below my left underarm. My wife wasn't feeling well, and I was worried about her (but she's doing better now). Raven wants to bark at every sound she hears outside and it's only the image of the poor, abused animals in the ASPCA commercials keeping me from beating her to a fare-thee-well. My feet are trying to cramp up like parrot claws, I'm getting hate tweets from clueless wingnuts who think Glenn Beck is the second-coming, and besides that...

They're out of Chocolate Dunkers at the Pizza Hut.

Oh well. I'll have to make do with the Cinna-sticks. A poor substitute. But I shall attempt to drown my sorrows in a stuffed crust, ham and beef, mushroom, extra cheese pizza.

It's days like the last few that make me kinda sorry I quit drinking.

MY SISTER BECKI IS A MEAN, MEAN GIRL!

And here's why. My Mom and I have this established tradition of calling each other during Green Bay Packers games. Luckily, yesterday's game was one that we got on FOX, but usually I have to watch NFL Red Zone to get updates. When the Packers score, I call my mother to celebrate.

Before the game yesterday, I called Muz to discuss it with her. And when we were done, an errant neuron in my diseased and corrupted brain misfired, and I believed that just flipping the phone shut would disconnect the line.

It didn't. And for 13 minutes my mother (the kind of person who waits for YOU to hang up before SHE does) listened to my regular conversation with Gail, my howls of outrage over the way the Detroit Lions got jobbed by the refs in their game with the Bears, etc. Then, I noticed the phone was still connected, so I hit the red "disconnect" button. My mother immediately called. "Did you know that for the last 13 minutes you were still on the phone?" I told her that I had just become aware of that fact.

My sister Becki always joins Muz to watch Packers games. When she got there, she sends me a text.

> *"i hear u don't know how to use your phone"*

First of all, I have no patience for people who text the letter "u" instead of writing out the word "you". It's TWO ADDED KEYSTROKES!   Lazy asses!

I responded.

"At least I have a phone, not a Cracker Jack prize."

My little brother Joe dubbed Becki's phone with that moniker.
   She responded.

"i know how to use mine... you worried muz to death"

Oh, how melodramatic. Mom could hear me talking and cursing the referee's decision in the Lions/Bears game. If she was worried, it was because she raised a son who uses that kind of language.

I responded.

"I thot flipping it shut hung it up. Sue me."

See, since she disrespected me by typing "u" instead of "you," I DOUBLED the insult by dropping 4 letters from the word "thought."

She responded.

"u thought wrong, dumbass"

And that's another thing. She never uses proper capitalization or punctuation in her text messages. Maybe her Cracker Jack toy keyboard doesn't HAVE that capability. Who knows.

I got the last word. Or so I thought.

"I have a brain disease. Nobody likes you."

Then, the Packers got their first touchdown. So I called Muz. I could hear Becki in the background, "Did Gail dial the phone for him?" I told Muz to tell Becki that THIS is why nobody likes her and she has no friends.

Next touchdown, I called again. This time, I hear Becki in the background, "Did RAVEN dial the phone for him?" Well that's not only MEAN, but it's SILLY! A border collie, no matter how intelligent, doesn't have the capacity to use or even comprehend cellular communications devices.

So, we left it at that.

Becki is a mean, mean girl. And if you should see her on the street today, I command you to throw apples at her.

HOW DOES ONE *FORGET* SOMETHING LIKE THIS?

(Bodily Function Alert: If talk about bodily functions, however tastefully described, horrifies you... skip this post.)

Monday morning. Shower time. But first, gotta go potty! Sat there for 10 minutes or so, staring at the pile of magazines Gail keeps in a little bin in front of the loo to keep her mind occupied while she conducts her business.

After the aforementioned 10 minutes, I think I actually said aloud, "Well... I guess I ain't gonna poop." I stood up, turned around to flush the john, and...

(Insert a sound effect of a dramatic nature here... something like a "dah-DAH-dah-DAAAAAAAAAH!")

There it was. At the bottom of the bowl. Mocking me with its very presence.

A dookie!

"HOW DID YOU GET THERE?" I asked it. The dookie, of course, had no answer. If it could speak and had shoulders, I assume it would have shrugged them and said, "The usual way, I s'pose."

Now, to be honest, there are days when I forget whether or not I've had a BM that day. But I usually find myself wondering about that in the mid-to-late afternoon. NOT MERE MINUTES AFTER DEPOSITING THE AFOREMENTIONED BM!!!

Ay yi yi!

COULD MMSE MEAN PD-D FOR ME?

I've been looking at a paper on the diagnosis of probable and possible Parkinson's disease dementia. There are several proposed criteria that must exist for there to be a diagnosis of suspected PD- D.

1. Ya gotta have Parkinson's disease. Check.

2. The Parkinson's had to become apparent well before the suspected dementia. Check. By about a decade.

3. The PD must be associated with a decreased global cognitive deficiency. Only one way to find out, and that's take a test.

There are some of these tests that just seem so dirt simple, but you can't administer them to yourself. You need to have someone give them to you. So I asked Gail to administer the Mini-Mental State Exam (MMSE). Then, I tried explaining what she needed to do and what I needed to do.

Gail has never been one for just doing something I ask without asking questions about it. This time, she wanted to know why I wanted to do this test if I already knew the answers. There was something in her tone of voice that made me feel like I was bothering her, so I told her to just forget it.

She asked again, "Why do you want to take this test if you already know all the answers?"

I told her that I did NOT know the answers, that some portions of the test required her to come up with a sentence telling me to do something, to make up three words and ask me to remember them, etc. and etc. And frankly, I was quite irritated.

And this is part of the problem. (We'll get back to the MMSE in a minute. Hang in there.)

On Thursday when our plane landed, Gail wanted to look in some of the little kiosks and stores to see if she could find a destination- related t-shirt or something. I reminded her of the last time we were at this airport, and I was so slow they had our luggage off the turnstyle and locked in an office by the time we got to baggage claim. Then I thought, well hell... we got our luggage LAST time so it won't hurt if she looks in a store or two, but she kept refusing every time I suggested it. I mistook this to mean she was angry with me. When we got to the car rental counter, I put my hand on her shoulder and began to tell her that I didn't know if we still had collision and comprehensive on our auto insurance, so we should probably get some sort of insurance for the rental and she pulled away from me saying I was hurting her shoulder. I didn't think I was pressing that hard, so I just said, "Fine," and turned around. She told me to "knock it off." I said "YOU knock it off. You've been mad at me since I said we had to get to baggage claim before they locked up our bag." She said the first time she had been mad at me all day was right that instant. And my mind flashed back onto this little bit of knowledge I picked up some time ago in my reading about Parkinson's disease dementia (PD-D).

> *Up to 40% of patients have visual hallucinations, usually benign, whereas more sinister symptoms, such as delusions, paranoid ideation, and delirium, become more frequent as the disease progresses. Delusions occur infrequently, but are upsetting for carers and relatives because they are often paranoid or accusatory in nature.*

Swell. Two flashes of paranoia in the span of less than a week.

Anyway, back to the MMSE. Like I said, it's a dirt-simple test, but you can't administer it to yourself. So Gail (quite cheerfully, actually) administered the test.

1. *What year is it, what season, what date, what's the day of the week, what's the month?*

   I screwed up the season. Twice. First I said, "Spring... no, no, wait... Fall." Gail said, "It's summer."

   D'oh. One point off already.

2. *Where are we now, state, county, town/city, hospital, floor?*

   Well, we're not in a hospital, we're in a house and I'm in the kitchen. Aced it.

3. Gail named three unrelated objects and asked me to repeat them. Car, Mail, Tree. I repeated 'em just fine.

4. I had to count backwards from 100, by 7's, stopping after the 5th attempt. I only got two right. Three more points off the total.

5. Gail asked me if I remembered the three unrelated objects. I got Car and Mail, but couldn't remember the word "Tree." One more point off.

6. She showed me a remote for the TV and a Magic Marker and told me to identify each, which I did with ease.

7. I had to repeat the phrase, "No ifs, ands or buts." Perfect.

8. *"Take this piece of paper in your right hand, fold it in half and put it on the floor."* Done, Done and Done!

9. She showed me a sentence she had written and I had to do what it said. She wrote, *"Pinch your nose."* I'm just grateful she didn't write, "Stick a knife into your throat."

10. I had to write a complete sentence with a noun and a verb. I wrote, "The dog ate the cat." Perfect.

11. I had to copy a picture of two intersecting pentagons. No prob.

My final MMSE score is 25. Here what the literature about PD-D says about 'dat!

> *Test proposed: MiniMental Status Examination (MMSE). The MMSE is a formalized mental status examination useful for identifying cognitively impaired patients and for characterizing PD-D. It is proposed because it is a simple and universally applied scale that can be easily and rapidly performed by a clinician in the office or at the bedside. Cutoff proposed: score - 26. A score of 25 or below is proposed because the MMSE is relatively insensitive to executive dysfunction. This cut off score was used in a recent pharmacological trial in PD-D. The MMSE is influenced by the effects of age and level of education. The recommended cut off is appropriate in patients below the age of 80 and in those with at least 10 years of formal education. In older or more poorly*

educated patients, reference to published norms may therefore be helpful in judging impairment in individual patients.

OK, so I scored below the cutoff. That means I meet criteria 1, 2 and 3. But that, by itself can't mean much, right? There are other factors to be considered. Right?

Of course.

Cognitive deficiency must be severe enough to impair daily life activities.

> *One cornerstone of the diagnosis of dementia is the evidence of an impact on daily living activities that cannot be attributed to motor or autonomic symptoms in case of PD-D. The examiner should ask questions about daily functioning such as the patient's ability to manage finances, use pieces of equipment, and cope in social situations. Appendix lists another simple assessment of the ability to organize independently the daily distribution of antiparkinsonian medication that may be suitable to determine an impact of cognitive changes on daily life, although this requires validation.*

OK, so I snapped at my wife twice in the span of a week and forget to take my pills unless reminded by an alarm to do so, and even then sometimes I still forget. I forget what I'm doing in the middle of a task. If I'm engaged in something and my attention is diverted, I have to backtrack mentally to figure out what the hell I was doing when interrupted. So #4? Check.

5. Impairment in more than one cognitive domain.

Well, let's see.

A. Attention.

- Serial 7's of the MMSE. The patient is asked to repeatedly subtract 7 starting at 100. As the test is aimed at assessing attention, the instructions should not be repeated. Cutoff proposed: At least two incorrect responses.

I got 3 wrong. So there's ONE cognitive domain.

B.   Executive Function.

One test is lexical fluency, for instance, naming as many words as you can starting with the letter "S" in 60 seconds. I tried this the other day and got 17. The cutoff is 9 or less. There's also the clock drawing test which I've also aced, so we'll say I'm fine with the Executive Function.

C.   Visuo-Constructive Ability

I drew the intersecting pentagons just fine. No problem with "C".

D.   Memory Impairment

The three-word recall test in the MMSE is the go-by. I missed one. And what does the literature say about THAT?
Cutoff proposed: At least one missing word. Missing one word in the free recall of the MMSE is considered sufficient to suggest the existence of a memory/retrieval problem.

OK, so that's TWO cognitive domains. And that fits the profile for PD-D. But that's not enough for a diagnosis, right?

Although behavioral symptoms are not required, the presence of at least one of the following behavioral symptoms (apathy, depressed or anxious mood, hallucinations, delusions, excessive daytime sleepiness) supports the diagnosis of probable PD-D.

So, we're noticing a trend?

1. TABLE 1. Algorithm for diagnosing PD-D at Level I

1. A diagnosis of Parkinson's disease based on the Queen's Square Brain Bank criteria for PD

2. PD developed prior to the onset of dementia

3. MMSE below 26

4. Cognitive deficits severe enough to impact daily living

5. Impairment in at least two of the following tests: Months reversed or Seven backward Lexical fluency or Clock drawing MMSE Pentagons 3-Word recall

The presence of one of the following behavioral symptoms: apathy or depressed mood or delusions or excessive daytime sleepiness may support the diagnosis of probable PD-D.

Well, dandy! Do I get a lapel pin?

Now this is for a provisional diagnosis of PROBABLE PD-D. For a DEFINITIVE diagnosis, you gotta take a lot more tests.

But these require a doctor's visit. I have one coming up next month.

And I have a headache.

JUST CALL HER MY "CARETAKING ANGEL"

I did a telephone interview this week for my day job. It was about "caretaking," how spouses who never bargained for the 24/7 nursing care of their loved one react to finding themselves in that position due to disease or injury.

Of course, I approach the story from the other side of the spectrum... Although I hardly need the 24/7 care yet (perfectly capable of tending to my own hygiene, etc...) I do need daily help with a lot of things. Primarily in the area of "getting around" and "remembering stuff."

When I gave up driving 17-months ago, Gail had to take those duties on to herself. And she doesn't like driving. I used to love driving. But I really don't miss it. Nor do I have the attention span to do it safely any more.

When we go shopping, Gail has to take care of the heavy stuff. And she's not the healthiest person in the world either, suffering from scleroderma as she is. But me? I could barely tote a 12-pack of soda from the shelf to the veggie aisle where Gail was salad-shopping.

And when we've gotten everything we need, she lets me go back out to the car to sit down while she goes through the checkout line.

When we're walking together, she's constantly at my side... just to my left, slightly behind me, watching for signs of stumbling. I really think she'd tear every muscle strap in her back if she ever tried to catch me in a fall, but there have been numerous time where I've started to wobble and she was there to put a hand on one shoulder or the other to stop me before I reached the tipping point.

I like to think I would do the same for her. I'm pretty sure I would. But you don't know until it happens.

I have no doubt in my mind that my former wife, known here as "Facebook user", would NOT have been able to handle it. She couldn't even stay faithful to me when I was young and healthy, so what would I expect from her when I'm older and having difficulties? I think my first wife would have been able to deal with it—from a technical point of view—because (from what I'm told) she was a physical therapist. But knowing her personality, she was the type that would have constantly blamed me for causing her extra work because I wasn't well.

Gail and I joke about it. Today in the store, I was waiting for someone to pass me on my right. Then Gail said, "Scoot over to the wall, Rat Boy." (See, as explained earlier, a rat stays close to the wall, feeling it with his whiskers. Gail likes me over by the wall to my right so she can protect me from my left.) I made my way over to the wall and said, "This is about as scooty as I get these days." We both had a good chuckle.

Over the past few days, I've been forgetful. Examples? "Is TJ here?" "No, he left. You said goodbye to him." "Oh, yeah."

I sneeze. I turn to Gail. "Bless me!" I say. "I did, I said 'God bless you.' You said 'thank you.'" Oh.

I walk into the kitchen to get ice cubes from the dispenser in the fridge. The glass overflows with ice cubes because I don't pull it out in time. Ice cubes on the floor. (The dogs used to love that. They'd dash in and get the ice cubes. But they had just recently enjoyed some "Frosty Paws" and their taste for cool treats had been sated.)

So, we deal with it. And it would be impossible to deal with if I didn't have my faithful companion, my best friend, a caregiving angel named Gail.

RIP BEDROOM FAN

It was a long, slow, lingering death. But our bedroom fan finally died last night at 10:28 p.m.

The fan had been ill for quite some time. When you turned on the switch, the blades would begin to turn, ever-so-slightly, then stop, then almost imperceptibly begin to move. The gears would catch and the blades would make a quarter-turn... then stop. Then slowly start again, but go a little further this time. And then it would stop, but not for as long, and the blades would begin to turn a little faster, a little further, a little faster, a little further, and then—generally about 10 minutes after turning it on—the fan would come to life, after making a couple complete revolutions with the blades, it would kick in and spin and spin and spin and provide the air movement (and white noise) we need to sleep well at night.

I admired the fan. It reminds me of me. It just would not give up. It would try, then freeze, then try, then freeze, then try, then freeze, then—slowly, oh-so-slowly—begin to execute its function. Every time the fan would kick in and run properly, I'd smile. If the fan could do it, I reasoned, so could I. There was hope.

Last night at 10:28, the fan began making a series of loud clanking noises. It was metal rubbing against metal. And it went on and on, despite our attempts to ignore it. Finally, we decided its suffering should not be allowed to continue and we turned it off for a final time.

(The lack of "white noise" proved to be a problem. Raven—who sleeps with us—could now hear every sound being made outside our bedroom window and had to "uff!" at it. I turned up the speed on the ceiling fan. It doesn't give out as MUCH of the "white noise" as the old fan, but it sufficed.)

Gail had a doctor's appointment this morning. Then she will stop by the Lowes and pick up a new fan. The old one will get a respectful burial in the trash.

Thank you, bedroom fan. You served long, you served well, you served when it would have been easier to just quit.

I will always remember and admire you.

YOU NEED *WATER* TO MAKE COFFEE!

Even back in the cowboy days, when they'd boil up a pot of coffee around the old cook fire, they needed water. This is a known fact. So when I made the coffee this morning, why did I forget the water?

Oh, I put the pot in the sink to wash it out. I filled the container with beans to grind. But that's not where the BEANS go... that's where they end up when they're GROUND! Ya gotta GRIND the beans FIRST! Shoot, even the cowboys knew THAT! So, I poured the beans from the container into the grinder, ground 'em up REAL good, then put 'em in the filter. Pressed the "strength" button to "strong", sat down and worked a little on my new book.

And maybe that's the problem. I got a bad night's sleep because of the book. I felt guilty about charging $20 for a thin little 156-page book. "NO!" I said, sitting up in bed. " I will sell it for $10! And I will make a BETTER cover design!"

I finally went back to sleep. And as I worked on the new cover design for the book, I wondered why I wasn't hearing any coffee-making sounds.

Then, Gail got up. I kissed her and told her that coffee was on the way. I looked at the pot... and...

(Insert your own sound effect, something like "da-DAH-da-DAAAAAAAH!")

The pot was still sitting in the sink. There was no water in the coffee maker. I hadn't washed the pot and filled the coffee maker.

So, I washed out the coffee pot, filled the coffee maker, pressed the "strong" button again, hit the "start" button. And sat down to weep.

Reason for Concern?

Let's be clear. I do not have a diagnosis of Parkinson's disease dementia. Yet. But there is reason for concern.

Let's sum up my various brain farts of the last 72 hours.

1. Monday morning, I was sitting on the potty before taking my shower. After a few minutes, I decided that I wasn't going to "move" anything that morning. I stood up to flush the john. There was a "dookie" in the bowl that wasn't there when I sat down. I went "poopy" and couldn't remember HAVING gone "poopy."

2. Tuesday. I made an online purchase of $16.16 -- but in the checkbook register, I wrote $19.19. Then, I bought a distribution package for my new book. And along with it, I thought I was buying a proof copy of the new book. The title was right there on the order form. The book I bought was NOT a proof copy of my new book, but another copy of my PREVIOUS book.

3. Today. Got up to make coffee. Poured the beans into the container where the grounds are supposed to go AFTER the beans are ground. "The beans don't go THERE," I said to myself, and then I poured the beans into the grinder. Took the coffee pot out of the coffee maker and put it in the sink to wash it. Ground the beans. Put them in the filter. Pushed the "strong" button for the coffee strength. Pushed the power button. Sat down to distribute e-mails, wondering why I wasn't hearing the sound of coffee brewing. Gail got up and I told her coffee would be ready in a minute, looked at the coffee maker and saw the pot was still in the sink. Washed the pot, filled it with water, poured the water into the coffee maker, made coffee.

This has all been coming on for awhile. In recent months, I've gotten into the shower with my glasses on, have sat down on my shower stool without bringing down the shower nozzle to where I could reach it to wash myself, have almost gargled with aftershave. I have to look very carefully at my morning pills to make sure I'm taking the right ones... not the night-night ones. I'm sure if I concentrated, I could come up with more examples.

I think I require careful watching.

YOU KNOW IT'S GOING TO BE A GOOD DAY WHEN...

1. You don't even open your eyes until 7:30 a.m.

2. When the dogs lie there respectfully and let you pet them instead of jumping on you.

3. You make the coffee in the correct order... water, beans, grinding, grounds, container, power, coffee!

4. You remember not only to take your pills when you get up, but at 10 am, too!

5. You change your "adult disposable undergarment" and see NO STAINS!

6. You can't really think of a decently entertaining blog entry, because everything is going along pretty well at the moment.

LESSONS LEARNED OVER THE PAST YEAR

I thought I'd share with you a partial list of things I've learned during my last year with Parkinson's disease. We'll start with things I've learned during my morning clean-up.

1. First thing in the morning, LOOK at your pills before you take them. I take five pills first thing in the morning. It would be wrong to just grab the first five pills I can get my fat, Parkinsonian fingers around and take them. I have to take the RIGHT pills or there will be trouble. I take a Stalevo (for PD), a Zoloft (for depression), a Metropolol (for blood pressure), a Lisinopril (which helps the Metropolol) and a

Prilosec (cuz I gots acid). That leaves three Stalevo in the pill box, along with an Ambien and two Klonopin. If I start the morning by grabbing two Stalevo, an Ambien and both Klonopin, I will need to force myself to throw up—or else just go back to bed until they wear off. And it won't be pleasant.

2. If you use a shower seat, make sure you have the flexible shower head on the floor and you are seated in the shower with the curtain closed before you divert the water to the shower head. If you are bent over the bathtub rim and turn on the shower head, you will get a blast of cold water on your back and neck that will run down your body onto the bathroom floor. This is not good. If you put the shower head on the tub floor and THEN turn on the shower head before getting in and closing the curtain, then you will have water EVERYWHERE. Also not good. Pay attention. Make a list. Do things in proper order and everything will work out just fine.

3. Wash everything. Then rinse everything. Set a routine. Start at the top, work your way to the bottom. Save the sensitive, naughty bits for last cuz they're dirty and you can wash your hands when you're done as the last part of the shower. Do not forget to rinse yourself all over. If you leave any area of your body soapy, you will be very uncomfortable later in the day. Learn from experience.

4. When in the bathroom, LOOK at the LABELS before you use things. Toothpaste and Preparation H come in similar tubes. This is not a mistake you will make more than once. But still, be careful.

5. You cannot put toothpaste on an electric toothbrush while the toothbrush is turned on. You will only succeed in getting toothpaste all over the sink, all over the mirror, all over your self. Leave the toothbrush OFF, apply the toothpaste, THEN turn it on.

6. If you have dysphagia and a balance problem, be careful gargling. If you tilt your head too far back, you will inhale some of the mouthwash into your windpipe. It will burn like

Satan's fire. If you close your eyes while tilting your head back, you will not only burn your windpipe, you will fall. Keep your head level, force that epiglottis to close by tucking your chin, gargle, then spit.

7. When using an electric razor, use the PRE-shave lotion BEFORE shaving and the AFTER-shave lotion AFTER shaving. If you use the aftershave lotion before you shave, all you're gonna accomplish is getting the blades all gunked up and you'll get a crappy shave. Then, when you apply the pre-shave lotion after you shave, it'll burn like a sonuvabitch. The PRE-shave has astringent properties that dry out the skin and make the whiskers easier to cut. The AFTER shave soothes the skin, which does not NEED soothing BEFORE you shave. Again, read the labels.

8. When shaving, shave the ENTIRE face. If you are distracted by something, like a dog barking or the glint from some shiny object, try to remember where you left off, start there, and finish shaving your face. If you leave a patch of face unshaven, it will look silly and bother you the rest of the day.

9. Adult diapers go UNDER the underpants, not over. I don't do this one much anymore. But early on, I would slip into a pair of Hanes or Fruit of the Looms only to look at my side and see a neatly-folded Depends sitting there waiting for me. These special undergarments are useless when worn over the standard underwear. Put the Depends on FIRST, and THEN the underwear.

I'm sure there are more of these hints, and I will share them as they occur to me.

SAY AGAIN?

Just got back from the store. Opened my passenger door, closed it, and began walking around the front of the car. I heard a voice. It was definitely Gail's voice. Loud and clear. From the back of the car.

"Are you done?"

"What's that?" I asked?

Gail looked up from gathering groceries from the hatchback. "What?"

"What did you just say? Am I done with what?"

Gail got a quizzical look on her face. "I didn't say a word."

She went back to gathering groceries.

I stood there, scanning the neighborhood. No one else was out.

I could hear nobody speaking. I looked again at Gail.

She had all the groceries and motioned toward the front door.

"Get a move on," she said.

"I DEFINITELY HEARD A VOICE! YOUR VOICE! ASKING ME IF I WAS DONE!!!"

She shook her had. "I didn't say a word." Now... Gail is not the kind of person to mess with me like that.

I stood there, listening and scanning for another moment, then headed for the front door.

EVER NOTICE HOW DEMENTIA AND DUMBASS START WITH THE SAME LETTER?

Like I said, I do not as of yet have a clinical diagnosis of Parkinson's disease dementia. But over the past year, I've been doing things that lead me to believe such a diagnosis is not far off.

This morning, for instance.

Got in the shower. Already had the shower head on the floor of the shower so I could pick it up and wet myself down while sitting on my shower chair. Sprayed myself down. Got to my face. Sprayed my face real good! Realized I was still wearing my glasses.

I have been taking showers since we got our first shower in 1970 (it was bathtubs until then). I've been wearing glasses since 1967. This marks the second time in a couple months that I have neglected to remove my glasses before getting into the shower.

Then...

After getting all soaped and scrubbed, I rinsed myself off. I do this from a seated position as well, since my eyes are closed and my balance is further compromised when I can't see. Stood up to put the shower nozzle back in its proper place. Opened my eyes. They stung! "I must still have some soap near my eyes," I surmised.

Not only near my eyes, all over my face, neck, head and hair. I had forgotten to rinse my head.

Yup! It's a slippery slope and I'm sliding down fast!

WHY THIS BOOK IS SELF-PUBLISHED

I've been marketing and marketing and marketing the basic idea for this book for YEARS! I've sent query after query after query to agents and publishers and MOST of the time I get no response whatsoever. SOME times I'll get a form rejection. OTHER times I get a come-on for a "editing scheme" where they'll look at your manuscript as long as you pay a stiff editing fee.

So the other day, I imagined meeting with an actual agent... in person. It went something like this...

Hey there, kid! So, you're a new writer are ya? Yeah, yeah, yeah... forgive me for the generalization. You've been writing for years, but other than print-on-demand and self-publishing, as far as the literary world is concerned, you're a "new writer." It's a tough world out there, kid. (OK if I call you "kid"? I know you're in your mid-50s, but I've never heard of you and we've only communicated by e-mail and, after all, I am a successful agent so you're lucky I had a cancellation today. I don't mean to denigrate, and I'm sure you're great at what you do for a living but you ain't a writer yet, kid. Not until you've been published.)

So, what's the pitch? Non-Fiction?

OK, then. I'll bite. What kind of non-fiction? I'm glad you didn't say "fiction" because these days we got two kinds of fiction, kid. Vampires and werewolves. We had that wizard

thing going for awhile, but when the actor playing the kid started collecting Social Security... well, you know... that genre kinda went belly-up.

What we're looking for is stories about celebrities with addictions, princes getting married and divorced, anything with Lindsay Lohan – you know, stuff people care about.

Parkinson's disease?

Humor? Satire? You say you wrote some funny crap about PARKINSON'S DISEASE?

Kid? Your last name Leno? Letterman? No? What network is your TV show on? No TV show? OK. What makes you think you can write funny stuff. I mean, if you could write funny stuff you'd be on TV, right?

Nah, I don't need to see your manuscript. Like I just said... you ain't on TV, and if you ain't an actor, you ain't a recovering alcoholic, you ain't a friggin' ex-circus clown with a heroin addiction and a pedophilia rap sheet, and your name ain't Seinfeld, Tim Allen or Larry the Whatzit Guy, you just ain't funny.

Got anything else? Were you a male prostitute? You weren't? OK, when you were mobbed up, did you push any buttons? You know, "whack" anybody? Not "connected," huh?

Kid, what do you have for me? And I don't wanna hear about the "funny stuff" again.

You volunteered for brain surgery to further the medical community's knowledge about how deep brain stimulation affects early onset Parkinson's disease. You wrote a book about the experience of getting a diagnosis. You take us into the operating room with you while you remained awake for a seven hour brain operation.

Well, OK, that explains the scars on your head. But as far as subject matter, we'll pretend anyone cares for a minute. What the hell is Parkinson's disease... oh, wait! YOU'RE MICHAEL J. FOX, RIGHT??? Oh, MAN! You've really let yourself GO, Mike... I mean, I loved you on "Back to th....."

You're NOT Michael J. Fox? Well excuse me, kid, but you clearly ain't Muhammad Ali or Brian Grant. And them is the only three people in America what's got this Perkyson disease yer talkin' about. So who's gonna buy your book?

You know, kid, I'll tell you this then I gotta cut it short cuz I got an appointment with someone who wants to pitch a GOOD idea—this 3-D CGI thing with characters so cute you could shit yer pants. Three big-eyed hamsters who have this hip-hop thing going except for the girl hamster who turns out to be this ball-busting Latina with an attitude...

Look. You seem like a nice kid. I'll share something with ya.

Ya wanna be a writer? Write something new. Write something that captures the imagination. Write something that no one has ever written before. Then convince an agent that it has been done—with great success—by many other writers who are now all rich. Write something that incorporates consumer products so we can get the product placement money. Write something with familiar characters in familiar situations doing things that nobody has ever done but somehow it all seems really familiar. And if you can toss in some girl-on-girl action, maybe even just some innuendo, that gives us something for the DVD release.

If ya ain't got nothing like that, something new that has been done to death but nobody's quite tired of it yet, something that the reader or the viewer will recognize right from the cover or from the opening scene although this time it's fresh and exciting, then you just ain't a writer anyone is gonna take seriously, kid.

But good luck. And no, I don't validate parking.

Sally, send in the idiot with the CGI hamsters. This is gonna be big. BIG, I tells ya!

You still here?

IT'S AN OUCHIE MORNING

Woke up about an hour earlier than usual. Back ache. More likely, a kidney ache. Past CT scans over the last few years have shown I have a large, non-obstructing kidney stone in my left kidney. No need to do anything about it since it ain't goin' anywhere. But some mornings, few and far between, my left flank gets all achey and I can feel the ureter that leads to my bladder.

So, at 5 am, got up, went potty, tried to lay back down but I was wide awake.

Got up again. This time, Raven "the Tattle Tale" walked me to the kitchen and looked very sadly at about 5 small turds Shiloh had deposited on the linoleum.

"What's all this?" I asked Shiloh, showing her the poo. Her ears went back as she lay on her bed with a "you have every right to kill me, but please don't" look on her face.

I picked up the mess, "Swiffered" the floor, took both girls out so they could go potty where good girls are SUPPOSED to go potty, then sat down at the computer and divided up the morning clinical trial information requests for the Patient Recruitment staff.

So... how's your morning going so far?

PD PATIENTS HAVE TROUBLE WALKING/TALKING

I first noticed this in my Parkinson's disease progression during my final 8-day "Droolfest" with my brain buddies in Nashville in early 2009.

We were walking from the Vanderbilt Medical Center North to a nice little restaurant and I realized it was difficult for me to walk and talk at the same time. The other fellas were chatting away, and I'd turn to say something—and almost stumble. And this was BEFORE I started having the serious problem with walking and balance. Now, clinical research indicates that this does not necessarily mean I am a stumble bum. (It doesn't say I'm NOT a stumble bum, either. In fact, the tone of the article is quite neutral on the subject of my stumble bummery.)

Today, I see this new study published.

A new Florida State University study found that older adults with Parkinson's disease altered their gait, stride length, step velocity and the time they spent stabilizing on two feet when asked to perform increasingly difficult verbal tasks while walking. But the real surprise was that even older adults without a neurological impairment demonstrated similar difficulties walking and talking.

A disruption in gait could place Parkinson's patients and the elderly at an increased risk of falls, according to the Florida State researchers.

No foolin'?

Francis Eppes Professor of Communication Science and Disorders Leonard L. LaPointe and co-authors Julie A.G. Stierwalt, associate professor in the School of Communication Science and Disorders, and Charles G. Maitland, professor of neurology in the College of Medicine, outlined their findings in "Talking while walking: Cognitive loading and injurious falls in Parkinson's disease." The study will be published in the October issue of the International Journal of Speech-Language Pathology.

"These results suggest that it might be prudent for health care professionals and caregivers to alter expectations and monitor cognitive-linguistic demands placed on these individuals while they are walking, particularly during increased risk situations such as descending stairs, in low-light conditions or avoiding obstructions," LaPointe said.

In other words, don't ask an elderly person or someone with Parkinson's to give directions or provide a thoughtful response to a complicated question while walking.

In fact, just leave me alone. (I'm kidding. I'm a kidder. I kid because I love.)

Actually, now that I'm having major difficulties walking with NO distractions, I find I have to stop walking completely to do almost anything. To get a tissue out of my pocket, to check my cell phone, no can do! Must concentrate on each step.

Gail makes me walk in front of her at the store. That way she gets to enjoy watching me fall. (SHE says it's so she can try to catch me, but WE know the truth... whoever WE is...) If she says something to me requiring a response, I have to stop. If I think of something I want to say to her, I have to stop.

So, once again, Medical Science has spent God knows HOW many gazillions of samolians to get answers to a question I would have HAPPILY answered for FREE! (Just give me a decent cut on the royalties from the paper you'll publish, and we'll call it even.)

So, if we're out walking, don't try to engage me in deep conversation...

Among older adults, falls are the leading cause of injury deaths, according to the Center for Disease Prevention and Control. They are also the most common cause of non-fatal-injuries and hospital admissions for trauma.

...unless you're TRYING to kill me.

LATEST RESEARCH SAYS I'LL DIE SOON–OR I WON'T

Just saw one of those REALLY helpful studies published recently in the journal Neurology. It purports to explain why some people with Parkinson's disease die earlier than others. Now, as we slog through this, let us keep in mind that Parkinson's—in and of itself - - is not a fatal disease. You die WITH it, not OF it. But when you fall and bust your hip and get pneumonia or choke to death on a big chunk of turkey leg cuz your swallowing muscles aren't working properly... well, dead is dead, no matter HOW you got there.

But according to THIS article...

1. How old you were when diagnosed is a factor in longevity.
   The older, the sooner and yada yada.

2. Average time from appearance of movement symptoms to death? 16 years. OH NO! I HAVE FIVE YEARS TO LIVE!

3. Average age at death? 81 years. OH NO! I HAVE 26 YEARS TO LIVE!

The study found that the risk of earlier death was increased about 1.4 times for every 10-year increase in age when symptoms began. People with psychotic symptoms, such as delusions and hallucinations, were also 1.5 times more likely to die sooner compared to those without these symptoms.

The odds of dying earlier were nearly two times higher for people who had symptoms of dementia in the study compared to those without memory problems. In addition, men were 1.6 times more likely to die earlier from the disease compared to women. Participants who scored worst on movement tests also had a higher risk of earlier death compared to those with the highest scores.

"...for every 10-year increase starting at WHAT AGE?" Huh? We'll assume that at 45, I'm on the lower range of that spectrum. I do have the occasional delusion or hallucination, so this study says I'm 1.5 times more likely to die sooner (sooner? Than WHO?) than those without those symptoms. I am also having memory problems, so that means I'm 2 times more likely (than WHO?) to die sooner (than WHO?) and being a man means I am 1.6 times more likely to suffer early death. Not sure where my movement scores lie, but they can't be all that good.

Now, I want to know are these scores consecutive? Cumulative? Concurrent? Do you add up all the risks (in my case, making me 5.1 times more likely—than WHO? -- to die early) or do you average the scores (making me 1.7 times more likely—than WHO? -- to die earlier (than WHO?), or do you just take the highest number and run with it, making me 2 times more likely (than WHO?) to die earlier (than WHO?)???

Well, gentle reader... after reading this article, one thing is crystal clear.

I am going to die in the near future. Or I am going to die 40 years from now. Or somewhere in between. So, make your plans accordingly.

MORE OF MY COMEDY CAVALCADE!

I generate comedy like rabbits generate little poo pellets.

Example: I'm getting into the shower this morning. As I've mentioned, I shower while seated because of my balance issues. That makes it necessary for me to take the shower head off its standard post and use the flexible shower hose to wash myself.

So, I get everything together. The water is just the right temperature, and I lean over to lift the piston that will divert the water from the faucet to the shower head when...

Ah! Ah! I stop myself. See, if I lifted the piston NOW, I'd get a splash of cold water on the back of my head from the water that's already in the flexible hose, and some of that water would certainly run down my back and onto the bathroom floor before I could get into the shower and close the curtain and THAT would be SILLY!

So, I reach up, grab the shower head, place it on the floor of the bathtub—facing up, mind you...

THEN I lift the piston!

WHEE! COLD WATER EVERYWHERE! In my face, on my chest, all over the bathroom floor as the happy little shower head sprays and sprays and sprays. See, what I SHOULD have done was wait until I was SEATED and the curtain was CLOSED before lifting the piston. But that would be the NORMAL way of doing it.

I swear to God, I'm my own Three Stooges comedy sometimes.

POSTSCRIPT: And if the above weren't enough, while I was putting the finishing touches on this post, sending out copies to various social media sites, etc...

I soiled myself.

Thank God for disposable adult undergarments (aka "diapers") but can you imagine the humiliation if I still worked in an office? With people?

SO, I'M A DYSFUNCTIONAL EXECUTIVE?

Just got home from my 4-month meeting with my neurologist. I seem to be doing OK as far as the motor symptoms are concerned. But the non-motor stuff seems to be on a downhill slide.

On the good side—I've lost weight. On the bad side—seems like the frontal lobes of my brain are involved in this thing now.

I described yesterday's fun in the shower with the nozzle and the wetness and the water going everywhere. That, and some other silliness of the recent past. He said this is suggestive of problems in the area of executive functioning.

The concept is used by psychologists and neuroscientists to describe a loosely defined collection of brain processes that are responsible for planning, cognitive flexibility, abstract thinking, rule acquisition, initiating appropriate actions and inhibiting inappropriate actions, and selecting relevant sensory information.

Uh-huh. What else?

Parkinson's disease causes problems with thinking and mood. These thinking disturbances occur early in the disease. The most common thinking deficits are in executive functions, which involve higher level thinking skills. These problems may lead to other difficulties such as, sadness and lack of impulse control.

Executive functions are a group of higher level thinking skills that involve planning and self-control. Most of the executive brain functions are controlled in the frontal lobes of the brain. This area of the brain is last to mature and the first to decline. Executive functions include the ability to develop strategies for a task that involves multiple steps, think ahead, switch from one task to another quickly, concentrate, control impulses, predict based on recognizing a pattern, think logically, choose what to do with incomplete information, pay attention to more than one thing at a time, decide things quickly and accurately, and change plans based on what is happening in the surrounding environment.

No shit?

The doc doesn't think it's actual dementia yet. Just executive dysfunction. But he did administer the Mini-Mental Status Exam (MMSE), and I scored a 22. I had trouble spelling the word "WORLD" backwards (I spelled it "WROLD" or, We're Old...) and I could only recall one of the three words I was supposed to remember. There may be some disagreement as to whether or not this denotes dementia.

Any score greater than or equal to 25 points (out of 30) is effectively normal (intact). Below this, scores can indicate severe (·9 points), moderate (10-20 points) or mild (21-24 points). The raw score may also need to be corrected for educational attainment and age. Low to very low scores correlate closely with the presence of dementia, although other mental disorders can also lead to abnormal findings on MMSE testing.

The rest of the visit was fine. I still fall when pulled backwards. I'm still remarkably non-rigid. I showed some tremor in my right hand that hasn't been noted before. And there are some new rules. Now, in addition to "not backing up" there's no more "bending over", which means that either the dogs will have to stand on their hind legs when I take off their collars when bringing them in from the yard, or else I have to sit down while doing it. I wonder which would work best.

Next visit, Feb. 15.

I HAVE ABSOLUTELY NOTHING TO SAY

I have absolutely nothing to say. How weird is that? I find myself staring at the computer screen, realizing that I haven't posted a single thing on this blog all day, and it dawns on me—I have absolutely nothing to say.

My mind isn't QUITE a blank. But it's close to it. I recorded and uploaded nine podcasts for work today. At this moment, a German shepherd is staring at me with an "I need to go outside" look in her eyes, but Gail said she'd take the pups out when she gets back from taking our neighbor to work. So I guess she can wait for a few minutes.

I have no new insights on anything today. Nothing new to say about my Parkinson's disease. Nothing interesting in the research news. Anything I could say about the political scene would be something I've said before, ad nauseum. Finished my podcasting at about 2:30, took a nap until shortly before 4. Now, I sit here, in the uncharacteristic position of having absolutely nothing to say.

Hah. Gail's home. She has the mail. Maybe something in there will spark a topic!

Nope. Nuthin' but crap.

The girlies are heading out into the cool, fall afternoon. I guess I'll go and sit in front of the TV and try to follow the plot line.

Oooh! Raven barked at something. Shiloh went to the window and started screaming. When she gets excited, she doesn't bark. Barking is for "alert". Screaming is for when she's all excited and stuff.

Typical afternoon. Is this what the French call "ennui"? Ah, the French. They have words for everything. Don't they just?

OLD PEOPLE? EEEEW! THEY'RE OLD!

I want to expand a little on my hypothesis that one reason there is no nationwide, publicized, "Jerry Lewis"- type effort to fund and find a cure for Parkinson's disease is—people don't want to look at older people.

To further this hypothesis, I submit two publications specifically targeting older folks.

First, let's examine the most recent issue of the AARP monthly magazine.

On the cover? A lovely photo of Kristen Bell (she's 30-years old), Jamie Lee Curtis (almost 52, selling yogurt on TV and looking great!), and Betty White (she'll be 89 in January, and in this photo it seems like her wrinkles have been airbrushed away).

They are featured in an article about "sex, love, and... staying hot!"

Hmmm. Most older folks would settle for affection, some good company and staying warm.

Let's open the magazine and look for old people.

Table of Contents page shows a 1971 picture of Milton Berle with Marlo and Danny Thomas. Nobody looking particularly old in THIS photo, and Uncle Milty and Danny have gone on to their maker. There's also a picture of Darryl Hannah, who will turn 50 in December. OK. Marlo is older, but well kept—and this is a 1971 photo. No old people here.

An ad for a rent-a-car establishment on page 9 shows a middle-aged couple. They're hiking up a mountain. He has gray fringes in his hair. She has white hair and nary a wrinkle. They are clearly youthful, vibrant and energetic.

I get winded hiking from the store to the car.

In the "You First" section on page 10, the five tips for the month "to enrich your life, starting now" are...

1. Drink wine.

2. Burn off some taxes (by installing insulation)

3. Catch a falling star (by watching a meteor shower in December)

4. Salute a vet. Veterans day, you know.

5. Go wild, by visiting your local zoo.

Hmm... nothing about things that I would think would be of concern to older folks—ways to avoid breaking a hip, for instance.

In the "What's New" section on page 13, the feature story is about how "old styles are back!" If you still have your glasses from the 1960's, they're COOL now! The picture... a young person wearing "cool" 60s glasses.

To be fair, there are articles with tips about handling diabetes, ads about not being too old to learn, some exercise tips, tips about claiming an adult child as a dependent, ads for "easy to use" cell phones, but nowhere in this issue—NOWHERE (outside of the picture of Betty White), is there an image of an older person looking like... AN OLDER PERSON!!! If you were a visitor from another planet and used the recent issue of AARP's magazine as a guide to human aging, you would be left with the impression that "older folks" are trim, thin, muscular, healthy, mountain-climbing, active and young!

Now, we turn our attention to a magazine you may have in your bathroom reading basket. A magazine that endeavors to sell stuff to older folks. The "Dr. Leonard's Catalog."

Let's look for older folks in here.

OK, an ad for a folding cane. Older folks use canes! But the photo with the ad? A woman, mid-30s, putting the cane into its pouch.

Ah! An ad for a triple-layer waterproof bed pad! We older folks sometimes, well, I wear "Depends" so I don't GET my mattress wet, but...

Oh. The ad has a picture of a woman in her early 40s. Sleeping comfortably. On the pad.

OH, WAIT! THERE'S AN OLD GUY ON PAGE 10! Oh. It's Jack LaLanne and he's selling his power juicer. Never mind.

On page 14, an ad for a "classic poplin driving cap" like the kind you see on the head of the old fart in the car ahead of you, driving 30 mph in the 55 mph zone with his right turn blinker on for the last five miles. But the ad has a photo of a guy, mid-30s, smiling like he's happy to be wearing an old guy's hat.

Now, who would use a "deluxe rollator"—a rolling walker that supports up to 250 lbs? According to Dr. Leonard, a beautiful young woman in her early 30s. That's who. And that guy in the "easy comfort lift chair" on page 21? 45-years old. Tops.

On page 20, a woman wearing a full upper-body "cotton terry bib" (cuz you know how messy we older folks are when we eat)? She's 30 if she's a day!

There's a "Carefree Comfort Floral Dress"—like the kind you'd see your gramma walking around the house wearing. Only on page 25 of the catalog, "Gramma" looks like she's 28.

I think I've made my point.

If we older folks can't stand looking at images of older folks in publications CREATED for older folks, then how can we HOPE that some day there might be a serious, nationwide awareness effort on behalf of folks with Parkinson's disease.

In the AARP magazine, all the older folks (the few I could find) were athletic and climbing mountains. With advanced Parkinson's disease, you sit staring blankly with drool on your chin, perhaps a tremor, you walk stooped and shuffling, you freeze in place, you fall. Hardly attractive. And there WERE no older folks (other than LaLanne shilling for his juicer) in the Dr. Leonard's catalog.

How in the hell can we get people to CARE about us when they don't even want to LOOK at us?

I'm open to suggestions.

THE DISEASE PROGRESSES

...although it seems kind of stupid to use the word "progress" in any form when discussing one's dance with Parkinson's disease.

I now find myself using my cane, even for simply moving around the house. This came about Monday when my addled midbrain was trying to negotiate the distance between Shiloh lying on the floor and the coffee table to see if I could pass through and I lost my balance, catching myself by planting both palms on the coffee table.

Gail looked up at me from the couch. "Where's your cane?"

"Over there," I said, pointing at its usual resting spot on the wall, knowing full well what she was driving at.

"Use it," she said. End of discussion.

And yeah, I find it helpful. I don't lose my balance as much. I rarely fall, but before using the cane in the house I lost my balance frequently. But this is such a small place, there's always something close by to grab onto.

MORE "PROGRESS"?

I wrote and recorded a podcast yesterday. You can hear all my podcasts, if you like, if you log into the Clinical Center's podcast site which is http://www.cc.nih.gov/podcast . Don't let the smooth, mellifluous voice fool you. I have audio editing software. I stumble over practically every sentence in the script. Once I get through a sentence without a mistake, I use it in the final cut. Sometimes, I have to splice together two or three attempts at the same sentence to get a complete sentence that doesn't sound like it's being read by Porky Pig or Popeye. But I get the job done.

The problem... where I'm seeing "Progress"?

There's a system in place for doing these things when you work from home. And in my current condition, it goes like this...

1. Get the raw audio of the person being interviewed. I have someone in Bethesda who does the actual interviewing. She sends me the audio and a transcript.

2. Decide what clips of the audio I wish to use for the podcast.

3. Using the audio editor, cut those clips from the raw audio, process them for volume, set aside.

4. Write my portion of the script. The easiest part of the endeavor.

5. Put together the whole script, e-mail it back to Bethesda to get final approval.

6. Once I get approval, I record my portion and produce the podcast bringing together all the elements—my voice, the interviewee, and the musical intro and outro.

7. Run the sound file through a program called "Levelator" to even out the volume.

8. Log onto my work FTP server and upload the finished soundfile and the transcript (for the hearing impaired).

9. The computer ladies put it on the test server. I give it all the once over and approve it. And they put it on the web.

Done.

Yesterday as I produced the aforementioned podcast, I kept getting "lost" along the way. I recorded my part of the script. Then I sat here looking at the screen, knowing I had to do SOMETHING... but damned if I knew WHAT!

I closed my eyes and concentrated. Blank.

Then it hit me. Gotta put my sound file into the multitrack screen of Adobe Audition, then add the soundbites from the interviewee.

Opened up the multitrack screen. Put my portion of the audio in place, as well as the opening and closing music.

OK, now what? Blank.

Closed my eyes. Thought real hard. Still blank.

AH! ADD THE SOUND BITES!

And where ARE these sound bites?

I have no idea. I puzzled and puzzled until my puzzler was sore.

AH! They're in the FLU PODCAST FOLDER!

There they were! I grabbed 'em and loaded them onto the multitrack screen.

Now, with everything right there in front of me, I was able to edit out all my stumbles and stutters and mumbles and "ummmm's" and pauses and hitches and put together a nice-sounding podcast. I mixed it all down to a single file.

OK, now what? Blank. My puzzler was still quite sore but I had to use it anyway. "Podcast recorded... must save it as .wav file." So I did. Brick wall again. OK... now what? "Must... put... .wav file into Levelator. Level sound!" Did it. The Levelator did its thing. OK... now what? Brick wall. Closed my eyes and thought real hard.

"Use Adobe Audition. Open newly created soundfile from Levelator. Save it in the "Files to be Uploaded" folder as

"CCRadio 102610." But not until you convert it into an .mp3 file."

OK, did it. Forgetting something... something... something... AH! PUT THE TRANSCRIPT IN THE FOLDER, TOO!

But wait, check the transcript and make sure you put the correct "run time" of the entire script cuz there's no way you could KNOW the total run time until the project is finished!

Did it. Now what? Blank.

Stared at screen. Screen offered no answer. Looked at the border collie at my feet. Raven didn't have a clue, either.

AH! GOTTA LOAD IT TO THE SERVER!!!

Logged on to the Clinical Center's FTP server, opened the podcast folder therein, opened up my "Files to Upload" folder, clicked and dragged the sound file and text file to the podcast folder on the Clinical Center's server.

Done. No. Not done. But what?

Ah! Write e-mail to computer gals, letting them know I've uploaded the podcast.

My neurologist describes the process I've just described as having trouble with executive functioning, which means the Parkinson's disease is now messing with the frontal lobes of my brain... the planning and decision making parts.

It's the same thing that makes me turn on the shower head with it laying on the tub floor, spraying water all over the bathroom floor. It's the same thing that almost made me pour freshly ground coffee beans into Gail's coffee cup. It's the same thing that makes me have to CONCENTRATE on which pills I'm taking. (5 pills in the morning means 5 SPECIFIC pills, not just the first 5 pills I can wrangle from the day's compartment in the pill box.) It's why I no longer handle the family finances.

And it's progressing.

Last night, Raven startled both of us with a VERY loud, sudden bark at something she saw outside. It so startled Gail she was nauseous. I didn't want my pill alarm at 8 pm to go off and startle her again, so at about 7:55 I got up and went into the kitchen to take my nitey-nite pills. I plugged in my cell phone to its charger, turned off my computer, went back into the living room, sat down, and remembered I had forgotten to take my nitey-nite pills.

And so it goes.

FUN WITH DEMENTIA

You know, as long as you're slipping into dementia anyway, you may as well have a little fun with it while you are still able. I suggest printing out this list and saving it for a day when you feel those first, subtle signs of dementia starting to creep in... that way you can refer to it because damned if you're going to be able to remember any of these suggestions.

1. If you're a man and you shave, leave about a silver dollar-sized patch of beard on one cheek or the other unshaved. (You choose the cheek.) When someone asks why you're doing that, you have a choice of responses.

    a.) "Oh, just in case. Just in case."

    b.) "Don't you worry about it. THEY know why."

    c.) Put a finger to your lips and say, "Ssssshhhh!" Then wink, point at the door, give the "thumbs up," and smile.

2. Every few minutes or so, ask your spouse, "When was the last time the dog was outside?" (Note: This is even funnnier if you don't have a dog.)

3. If your motor skills allow you to do so, bake a pie. Leave it on top of the refrigerator. Don't allow anyone to touch it. Refuse to answer questions about it for three days. Then, after three days if someone asks, shout at the top of your lungs, indignantly, "Because JESUS is coming back and it's an established FACT that he likes PIE! And I'll be DOGGONED if I'm gonna let this family be damned to eternal fire and damnation because nobody remembered to make a frickin' PIE!"

4. Put the TV on "The Weather Channel." If the forecast is for sunny skies, applaud wildly! If the forecast is for rain or snow, weep inconsolably.

5. Sit in your recliner all day. Don't say a word. Keep a blank stare on your face. Don't move. If it's a rocking recliner, feel free to rock but vary the speed of your rocking from very slow to very fast.

Don't respond to anyone. If you are offered food, eat it but don't say a word. Put the plate on the floor when you are done. Watch the evening TV programs with a blank expression and utter silence. Then, at bedtime, stand up, stretch, yawn and scratch yourself and say, "Well, another day, another dollar!" Then trundle off to bed.

This should be enough to get you started. And if you're lucky, these actions will get you shipped off to a nice residential care facility where—if you're not REALLY all THAT demented— you'll likely end up running the joint.

And remember, if you let Parkinson's disease kill your sense of humor, it'll take your humanity with it.

OBSESSING OVER ATROPHY

OK, so I'm obsessing over yesterday's discovery that I've had "diffuse brain atrophy" since 2007. Gail said so. She's the type of person who, when there's something wrong with her, will say, "Meh... let me know when it kills me." And I respect that. I really do.

"Arrow through my liver, you say? So that's that stinging feeling I noticed awhile ago. Oh well. Saw it off at the ends and I'll get the vacuuming done."

She's a tough, rugged, pioneer woman. Me? I'm the kind who wants to know every single detail about the condition because I figure the more I know the more I can ask my doctor, the more straight information I can get from him, and the better able I am to share the information with the people who read this blog who ALSO have Parkinson's disease and might learn something from MY experiences. So if that's "obsessing..."

318 BY BILL SCHMALFELDT

I guess I'm obsessing.

Anyway... it dawned on my as I was going to sleep last night that I had a brain MRI just a bit more than a year before the MRI that declared I had mild, diffuse atrophy of the brain. The earlier MRI, done on Feb. 8, 2006, came back with this report.

NORMAL MRI, Feb. 8, 2006 I don't have copies of the one they did in 2007.

 "FINDINGS: The brain stem and cerebellum are unremarkable. The internal auditory canals are synmetric. There are no temporal bone erosions. No mass, hemorrhage or infarct seen. The ventricles and cortical sulci are normal in size. There is no midline shift. The visualized paranasal sinuses are clear.

IMPRESSION: Normal cranial MRI."

So, 16 months later, almost to the day, I have ANOTHER MRI (after having the bone marker/frame anchor screws inserted into my skull) and the results are just a little different.

"FINDINGS: There is some mild atrophy of the brain. Normal arterial flow voids are present. There is no evidence of abnormal extraaxial fluid collection or midline shift. No abnormal areas of contrast enhancement are evident. Four screws are present in the outer table of the calavarium (fancy word for "skull" or "haid bone").

IMPRESSION: 1. Limited MR done prior to deep brain stimulus placement. 2. Diffuse atrophy"

So... being the logical person I am (or that I think I am, because who the fuck knows with my brain shrinking away to the size of a walnut), if THAT much change was apparent in 16 months, what's been goin' on under the ol' calavarium in the 41 months SINCE the MRI?

No way to know for sure, since I can never have another MRI because of all the metal and junk in my brain and chest (I am more machine than man).

But it does cause one to wonder. Or, "obsess," if you will.

SINCE I LAST WHINED ABOUT MY PD...

At 3:30 this morning, the calf of my right leg balled up on the side and would NOT loosen up. It was like having a golf ball on the outside of my right calf. Usually when that calf cramps, I can relax it by moving my foot in a certain manner. This morning, my calf told my foot to go fuck itself. In fact, it decided to turn my foot FOR me! I COULD NOT MOVE MY FOOT!

(See, this part is funny cuz Gail said, "Why don't you use the Ben Gay with the little massaging nubs on it? Maybe THAT will help.")

I BEAT MY CALF WITH MY FISTS, AND IT WOULD NOT LOOSEN UP!

I laid on my back, my right leg in the air, rubbing it, kneading it, smacking it with my closed fist, and IT WOULD NOT LOOSEN UP! In fact, it seemed to ENJOY it!

"COME ON, FAT BOY! THAT ALL YOU GOT? THAT ALL YOU GOT? BRING IT ON, YOU DICKLESS WONDER!!! HAHAHAHAHAHAHA!"

So, I got out of bed and tried walking on it. I had to walk on the outside of my right foot since my cramp had the foot twisted in that direction. Trying not to wake Gail, I walked back and forth slowly across the room.

Every time I got close to the door, Raven would get up — thinking that we were going out. I'd walk back toward my bed, she'd head back to her sleeping pad. Back to the door, Raven gets up. Back to the bed, Raven lies down.

Then went on for about 20 minutes. Then my calf yawned and said, "Well, I guess that's enough for now." It loosened up, I got back into bed, and fell back to sleep where I dreamed about doing dishes until I woke up at 7.

My calf muscle is STILL sore. And when I took a nap this afternoon, when I got out of bed, my calf cramped up again. But just for a moment.

"Just a reminder, fat boy," it said. "Just a reminder."

Oh, yeah…

When I went to get my second cup of coffee this morning, I took my cup over to the sink and turned on the faucet. "No!" the ever-decreasing working part of my intellect said. "Coffee no come from faucet. Coffee come from coffee pot. Pour coffee from pot, not sink."

Best advice I've had all day.

BAD BRAIN! DO DUMB THING!

Bad brain! You do dumb thing. Why you so dumb, brain? Why?

I didn't get back to sleep after all. I went back in directly after finishing the previous entry, thinking that since I had solved my memory problem I should be able to drift right off to sleep. No such luck. So, at 3:30 I got up and watched a half hour of Robot Chicken on "Adult Swim." My eyes felt heavy, so I went back to bed. Still no sleep. So, I got up at about 4:40, took the dogs outside, and decided to do some reading up on my sleep medication, the generic version of Ambien.

I was surprised by what I learned. I know it's meant for short-term use, by that I mean 7-10 days. They say that Prilosec shouldn't be used for more than 14 days, but on day 15 yer gonna have heartburn again if you stop taking it. But I have noticed over the past couple weeks that I don't get to sleep quite as quickly as I had when I first started the Ambien at 5mg, then had my dosage increased to 10mg. The literature on Ambien (zolpidem tartrate) says a person can build up a tolerance to the

drug after long-term use. And then, you might as well just plug
the pill into one of your ears for all the good it's going to do.
And continuing to use it can lead to a physical dependence. And
if you stop suddenly, you can get mild withdrawal syndromes —
like rebound insomnia and such.

Well, I decided that I would cut back on the Ambien starting
tonight. I would take half a pill a night for the next week, then
cut down to nothing.

Right now, it's a bit after 9 am. I just got scolded for not clearing
a tissue out of one of my PJ pockets. I'm supposed to "try
harder" to remember to check my pockets when I take my pants
off. Sure. I'll try harder. To remember. I just noticed a few
minutes earlier that the main reason (probably) that I couldn't
sleep last night (she just found another tissue in another pair of
pants… whoops!), was that I FORGOT TO TAKE MY NIGHT
TIME PILLS!!!

Oh, I retrieved them from their spot in the pill box. I put them in
the little green shot glass by my chair so I wouldn't have to get
up to get them when I heard my computer alarm go off — which
is the only way I remember to take a pill anymore. But I must
not have heard the alarm, because there they were… in the shot
glass by my chair about 20 minutes ago. Two little green 1mg
clonazepam pills which are supposed to KEEP me asleep and
help with the REM sleep behavior disorder, and one little white
10mg zolpidem tartrate (Ambien) pill — which is supposed to
PUT me to sleep.

This means a revision in my plans. I've already gone one night
without the zolpidem. I've had my sleepless night, promised by
the literature when stopping cold turkey. I may as well just use
the damn things like I'm supposed to use them… not as an every
night thing, but for nights when I can't sleep. Henceforth, after
giving my system a couple days to completely get this shit out of
my system (thankfully, the half-life of zolpidem is incredibly
short… given the fact that I took my last one 36 hours ago and
the half-life is 2.8 hours (more or less), my blood plasma level of

zolpidem should be somewhere around 0.01220703125 of a therapeutic dose by now. So if I'm gonna have withdrawal, I'm already having it. So, after about a week or so, if I reach 11pm and can't sleep by then, I'll get up and grab a zolpidem. The way I'm supposed to. (Might take a shot of Nyquil to help put me to sleep… the clonazepam (generic Klonopin) should keep me there once I get there.

Bad brain. Naughty brain.

Oh, and I forgot to snap down the lid on the coffee creamer when I poured my first cup this morning. Gail got my second cup and shook the creamer bottle. Creamer everywhere.

No more dumbass shit from you today brain. Please?

LEARN TO ENDURE STUPIDITY

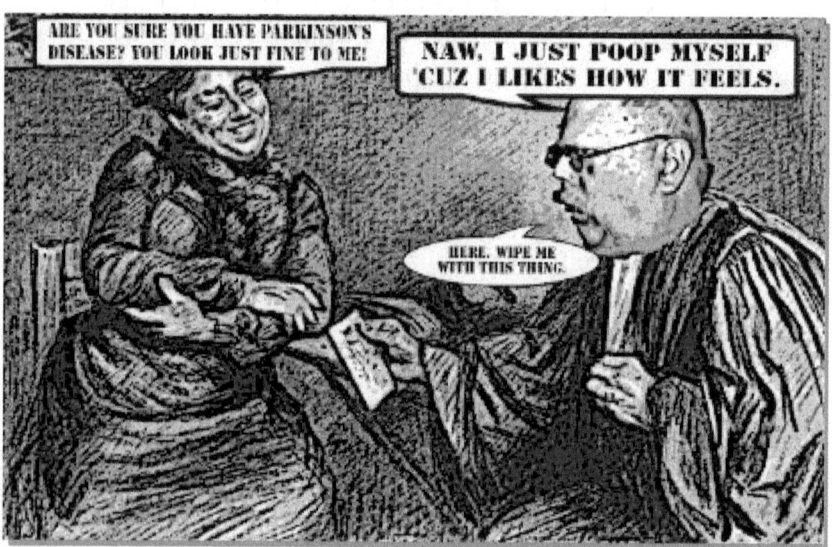

You will endure much stupidity early in the course of your waltz with Parkinson's disease. You will continue to encounter this stupidity when your meds are still working well in the middle course of the dance. I'm talking about the people who, when you tell them you have Parkinson's (or that someone you love has it), reply… "Oh, but he looks FIIIIIINE! Doesn't he look FIIIIIIINE? He looks FIIIIIIIINE!!! Are they sure it isn't something else?"

Now, from the person with Parkinson's (PWP) point of view, there are many snappy answers that used to rush to my lips when someone would tell me how great I looked. I will share them with you, if you promise to keep them to yourselves.

1. Thank you. I feel like shit.

2. Oh, that's just because my meds are working. You can hardly notice a thing when the meds are working. Tomorrow, I'll skip the meds so you can come watch me shake like a leaf and drool on myself.

3. I sure wasn't fine this morning, when I was so constipated from this PD that a large, backed-up bowel movement the consistency of a piece of moist drift wood had to break through an anus that wasn't up to the task because the PD wouldn't let all the proper muscles relax. It was like "The Incredible Hulk" busting out of a police station. And BLOODY! Look at my cell phone. I took pictures. Look. *LOOK*, God Damn You! *LOOK*!!!

When they say stupid stuff like, "Are they sure it's Parkinson's? You look FIIIIINE!"

1. Well, my neurologist says it is. Personally, I was hoping for Lou Gehrig's disease, but whatchagonna do?

2. We haven't explored the possibility of demonic possession yet. Could you recommend a good exorcist?

3. Nah. I'm just lying about having PD for the sympathy I get from all the hot babes at the swinger's clubs!

Caregivers, you will deal with stupidity like… "Are you sure it's PD? I saw him walking yesterday and he wasn't even limping."

1. Yeah? Well, I saw him first thing this morning before he took his meds and had to struggle to get out of bed. Then he knocked over his coffee cup and had to change his clothes. But we're happy that he can look so good for YOU! We wouldn't want to make YOU uncomfortable.

2. I know. I'm grateful for the times when his meds are working well and he can walk without falling.

3. I told him the same thing yesterday. We were at a movie and when we went in, he was just fine. But his meds wore off during the show and I had to help him out of his chair and hold his arm while we shuffled to the car. I told him, "Why are you always trying to make such a damn fool of yourself by having Parkinson's disease symptoms in public?" Then he started crying — that's another symptom, they cry easily — so I told him to quit being such a big damn baby and I just walked ahead of him and waited until he got to the car on his own. I mean, who wants to be seen with someone like THAT, right?

No, the best thing to do is to try to explain why your PWP looks good now but could change at any moment, until the person you're talking to gets a glassed-over look in his or her eyes and changes the subject to the elimination round of American Idol.

Now, one of the few good points of being more advanced in the condition is that people stop with the stupid remarks. Even when your meds ARE working, you can still tell that a Parky is a Parky at that stage.

But this is why, here at the advent of yet another Parkinson's Disease Awareness Month, we need a REAL awareness campaign to TEACH people about PD, especially in its early stages. With a little education, maybe we can stop some of the stupidity.

I will hold my breath waiting for that to happen starting…

Now!

THERE WILL BE DAYS LIKE THIS

There will be days when you can't really put your finger on what the problem is, but somethin' ain't right.

Slept like a baby last night… not as well as Saturday night, but I wasn't operating on 36 hours without sleep like I was on Saturday.

I'm not feeling unwell.

I'm not feeling anxious.

I'm not feeling sad, moody or depressed.

I'm just not — feeling.

Does that make any sense?

I joked around this morning with some of my former co-workers about how they were dealing with rush hour Monday traffic while I was sipping coffee in my jammies. The thing of that is — that's pretty much my life now. Other than my twice-weekly trips to physical therapy and our Sunday grocery shopping, that's the extent of my contact with the outside world.

And that's OK with me! I have no problem with that. It doesn't make me sad or happy or anything, really.

It is what it is.

It's just another day for Parky Bill. Some days are glorious. Some days are, "meh!" And some days are — nothing.

I did just have a nice lunch… some Jack Daniels pork riblets with white-cheddar mashed 'taters. So that was good. And I didn't choke on any of it, so that's good too.

Now I'm ready for a nap, which I can't have because the sleep instructions say I shouldn't do that if I want to sleep well at night. And they're DOCTORS. These are smart guys and gals. They don't give MDs to chimps. And if they ever start doing that, well, that's not a future I want any part of.

It's a day like any other day. Like every other day? Sorta. But not really. Just kinda.

Did any of that make sense?

I SLEEP, THEY STUDY

I sleep while they study me. That's why it's called a "sleep study." It was as simple as that. Well, not quite.

First I had to be covered with a buttload of wires. Then I had straps around my chest and abdomen to measure the "effort" of my breathing. They had electrodes on my scalp, electrodes on my face, a thing to measure the temperature of the air I breathed in compared to the air I exhaled. Electrodes attached to measure my heart rate. Electrodes to measure my leg movements.

By the time they were done, I was more electrode than man!

But the results were fairly good. I don't have sleep apnea. When I'm in REM Sleep, I take longer pauses in my breathing, but my pulse oximetry didn't dip any lower than into the 80s, so no need for a CPAP machine or anything like that.

The clonezapam is doing its job. I didn't lash out at or holler at anything last night, which is good. The tech woke me up at 5, just as I was cycling out of one REM sleep zone and getting ready to dip back into another.

So... one less thing to worry about. The clonezapam and

Ambien are doing a good job getting me to and keeping me asleep.

And if you listen very carefully, you can hear FM radio in your head when you're all wired up like this.

Kidding.

It's amazing, really. You would think it would be hard to sleep with all this crap stuck to you and in an unfamiliar bed. But the bed was comfy and after awhile you barely notice the electrodes.

Now there will have to be an extensive poring over the results, how much was I asleep vs. awake, how much time in REM, how much in the other stages, what does it all mean...

Still, glad I don't have sleep apnea — just some minor shallowness of breathing which I think is alleviated when I sleep in my adjustable bed with my head raised. And I'm glad this test is over with one less thing to worry about.

WHEN YOU WANDER INTO THE KITCHEN AND FIND YOURSELF STANDING AT THE COUNTER, WONDERING WHAT THE HELL YOU'RE DOING THERE, JUST STAY PUT. IT'LL EVENTUALLY COME TO YOU

As your disease progresses, if you are like 80 percent of Parkies, somewhere along the way you will lose your mind.

OK, that's not true. But a condition called Parkinson's disease dementia does affect a goodly portion of our number. It's like Alzheimer's to a degree, that is where protein strands gum up the brain's nerve synapses, but the memory problems aren't nearly as severe. You will not forget who people are. You might have trouble with name recall and such. Think of it this way... if you have PD-D, it's like your boss told you to file away a memo where you can retrieve it later. A couple days later he asks for the memo, and you don't recall where you filed it. "Did you file it under 'M' for 'memos'?" your boss asks. "Oh yeah, that's exactly what I did," you will say. See, it's not like Alzheimer's where your boss hands you a memo and you make a paper plane out of it and stuff it down the back of your pants. You can recall info, but sometimes you need to be reminded where you put it.

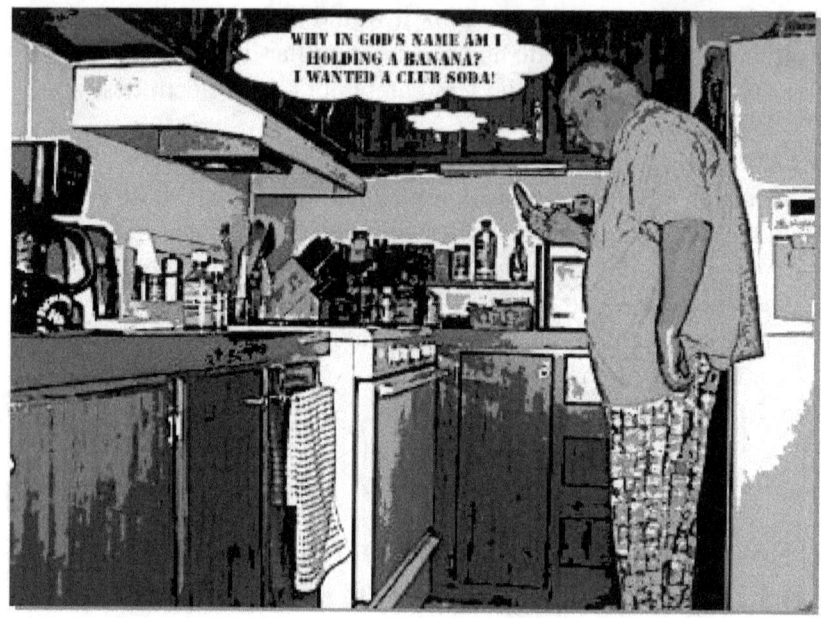

Another fun part of it is what they call "executive dysfunction." It's the whole decision-making thing, planning ahead. With PD-D, that part of your brain gets impaired. That's why on more than one occasion I've found myself standing in the bathroom with my toothbrush and a tube of "Preparation H" and had to think real hard about it. "This ain't right. This ain't right at ALL!" I have also nearly gargled with cologne. I have emptied a grinder full of freshly ground coffee into Gail's coffee cup. I have taken my pills (when I remember to take them,) dumped the leftover water from the glass onto the kitchen counter, then put the glass into the sink. Yesterday I slid a SD memory card into my computer's CD/DVD drive. Thankfully, I still have enough working neurons to have (after a nap) formulated a plan to put duct tape, sticky side out, on a long card, wiggled it around in the drive and pulled out the card.

So, my advice. When the time comes and you find yourself walking into your kitchen, reaching the counter, staring at it blankly and wondering just what the hell you came into the kitchen to get, just stand there for a little while. Try to let your mind go blank. It'll come to you. Eventually.

MORE WEIRD DREAM THEATER

As I've said time and time before, vivid dreaming is part and parcel of Parkinson's disease. Some are weirder and more vivid than others.

Gotta write this one down quick before the details fade.

I was on my way home from… somewhere. Japan, maybe. I was on an airplane. The pilot was Andy Griffith. Not the young, Sheriff of Mayberry, the doddering old one post-Matlock. He had a co-pilot. It wasn't Barney. Some time after we took off, Andy landed the plane on a railroad track so that the co-pilot could jump out of the plane, dash over to a locomotive that was waiting for him to be its engineer.

We took off again, and I couldn't help but notice we were flying real low the whole time. When we landed, Andy's wife let us in on the joke. We had been flying at normal altitudes the whole time, but she and Andy had videotaped a time when they went out in their private plane and flew under highway overpasses and around tree lines, etc., and fed the video into our windows which, as it turned out, doubled as video screens.

I got out of the airplane, and I was in a train yard. But this was OK… I'd just walk along the tracks until I got to my hometown of Clinton, Iowa where my Mom and Dad were waiting for me.

Along the way, I felt something bite my left forearm. By the time I got home and I took off my shirt, my whole right forearm was a bunch of pink and purplish pustules. Mom came over to look at them, but told me I had to be quiet because Dad was still sleeping.

Now, the pustules started wriggling and bursting from my forearm. I was starting to get them on the backside of my hand and on my chest and legs as well. Mom wondered if it was poison ivy.

But the little pink and purple pustules would wriggle out of my body and — pop! — float in the air like little balloons until they would pop into a little cloud of white dust. I guess they were spores, because Mom started getting them, too.

I managed to grab a couple of the little things as they popped out of my arm and examine them. They were light, air-filled little balloons, but if you looked closely you could see two little eyes and little mouths — sorta like grubs.

As more of them popped out of me, my skin started to clear up. So did Mom's. I rubbed my forearm and a bunch of white dust fell off of it. I decided I needed a shower. So I got out of bed and saw the bathroom door was closed. Turns out dad was in there. So, walking hunched over, I festinated (took a bunch of tiny running steps) and fell foward. Mom came to my assistance.

Then, I woke up.

And... SCENE!

IS IT HELPING, OR JUST BUSY WORK?

Physical therapy (Round II) starts a week from today. Sometimes I wonder if these treatments are actually supposed to be helping, or if they're just "busy work" to keep me occupied while I continue to deteriorate.

I just had my sleep study a couple nights ago and I'm glad I did it. I've wondered whether or not I have sleep apnea and it's good to know that I don't.

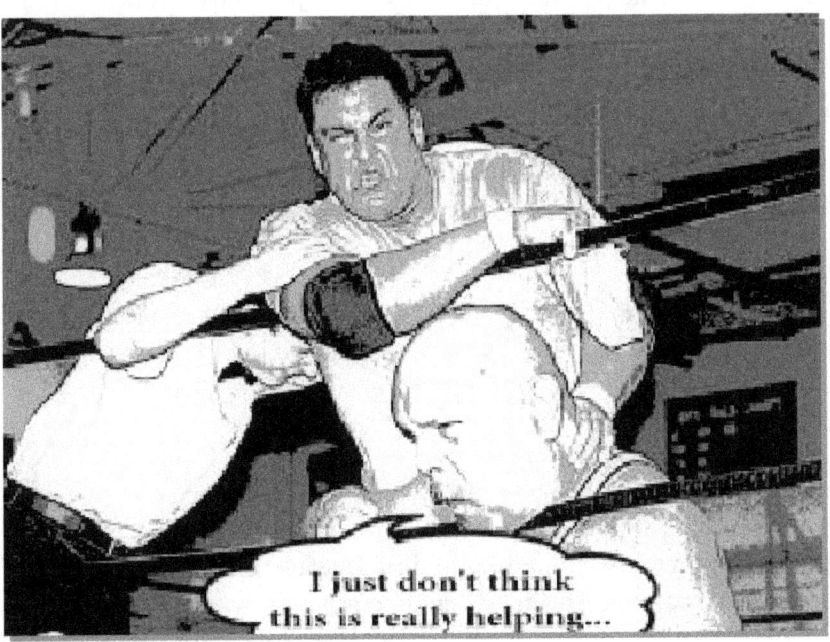

I just don't think this is really helping...

But Parkinson's disease is a PROGRESSIVE disease. If I could write a motto for the disease for newly-diagnosed folks to read, it would be this:

"It Is Going to Get Worse!"

So, I wonder what's the benefit to be had by "gait training" and "balance work" in Parkinson's disease.

Oh, don't get me wrong. I'm going and I'm looking forward to it. But I had a round of PT last year. They taught me tricks that I use to this day. But I still wobble. I still take tiny, shuffling steps unless I really concentrate and then when I take larger, longer steps I'm more likely to freeze in place. My balance is terrible. I still fall from time to time.

And, as far as I can tell from the literature on Parkinson's disease that's all pretty much "par for the course" for someone 11-years into this thing.

So… will the PT help in the long run? Or is it just "busy work?"

I guess it's all in how you look at it.

If you undergo a course of PT with PD and think that you're going to come out of it walking straight and tall with a long, quick stride and your problems are over… you're wasting your time.

If you go into it with the idea that the therapists KNOW what to expect in the course of your disease and their job is to give you the best tools to deal with your individual challenges, then it's well worth the time and effort.

Because of PT, I know how to turn around without falling. Because of PT, I can recognize when my center of gravity is beginning to tip to the point of no return. Because of PT, I no longer have a painful, frozen left shoulder.

No telling what I'll learn this time.

So, let me amend that motto I suggested earlier.

"It's Going to Get Worse. But There Will Be People to Help You."

Take advantage of every trick, every tool, every weapon you can put into your arsenal to fight this thing.

Nobody's gonna do it for you.

MY BRAIN IS BEING NAUGHTY AGAIN

My brain is being naughty again. This morning after doing my morning "business", I realized I would have to change the toilet paper roll before I concluded the paperwork. See, Gail has this charming habit of leaving about a turn and a half on an otherwise empty roll. That leaves enough tissue on the roll with which to blow one's nose, but nowhere NEAR enough to do that which needs to be done following "morning business," I don't CARE what those cartoon bears say in the Charmin ads. I NEED PAPER, and plenty of it!

So, I removed the rest of the tissue, blew my nose (mustn't be wasteful), and put the empty roll on the sink counter. I reached under the sink, got a fresh new roll, put it where it belongs, and concluded the paperwork to my satisfaction.

Got off the throne, looked at the empty roll on the sink counter, and did what every good boy who cleans up after himself does.

I tossed it into the toilet bowl.

"NO!" the shrill and thin, ever-harder-to-hear, still-working parts of my withering frontal lobes shrieked! "Toilet paper go in TRASH bucket! NOT in TOILET!"

So, I fished it out of the bowl, tossed it in the trash, flushed the bowl, finished my other morning ablutions and went to get dressed. Gail and I had an appointment this morning. We're getting blood drawn in advance of appointments with our family practice doctor next week.

I went into the bedroom, where I had already tossed everything I would need for the day onto my bed. Pants, shirt, absorbent adult undergarment, regular underwear (which helps keep the aforementioned absorbent adult undergarment in place), socks and belt.

The final act of getting dressed is the buckling of the belt. After which, I turned toward the bed… and there they were. My underwear.

"NO!" the faint, reedy, haunting voice of my shrinking, still-working executive functional brain area moaned. "Underwear go over diaper! Not on bed! Take off pants! Put on underpants!"

I did as I was told, met Gail in the living room, we got into the car and went to get our labwork done.

Then... breakfast.

WHOOPS! I DID IT AGAIN!

Whoops! I did it again. Lost my balance out in the yard, fell on my ass, bruising my right in the process. Were it not for the padding that my neurologist INSISTS that I get rid of down there, I could have been hurt more seriously.

Here's what happened.

See, most of the folks in this trailer park own dogs. Unfortunately, most of the dogs in this trailer park are SMARTER than their owners and they run free pretty much whenever they like. Two in particular have been a pain over the last couple days. They're nice, sweet dogs who wouldn't hurt a fly, but Raven thinks ALL dogs (other than Shiloh) are going to try to HURT her like that damn across the street has time after time. Shiloh just likes to scream and scream at them.

So, our dogs had an urgent need to use the yard. So, one at a time we took them out... Gail standing with a shovel to ward off intruders, me holding the leash and trying to keep each dog on task.

Raven had to posture and growl and bark and bristle, but she finally DID pee, then scratched the dirt to show she meant business. I had to get Gail's help to drag her back to the steps.

Shiloh wanted to run and sniff and run and sniff, and then the dogs came back, so Shiloh wanted to run over to where they were. She peed, turned and ran to the front of the yard. I turned as well... and lost my balance.

"YIPE!"

The sound came from Shiloh, not me. My falling "startled" her.

"Uh, Gail? A little help?" I asked from my back with my head on the downhill side of a gentle slope in the yard.

She helped me up, and that is when I noticed my knee hurt. My right forearm and hip hurt as well. So did my left shoulder.

Limped back into the house to assess damage. Just a small abrasion on the knee. Felt my hip and noticed a big lump right above the point where my femur attaches to the hip. The lump has gone down, but this baby still stings and is no doubt going to bruise up quite nicely.

I've always felt that when you fall off the world, the best thing to do is get right back on it. So Gail and I went shopping.

WHY WE NEED BETTER PD AWARENESS

Gunther von Hagens, the anatomist behind the "Body Works" plastinated corpse exhibitions, announced the other day that he has , he's had it two years, he's noticed his hands getting clumsier and his speech getting more difficult, and therefore by his own calculations he will be dead in seven years.

HOGWASH!

First of all, his symptoms for two years post-diagnosis at his age ain't all that bad!

Secondly, YOU DO NOT DIE OF PARKINSON'S DISEASE! You die WITH it. You CAN die from COMPLICATIONS of PD, like inhaling a milk shake because your epiglottis didn't close in time, or falling and cracking your skull, or breaking a hip and lying around in bed and getting a pulmonary embolism or pneumonia. But it won't be the PARKINSON'S that kills you.

And the fact that this man, an anatomist, calls a press conference widely covered by the European press which, like their American counterparts, wouldn't know a "fact check" if it bit them on the ASS, and says "I will be dead in seven years..." really hurts our efforts to get accurate information out there.

Imagine the impact a statement like that has on a less-than-well-informed Parkinson's patient or his/her caregiver!

"Goodness! HE has Parkinson's! He says he'll die from it in seven years. And he's a DOCTOR of some sort. What are MY chances?"

Bullshit, bullshit, bullshit, BULLSHIT! For God's Sake, look at Michael J. Fox. 20 years post diagnosis and he still plays golf! Even poor little me, 11 years post-diagnosis and I'm still RELATIVELY functional and CERTAINLY not planning to DIE any time soon.

But... I knew people would believe von Hagens. If you follow me on Twitter **(and if you don't, what's your problem? http://twitter.com/ParkyBill)** , you see this little discussion I have going with a perfectly well-meaning, probably very nice little real estate attorney who reposted the von Hagens story last night. I responded by saying that nobody dies FROM Parkinson's and we should not help this guy spread his drama.

She responded that I should walk a mile in von Hagens' shoes before judging him.

Well, that got my dander up a bit. Lady, how many miles can you walk in 11 years, cuz that's how long I've had this thing. So, I pointed her to the blog post from earlier in which I listed several stories where the reporters write that von Hagens is dying, has been given seven years to live, etc. and etc. She responded.

"We have no way of knowing if he is right or wrong."

MISSING THE POINT ENTIRELY!!! How can he self-diagnose when and how he will be incapacitated? Most people with PD are older than I was when diagnosed, but I've remained on the job for 11 years (I am filing for early disability retirement, but that's because executive dysfunction and speech problems are setting in). Again, the less-than-well-informed Parky or caregiver sees this and says, *"Holy God! He only has SEVEN YEARS?? And he's YOUNGER than I am. Martha! Call the funeral home!"*

So, I wrote back asking if she even bothered to read the link I sent in which the news media was reporting that "Dr. Death Says He's Dying." She responded.

"Von Hagens isn't responsible for what the press is saying about him."

AGAIN, MISSING THE POINT!!! The HEADLINES say "VON HAGENS DYING FROM PARKINSON'S!" Is von Hagens out there CORRECTING this horrible misconception? Is he holding press conferences to say, *"The reporters misunderstood what I said. I merely said I expect to be totally incapacitated in seven years, based on my own research (which is STILL bullshit)"*?

No. He isn't. Because he's a Drama Queen!

So, I sent this very nice lady quotes from the selected news articles, all of which say "von Hagens claim he is dying from Parkinson's." These, again, are articles that will be read by less-than-sophisticated folks who know little to nothing about their illness other than that they've been diagnosed with PD. *"OH NO! SEVEN YEARS? And then you're DEAD? Or TOTALLY INCAPACITATED? I've had it for 5 years! Martha! Call the nursing home!"*

This very nice lady, whose husband has PD, has had it for 8 years, who says she KNOWS PD isn't fatal, still defends von Hagens and his headline grabbing scare mongering. I suggested that I wouldn't lecture her about real estate law, and she shouldn't lecture me on Parkinson's disease.

@ParkyBill Never said a word lecturing you about PD & you're really being a jerk;huz having it 8 yrs doesn't make me an expert

& I don't judge others

Well, if trying to stop the spread of disinformation makes me a
jerk, then I'm a jerk. You would think someone with a spouse
with PD would understand that. It's not a case of "judging
others." It's a matter of telling the truth.

Those who prefer the lie to the truth? Damned if I know what to
say about them.

You want ACCURATE info about PD, including prognosis, life
expectancy, etc.and etc.

I find it's best to KNOW what you're talking about before
shooting off your mouth about something. Don't you?

So, I offer this "open letter" to Professor von Hagens...

Sir:

**We all love your "Body Worlds" displays, even though some
of them show you to have pretty quirky if not downright
"questionable" tastes. Posing your plasticized corpses in
sexual positions, for instance. I mean, if you're the corpse
and the other corpse is attractive, who wouldn't like THAT?
But is that something we want the KIDS to see?**

**No, sir, my beef with you is that since you announced several
days ago that you have Parkinson's disease, you've had it for
two years, therefore by your own research *you have seven
years to live,* people are reporting this supposition of yours as
if it were fact! You need to knock that crap off. People read
these stories and think their doctor has been lying to them!
"I HAVE PARKINSON'S! AND THIS GUY'S A DOCTOR!
IF HE'S DYING, THEN SO AM I!!!!"**

**You're scaring people. Even more than you do with your
basketball playing corpses with their skulls split open to show
their brains.**

"Your Own Research?" **Sir.** As an employee of the National Institutes of Health, I have pretty much the entire National Library of Medicine at my disposal. As a person who has been dancing with this exquisite little inconvenience for 11 years and hasn't died yet, let ME tell YOU what MY research says.

Parkinson's disease is NOT fatal!

I'm sorry, did you miss that? I'll say it a little louder and cite some examples of eminent scientists who agree with me.

<u>Parkinson's disease is not fatal,</u> but it reduces longevity. The disease progresses more quickly in older than younger patients, and may lead to severe incapacity within 10 to 20 years. Older patients also experience freezing and greater declines in mental function and daily functioning.

<u>Parkinson's disease is NOT fatal.</u> It is NOT infectious. It CANNOT be transmitted to other members of the family.

<u>Parkinson's alone is not fatal</u> , but it can bring about events, such as choking and falling that may become deadly. It progresses slowly. The symptoms may make daily routine activities difficult.

<u>Although Parkinson disease</u> itself is not fatal, it increases the risk of dying from PD-related complications, such as falls, choking, or pneumonia.

Again, it is important to remember that progression is slow and that available medications may manage symptoms for a significant period of time.

And THESE snippets are just from non-scholarly sources that are available to EVERYONE.

So, sir, you need to stop telling everyone with a microphone and a note pad that you're "dying" from "Parkinson's." These are REPORTERS you are talking to. As such, they're not USED to doing research and fact checking. They will write down whatever you say as if it was God's word from the Mount, print it verbatim or put it right on the air as if it were true.

Terminally-ill 'Dr. Death' to display own body

The German anatomist dubbed "Dr. Death" who has turned stomachs worldwide preserving and displaying dead bodies, said Wednesday he is terminally ill and plans to exhibit his own corpse.

Gunther von Hagens, 65, told the Bild mass circulation daily he is suffering from incurable Parkinson's disease and intends to have his dead body put on display to "welcome" visitors to his exhibition.

BODY WORLDS Creator, Anatomist Gunther von Hagens Reveals His Two Year Life-Changing Battle With Parkinson's Disease

"This disease has led me to an existential bewilderment. According to my research the average duration of the disease and disability is about nine years. Since I was diagnosed two years ago, I can realistically expect seven active working years before I become totally incapacitated," he told the assembly.

Dying Body Worlds inventor wants to become part of exhibit

Gunther von Hagens, the German anatomist who created the controversial Body Worlds exhibition of preserved corpses, has announced that he is dying and wants to become part of the exhibit after his death.

Physician, plastinate thyself: von Hagens reveals he's dying – and wants to be preserved

His preserved dead bodies have spooked, captivated and disgusted the public. Now, Gunther von Hagens, pioneer of the controversial Body Worlds exhibitions, has added future plans to display his own corpse after being diagnosed with Parkinson's disease.

Plastic bodies Prof Gunther von Hagens dying

A MACABRE professor who preserves human bodies with plastic said he is dying and will go on display at one of his grim exhibitions.

Anatomy expert Prof Gunther von Hagens, who caused outrage in Tyneside when he displayed an exhibition of dead bodies in Newcastle, said he has been battling Parkinson's disease for two years.

The German-born pathologist has been given seven years to live and wants to have his body preserved using his plastination technique.

'I'm dying, so put MY body on show': 'Dr Death' Gunther von Hagens plans grim farewell in one of his own corpse displays

65-year-old reveals he has Parkinson's Disease and seven years to live

The professor behind a shocking exhibition in which corpses are displayed stripped of their flesh has revealed he is dying – and wants his body to be put on display.Self-styled 'Dr Death' Gunther von Hagens is suffering from Parkinson's Disease and has been told he has seven years to live.

HUH? *WHAT?* WHO gave you "seven years to live?" What neurologist in his right mind would TELL you such a thing? Dude… you have PARKINSON'S disease. Not pancreatic cancer, not esophageal cancer, not mesothelioma. You have a CHRONIC, but not FATAL disease! Even by your own description, after two years, it's not even that BAD yet!!! I've had it 11 years, brother, and I'm still standing upright and exchanging oxygen for carbon dioxide and stuff.

If you told reporters that Parkinson's disease results in growing a fucking *UNICORN* horn, they'd write "Body World Creator to Grow Unicorn Horn."

It helps if you know what you're talking about, sir. And you, clearly, do not in this regard.

I do, however, admire your desire to plastinate yourself and include your corpse in your collection... unless it turns out to be some sort of Twilight Zone episode where the museum closes at night and all the corpses come to life to tear your plastinated corpse apart, leaving the security guards scratching their heads in the morning.

And none of this dampens my desire to be part of your display myself some day. Maybe you and I could be in a classroom setting. My corpse could be the teacher. You would be the student at a desk. Your opened skull would be empty because I would be holding your plastinated brain teaching it about Parkinson's disease and why it's important NOT to scare people who already are already worried and concerned about their conditions.

That would be cool.

EXECUTIVE FUNCTION, WHAT'S YOUR FUNCTION?

It's not like Alzheimer's. The mechanism is similar, but the results are different. Parkinson's disease dementia does affect the brain's cognitive processes, mainly in the area of executive function. See, when you have trouble with **Executive** Function, it doesn't necessarily indicate a problem with **MEMORY**.

The official definition of EXECUTIVE Function is...

Executive functions are necessary for goal-directed behavior. They include the ability to initiate and stop actions, to monitor

and change behavior as needed, and to plan future behavior
when faced with novel tasks and situations. Executive functions
allow us to anticipate outcomes and adapt to changing situations.
The ability to form concepts and think abstractly are often
considered components of executive function.

I used to have me all KINDS of executive function! Time was
when I could go from writing a podcast to answering the phone,
to dealing with a media query, back to the podcast writing,
answer a question from someone else, look up a file on the
computer, get back to writing the podcast and not miss a beat.
Those days, sadly, are behind me.

It's called "executive   *dysfunction*" and it's part of the colorful
tapestry that makes up Parkinson's.

Executive function is an interrelated set of abilities that includes
cognitive flexibility, concept formation, and self-monitoring.
Assessing executive function can help determine a patient's
capacity to execute health care decisions and with discharge
planning decisions. With executive function impaired,
instrumental activities of daily living (accounting, shopping,
medication management, driving) may be beyond the person's
capacity even though memory impairment is mild. The person's
capacity to exercise command and self-control, and to direct
others to provide care, becomes diminished. Executive
dysfunction is one element in the DSM-IV criteria for the
diagnosis of dementia and occurs in all dementing diseases.
NOTE: Patients with impaired executive function need not have
impaired memory.

It's precursor to PD-D. It makes it very, very difficult to drop
one task, go to another, then pick up again.

There's more fun involved, too!

I just went over to mute the TV so I could record the Rec
Therapy podcast for my work. One of my dogs was pointing at
the door like she wanted to go out. So I pointed the TV remote at
the door and hit mute. I wondered why I could still hear the TV.

Then I realized the remote has to be pointed at the TV, not the door.

I've already written about these, but the other day, while taking a pill, I put the pill under the stream of water instead of putting the water in the glass. More recently, I filled the glass, took the pill with the water, dumped the water on the counter, then put the glass into the sink.

Also today, I'm standing at the sink, getting my 10am Stalevo 100. I see one of those little flies one sees around rotting fruit. I ask Gail if she can see it. I look again, it's gone. That's when a big housefly landed on the screen outside, then flew away. It was 27-degrees outside. That had to be one hardy fucking fly to be out buzzing around in sub-freezing weather.

I've been seeing flies a lot lately… usually out of the corner of either eye. They buzz by and vanish.

Yessiree PETE!

In the meantime, I'm speaking in a series of grunts and hand signals that, thank God, my bride of 23 years understands. God, how I love her.

Not a good day. Not at all. But the odd thing is, I'm in a good mood. Funny thing, that.

HOW TO TELL IF THE BUGS ARE REAL

While taking my shower this morning, it sure seemed like there were more than the usual amount of bugs in the bathtub with me.

(BTW: The "usual number" is "03.)

But I've been having these "illuuuuuuuusions" lately (some might call them hallucinations), a lot of them involving flies, bugs and other creepy-crawlies. Usually, I'll be sitting here at the computer and one of those little flies you see around rotting bananas sometimes will buzz by.

How can you tell if that fly is real?

If you look right at it and it isn't there, it wasn't there in the first place.

Last week, a big horsefly, about an inch in length, landed on the outside screen of our kitchen window.

How do I know whether or not THAT fly was real?

It was 27 degrees outside. A REAL horsefly would be frozen solid, not landing on the outside screen of my kitchen window only to disappear when I looked directly at it.

Back to this morning's shower.

I was noticing a lot of black, moving little dots on the bathtub floor. When I would look directly, they would vanish.

This means one of three things.

1. I was dirtier than usual when I took my shower, and the black dots were crud being washed off my body.

2. I had more bugs on my skin than usual, and they were washed down the drain before I could get a good look at them.

3. They weren't there in the first place.

Now, a lot of this depends on how clean of a house you have. Gail would cut all our throats if we let things get dirty enough for bugs to thrive. If you live in a house that usually has bugs and you're not sure if you're seeing real ones, try crushing one. If you have crushed bug on your hand, it was real.

Now lizards... different story all together. I saw a lizard dart under my shower seat once. I decided I didn't really NEED to get up and look under my seat as we don't live in Florida any more. (Did I ever tell you how I once discovered an actual scorpion in my dishwasher when we lived down there? And that was BEFORE I was diagnosed with Parkinson's disease.)

NICE. I JUST FELL. AGAIN.

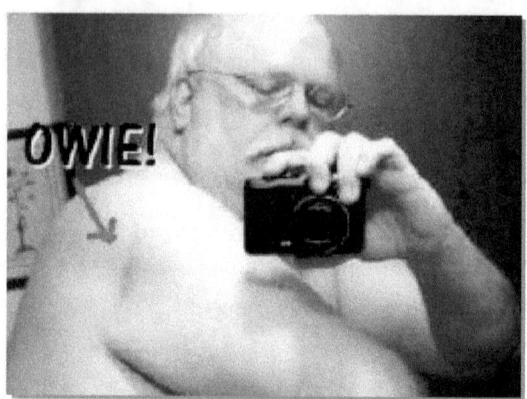

Moments after the last post, Gail left to take our neighbor to work. My German shepherd Shiloh started hounding (hah!) me about being taken outside. She is relentless, so I finally got up to take her out. Put on my shoes, disconnected the choke collar from the leash and turned to where I thought she was, but she had circled around to my other side. This surprised me, I lost my balance, fell into the hallway, bashing my right upper arm and right side of my tummy into the corner of the wall at the entrance to the hallway.

Bruising up nicely, thank you.

I think I'll let Shiloh sit outside until they have to chip ice off of her.

WELL, THAT WAS HUMILIATING!

My first clue that the brain wasn't clicking on all cylinders today was when I was shaving and I caught a brief glimpse of Gail

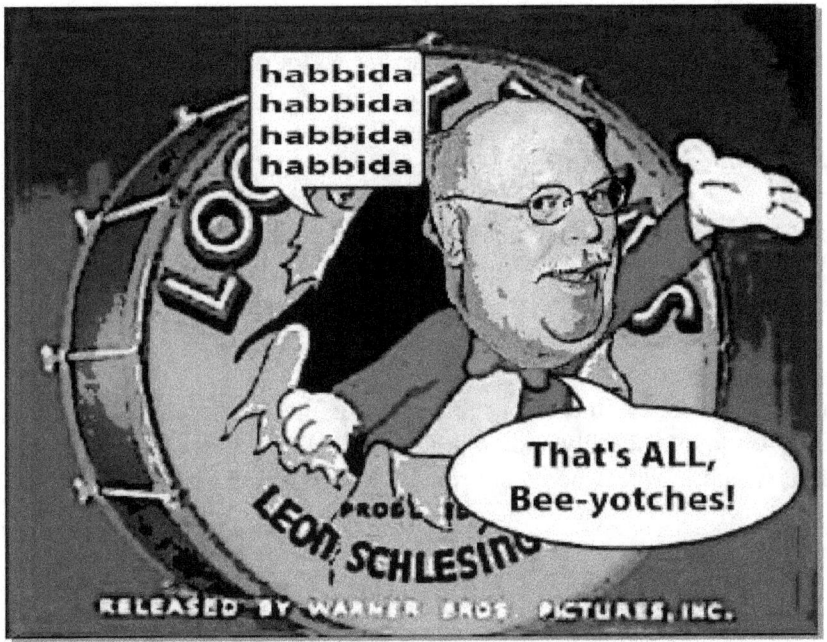

standing just off to my left. I turned. No Gail. I imagined her being there.

Then, there was our usual Monday teleconference where we all talk about our ongoing projects and such. At first, I spoke slowly and carefully and was able, I think, to communicate what I've been up to here in the Elkridge, MD branch of the NIH Clinical Center Office of Communications, Patient Recruitment and Public Liaison.

Usually, after I say my piece in these things, I try to just lie there and listen on the blue
tooth and not make an ass of myself. But then our Presidential Intern *(or whatever her title is)* mentioned that her next assignment would be with my old pals Calvin, Wally and Joe over at the Office of the Director's NIH Radio department.

All I wanted to say, when Sara said she would be in good hands over there, is "I concur. They're great guys and you'll learn a lot."

What came out of my mouth was something more like,   *"habbida habbida habbida habbida...."*   I paused to let my brain reset as the teleconference sat in silence. Tried again.   *"Habbida habbida habbida habbida..."* and I just gave up. Finally, during a pause, I managed to say, "What I was trying to say was, "I concur.""

Jesus, how embarrassing. I mean, Gail's used to it. When I can't talk, I can generally get my point across using hand signals or she knows what it was I was trying to say. Try doing that on a phone conference.

Oh, Parkinson's. Thou art a bastard. You've already stolen my ability to move smoothly and walk unaided. Now you've stolen that of which I used to be most proud... my speaking ability.

A SCARE I CAN'T REMEMBER

Might have to talk to the doc about this thing again.

I mentioned previously that I woke myself up getting out of bed the other day. Almost stepped on one of the dogs.

Yesterday, Gail informed me that it was about 5:30 in the morning (just about the same time I tried to crawl out of bed a few days earlier) I gave out with a little girlish scream as if something were scaring me. Or trying to touch me with a booger. Or something.

Damned if I know. I don't remember the dream.

At any rate... me no likee!

CHAPTER 7

End Game – In a Manner of Speaking

HANGING IT UP – THE PROCESS BEGINS

After talking it over with Gail and giving it a lot of thought, I've decided to begin the process that will result in my taking disability retirement under the Federal Government's disability retirement plan.

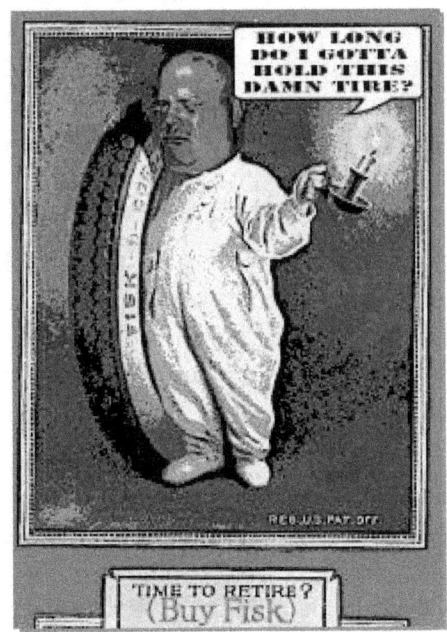

I've printed out the excellent form the Parkinson's Action Network provides and have asked my neurologist to fill in the parts he's required to fill in. I've also asked for the records that the Office of Personnel Management say he will have to provide. I've made the same request of the good folks at Vanderbilt who plugged holes in my brain three years ago. Odessa says she'll have a release for me to sign and get the stuff right in the mail.

In my note to my boss, I said...

I wanted you to be the first to know (other than Gail, of course) that today I've gotten the ball rolling towards seeking disability retirement. I know that it's a lengthy process, so I wanted to get the paperwork in play while I still have a few crispy cookies in the cookie jar, so to speak. I've asked my doctors (here and in Nashville) to provide me with the information I'll need to make a formal application, and I expect to do so relatively soon.

You've no doubt noticed a decline in my production and performance. In addition to the motor symptoms of Parkinson's disease (the walking, the balance difficulties etc.), the disease has started to interfere with my brain's executive functioning (planning, decision-making, task-shifting). You've heard how it affects my speaking, and I've found myself making silly, idiotic mistakes – mostly non-work related, like pouring coffee grounds into Gail's cup or trying to make coffee without adding the water, and a mess of other stuff I write about in my blog. In an e-mail I sent you earlier today, on proofing it, I saw that I had typed the word "the" three times in a row. I'm forgetting things, I'm easily distracted, I'm beginning to experience auditory and visual hallucinations (nothing scary, stuff like rabbits where there are none and waking up to the sound of an old fashioned phone ringing). My attention span is suffering and I'm losing my ability to concentrate. And most afternoons I get hit with a wave of fatigue that requires me to take a nap.

Meeting with my neurologist two weeks ago, he said that this is a sign of "executive dysfunction" which is one of the early harbingers of "Parkinson's disease dementia." He doesn't think it's "frank dementia" just yet, but it's progressive, it's insidious and it creeps up on ya!

I'm not looking for sympathy or for anything other than you've already so generously provided. If my condition were to stabilize, I'm sure I could sit here for years and continue to crank out podcast after podcast. But I don't want to wait until I really start to stink up the joint before making a graceful exit. I don't wanna be a Brett Favre, in other words. :)

I'm sure I'm still good enough to take the snaps and get the ball down the field. But I don't want to wait to be TOLD I have to hang it up. I wanna go on my own terms. It means a cut in salary—I'll get roughly 2/3 of my top 3 yearly incomes, averaged. I don't expect this to happen until summer or early fall, the way it takes these guys forever to make decisions. I also have to file for Social Security Disability Insurance, but it's not necessary that I be approved to get disability retirement.

So, I'll keep y'all informed and let you know how it goes. This will be a long, strange trip indeed.

AND WHEN THE END COMES, AS IT MUST

I've seen their commercials on TV from time to time, and I've always said to myself that I should get more information about it. Now, I have. And when the day comes—as it surely must— where I shuffle off this mortal coil, my body will be donated to medical science through a company known as "Anatomy Gifts Registry."

I just filled out a lengthy application, with repetitive questions, and put it in the mail. If I'm accepted, Gail and I will each get embossed cards that explain what to do with my mortal husk once my eternal soul has winged its way wherever it's going. Here's what we're supposed to do...

Once a death occurs and is pronounced, contact AGR ... An AGR representative will verify the consent method ... and will immediately make arrangements with a mortuary transport organization to pick up the body and transport it to our facility. Do not call a funeral home. AGR has contracted organizations throughout the US that are familiar with AGR's process.

AGR, will make timely arrangements to register the death with your State Department of Vital Records.   Experienced AGR personnel can assist family members with obtainingthe certified copies of Death Certificates.

Not that I'm expecting that happy day of blissful escape to come anytime soon, but it never hurts to be prepared.

Since I was diagnosed in 2000, it's been my intention to donate my brain after I die for furtherance of the Parkinson's disease knowledge base. By donating my entire body, hopefully there is stuff to be learned about PD's effect on the rest of the body as well. And this agency has a new, state of the art facility. So it's not like I'm gonna get segmented at Satriale's Pork Store, like on "The Sopranos"!

The advantages of this new establishment are not limited to only the scientists and doctors utilizing the facility. The donors and their families, whose participation has helped advance science and medicine, will also benefit. Participation in the AGR program, throughout the many years it has been in existence, has always translated into being part of a new and innovative way of helping to advance medicine and allowing for donors to make an impact on the health and welfare of millions of people. The development of this new teaching tool will further advance medical and scientific learning and acknowledge and highlight the generosity and sacrifices made by donors and their families.

Whatever isn't used in research is cremated and sent to your next of kin.

If this sort of thing appeals to you, check out the website. I think it's a great way to leave a lasting legacy. And it's comforting to think that I'll still be assisting in the search for a cure even after I'm playing a harp on a cloud somewhere.

STUFF AND NONSENSE

Here's where we report on stuff that's happened over the last few days that don't merit their own post but are marginally interesting nonetheless.

Gave myself three self-administered PD symptom assessments over the last day. They all say about the same thing.

In the PDQL (Quality of Life), my total score is 80. Higher scores are better. The best info I can find online is that the overall PDQL of patients in group 1 (independent, activities a bit slower) had a mean score of 137, patients in group 2 (slightly dependent, activities considerably slower) had a mean score of 118, and patients in group 3 (dependent, needing help or care) had a mean score of 98. So I guess I'm in the lower end of group 3, although I do tend to take pretty good care of myself in such tasks as dressing, hygiene, etc. I'm slow, but I can still do it.

The PDQUALIF, which oddly enough ALSO means Parkinson's Disease Quality of Life), I had a total final score of 58.66 which places me right over the edge Class IV in the 5-point UPDRS. (IV= Symptoms on both sides of the body and moderate difficulty walking.) Class V means bedridden.

AND, I checked myself out on the Webster Scale, which gave me a final score of 19. That's at the upper edge of "moderate" with "Severe or Advanced" starting at 21.

The last time I took the PDQ-39 (Parkinson's Disease Quality of Life Questionnaire), I had a final score of 55.055, which is well over the line between H&Y III and IV.

So that's where we are today.

Got a call from my boss this morning warning me that she was filling out my yearly eval, and to support my request and her support for my disability retirement. She said that meant she would have to mark me as "unsuccessful" in a few areas and she felt crappy about it. I told her I figured it would have to be done what's the point of getting a disability retirement if you can do all your duties "satisfactorily." After all, my last two evals were "exceptional." I know there are things I can't do that I used to be able to do. No hard feelings.

Took the dogs out last night. Raven first. She did her business, including #2, and came back into the house. Shiloh, however, diddled around and diddled around and diddled around acting like she was GOING to poop, but didn't and eventually came back to the house. I sat down on the recliner. Raven took a spot in front of Gail's feet by the couch and stared at me. A few minutes later, I hear…

"grrrrrrrrrrr……"

I look down, and Raven's giving me the "stink eye." I asked what was wrong, what did I do, what did I forget….

I FORGOT TO GIVE HER THE TREAT SHE GETS FOR

GOING POOPIE!!!

It took her awhile, but she forgave me.

STICK A FORK IN ME

March 13, 2011

At the stroke of midnight this morning, I went from a pay status to the retired rolls.

Huzzah?

The next order of business will be to do what I can to get my Social Security Benefits started. Shouldn't be a problem. I'll re-send everything I sent before along with the letter I got Friday from OPM with this relevant statement...

"In reviewing your medical records we have found you to be disabled for your position as a Writer due to Advanced stage of Idiopathic Parkinson's Disease."

I need to withdraw my funds from the TSP that I have been pretty much ignoring... between that and the unused annual leave that will show up in one future paycheck or another, we might have close to enough to pay off the car, which will eliminate $582 from our monthly outgo.

I've already sent forms to OPM proving that I had filed, but was turned down for SSDI. Now I have to do it again, and this time, cuz I'm no longer on a work status, it should go through.

But many and mysterious are the ways of the government.

I know.

I used to work for 'em!

AFTERWORD

Like I said at the outset of this book. I'm Serving Notice!

I plan to get in contact with as many Parkinson's advocate groups as possible and offer my services as a speaker. I'm still loud, although slurry and stuttery. And I'm still a decent writer.

I am going to try my level best, using whatever energy I have left for however long I have to raise awareness about Parkinson's disease, and to raise money to fund the research.

If we wait for the government, it ain't gonna get done. Now that the conservatives are back running the show (at least in the House of Representatives, although in the White House and Senate, they roll over on their backs and shoot a little jet of "fear pee" when a Republican walks by), it's gonna be a long time before we get resumed federal funding for embryonic stem cell research. Religious superstition will once again take precedence over medical science.

My job will be to convince as many people as I can that this is NOT a natural occurrence of aging, and that even though most of my fellow Parkies are elderly, they deserve a good quality of life. Most of all, I want to convince folks that if they fund research, the day may come – sooner rather than later – when a definitive CAUSE is found for what they currently call "idiopathic" Parkinson's disease. Once they know for sure what CAUSES it, it's easier to work on ways to KEEP IT FROM HAPPENING!

My job will be to present Parkies as alive, vibrant, intelligent folks who are worthy of support. If I'm successful, perhaps someday we will have a MEANINGFUL Parkinson's Awareness Month where the media FOCUSES on our plight and WORKS towards highlighting research and funding the cure.

If I'm not successful, I'll either be dead (and, if I have my way, on display somewhere) or demented.

Either way, my problem will be solved. But what will we leave for the 1.5 million Americans (probably more by then) who

HAVE the disease and the 50-thousand (also likely to increase) who get the diagnosis this year, next year, the year after that?

Your mom? Your dad? Your gramma or grandpa? Your brother or sister?

Maybe even... You? Will you wait to care until then? Or will you start to care now?

AFTER-AFTERWORD

It's been a half-year since the initial publication of this expanded volume. In that time, as you've read, I retired from government service. I currently spend my time blogging, writing for the online newspaper Examiner.com, and generally trying to right the wrongs of the right wing by writing.

My walking has gotten far worse in the intervening months. I lose my balance very easily. My Porky Pig stutter has its good days and its bad days. It's just like the disease itself.

Some days are great.
Some days suck.
Most days are OK.

On October 28, 2011, I may have finally had that mini-stroke that they were so concerned about back in late 1999 and 2000. This happened after working out on my treadmill. I felt weak, had pins and needles on my right side, blurry vision in my right eye, and trouble speaking.

Spent the night at Howard County Memorial Hospital where they did a CT scan... and for the first time, I see the work they did on my noggin back in 2007!

At first we thought it might just be a TIA (transient ischemic attack) – sort of a "temporary" stroke – but since I didn't recover full function – still weak on the right, still some speaking difficulties – Dr. Grill fears I may have had a minor stroke.

As I write this, it is a Thursday afternoon. On Monday, I will have an MRI.

Yeah. I know. I said I could never have one of those. Apparently I can. Dr. Grill will "zero-out" the settings of my devices, and then, I guess, I'm good to go.

In the meantime, I'm having sharp, ice-pick headaches on the left upper temporal side of my head. Dr. Grill suspects (although I doubt it) that it might be something called "temporal arteritis," which is defined as *"...inflammation and damage to blood vessels that supply the head area, particularly the large or medium arteries that branch from the neck and supply the temporal area."* But that would supposedly be tender to the touch, and this is not. It just comes and goes of its own volition. Monday, it was an all day thing, every few minutes or so. One attack each day yesterday and the day before. Today, I'm getting them again at intermittent intervals.

Monday, we'll see whether or not I had a stroke. Want the results?

Check out my blog at http://billschmalfeldt.com.

See ya!

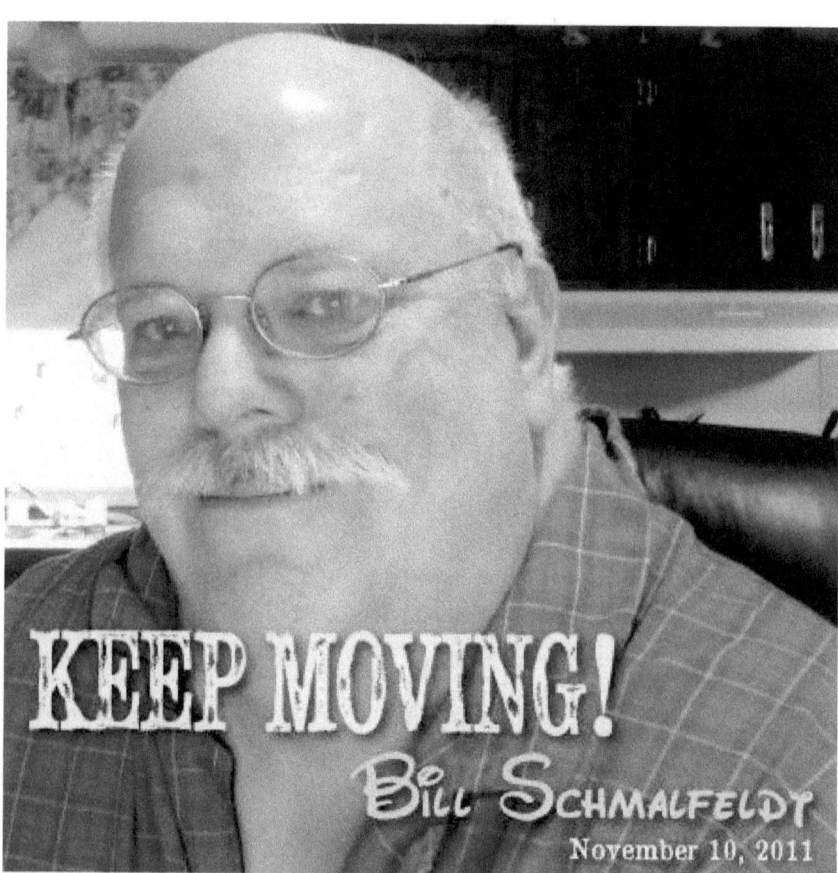

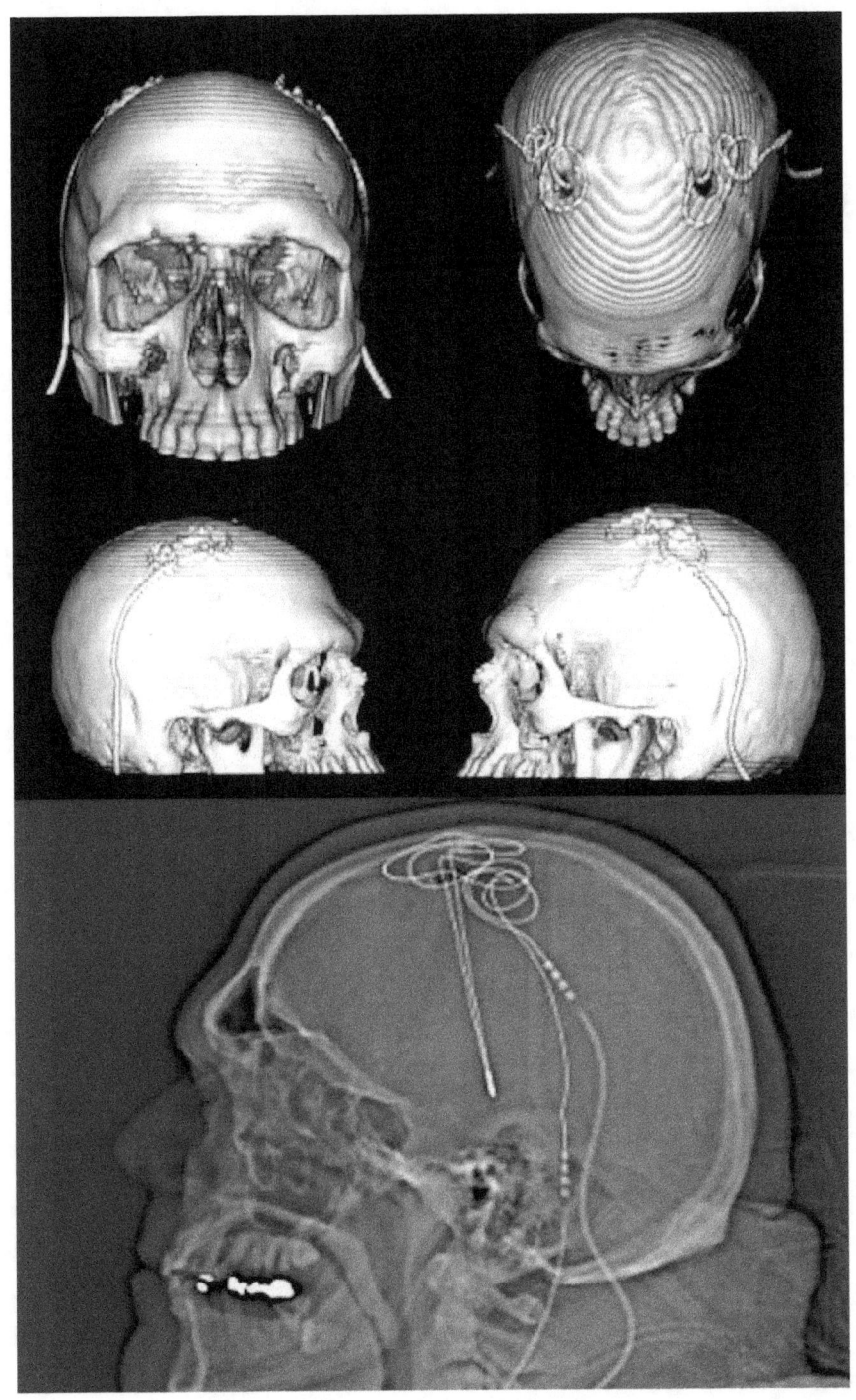

The stuff they put into my head on June 13, 2007, as seen via CT Scan on

Oct. 28, 2011.